ORTHOPEDIC CLINICS OF NORTH AMERICA

www.orthopedic.theclinics.com

Sports-Related Injuries

October 2016 • Volume 47 • Number 4

Editors

JAMES H. CALANDRUCCIO
BENJAMIN J. GREAR
BENJAMIN M. MAUCK
JEFFREY R. SAWYER
PATRICK C. TOY
JOHN C. WEINLEIN

ELSEVIER

1600 John F. Kennedy Boulevard • Suite 1800 • Philadelphia, Pennsylvania, 19103-2899.

http://www.orthopedic.theclinics.com

ORTHOPEDIC CLINICS OF NORTH AMERICA Volume 47, Number 4
October 2016 ISSN 0030-5898, ISBN-13: 978-0-323-46321-8

Editor: Jennifer Flynn-Briggs
Developmental Editor: Kristen Helm

Orthopedic Clinics of North America (ISSN 0030-5898) is published quarterly by Elsevier Inc., 360 Park Avenue South, New York, NY 10010-1710. Months of issue are January, April, July, and October. Business and Editorial Offices: 1600 John F. Kennedy Blvd., Suite 1800, Philadelphia, PA 19103-2899. Customer Service Office: 3251 Riverport Lane, Maryland Heights, MO 63043. Periodicals postage paid at New York, NY and additional mailing offices. Subscription prices are $310.00 per year for (US individuals), $653.00 per year for (US institutions), $365.00 per year (Canadian individuals), $797.00 per year (Canadian institutions), $450.00 per year (international individuals), $797.00 per year (international institutions), $100.00 per year (US students), $220.00 per year (Canadian and international students). Foreign air speed delivery is included in all *Clinics* subscription prices. All prices are subject to change without notice. **POSTMASTER:** Send change of address to *Orthopedic Clinics of North America,* **Elsevier Health Sciences Division, Subscription Customer Service, 3251 Riverport Lane, Maryland Heights, MO 63043. Customer Service (orders, claims, online, change of address): Elsevier Health Sciences Division, Subscription Customer Service, 3251 Riverport Lane, Maryland Heights, MO 63043. Tel: 1-800-654-2452 (U.S. and Canada); 314-447-8871 (outside U.S. and Canada). Fax: 314-447-8029. E-mail:** journalscustomerservice-usa@elsevier.com **(for print support);** journalsonlinesupport-usa@elsevier.com **(for online support).**

Reprints. For copies of 100 or more, of articles in this publication, please contact the Commercial Reprints Department, Elsevier Inc., 360 Park Avenue South, New York, NY 10010-1710. Tel.: 212-633-3874; Fax: 212-633-3820; E-mail: reprints@elsevier.com.

Orthopedic Clinics of North America is covered in *MEDLINE/PubMed (Index Medicus), Cinahl, Excerpta Medica,* and *Cumulative Index to Nursing and Allied Health Literature.*

PROGRAM OBJECTIVE

Orthopedic Clinics of North America offers clinical review articles on the most cutting-edge technologies and techniques in the field, including adult reconstruction, the upper extremity, pediatrics, trauma, oncology, and sports medicine.

TARGET AUDIENCE

Practicing orthopedic surgeons, orthopedic residents, and other healthcare professionals who specialize in orthopedic technologies and techniques for adult reconstruction, the upper extremity, pediatrics, trauma, oncology, and sports medicine.

LEARNING OBJECTIVES

Upon completion of this activity, participants will be able to:
1. Review sports-related injuries to the upper extremity in pediatrics patients.
2. Discuss pricing, quality, and reliability of care in treatment of sports-related injuries.
3. Recognize orthopedic management techniques for sports-related injuries to the lower extremity.

ACCREDITATION

The Elsevier Office of Continuing Medical Education (EOCME) is accredited by the Accreditation Council for Continuing Medical Education (ACCME) to provide continuing medical education for physicians.

The EOCME designates this enduring material for a maximum of 15 *AMA PRA Category 1 Credit*(s)™. Physicians should claim only the credit commensurate with the extent of their participation in the activity.

All other health care professionals requesting continuing education credit for this enduring material will be issued a certificate of participation.

DISCLOSURE OF CONFLICTS OF INTEREST

The EOCME assesses conflict of interest with its instructors, faculty, planners, and other individuals who are in a position to control the content of CME activities. All relevant conflicts of interest that are identified are thoroughly vetted by EOCME for fair balance, scientific objectivity, and patient care recommendations. EOCME is committed to providing its learners with CME activities that promote improvements or quality in healthcare and not a specific proprietary business or a commercial interest.

The planning committee, staff, authors and editors listed below have identified no financial relationships or relationships to products or devices they or their spouse/life partner have with commercial interest related to the content of this CME activity:

Afshin A. Anoushiravani, MD; Gonzalo Barinaga, MD; Eric N. Bowman, MD; Jennifer M. Brey, MD; Monique C. Chambers, MD, MSL; Aristides I. Cruz Jr, MD; Eric W. Edmonds, MD; Matthew D. Ellington, MD; Mouhanad M. El-Othmani, MD; Peter D. Fabricant, MD, MPH; John J. Feldman, MD; Jennifer Flynn-Briggs; Anjali Fortna; Theodore J. Ganley, MD; Michael C. Greaser, MD; Daniel Hatz, MD; KY M. Kobayashi, MD; Mininder S. Kocher, MD, MPH; James E. Moyer, MD; Premkumar Nandhakumar; Jason Patton, MD; Barry B. Phillips, MD; Khaled J. Saleh, MD, MSc, FRCS (C), MHCM, CPE; Zain Sayeed, MSc, MHA; Steven H. Shaha, PhD, DBA; Kevin G. Shea, MD; Richard B. Siegrist, MBA, MS, CPA; Megan Suermann; Megan Walters, MD; Peter K. Wong, PhD, MSc, MBA, RPh; Hussein A. Zeineddine, MD.

The planning committee, staff, authors and editors listed below have identified financial relationships or relationships to products or devices they or their spouse/life partner have with commercial interest related to the content of this CME activity:

Chance J. Henderson, MD, LTC USAF's spouse/partner has stock ownership in, and receives royalties/patents from, S.E.G-WAY Orthopaedics Inc.
John Weinlein, MD receives royalties/patents from Elsevier.

UNAPPROVED/OFF-LABEL USE DISCLOSURE

The EOCME requires CME faculty to disclose to the participants:
1. When products or procedures being discussed are off-label, unlabelled, experimental, and/or investigational (not US Food and Drug Administration [FDA] approved); and
2. Any limitations on the information presented, such as data that are preliminary or that represent ongoing research, interim analyses, and/or unsupported opinions. Faculty may discuss information about pharmaceutical agents that is outside of FDA-approved labelling. This information is intended solely for CME and is not intended to promote off-label use of these medications. If you have any questions, contact the medical affairs department of the manufacturer for the most recent prescribing information.

TO ENROLL

To enroll in the *Orthopedic Clinics of North America* Continuing Medical Education program, call customer service at 1-800-654-2452 or sign up online at http://www.theclinics.com/home/cme. The CME program is available to subscribers for an additional annual fee of USD 215.

METHOD OF PARTICIPATION

In order to claim credit, participants must complete the following:
1. Complete enrolment as indicated above.
2. Read the activity.

3. Complete the CME Test and Evaluation. Participants must achieve a score of 70% on the test. All CME Tests and Evaluations must be completed online.

CME INQUIRIES/SPECIAL NEEDS

For all CME inquiries or special needs, please contact elsevierCME@elsevier.com.

EDITORIAL BOARD

CONTRIBUTORS

AUTHORS

AFSHIN A. ANOUSHIRAVANI, MD
Clinical and Translational Research Fellow,
Division of Orthopaedics and Rehabilitation,
Southern Illinois University School of
Medicine, Springfield, Illinois

GONZALO BARINAGA, MD
Senior Resident, Division of Orthopaedics and
Rehabilitation, Southern Illinois University
School of Medicine, Springfield, Illinois

ERIC N. BOWMAN, MD
Resident, Department of Orthopaedics,
University of Tennessee-Campbell Clinic,
Memphis, Tennessee

JENNIFER M. BREY, MD
Assistant Professor, Department of
Orthopaedic Surgery, Kosair Children's
Hospital, Children's Orthopaedics of
Louisville, University of Louisville, Louisville,
Kentucky

JAMES H. CALANDRUCCIO, MD
Assistant Professor, Department of
Orthopaedic Surgery and Biomechanical
Engineering, University of Tennessee-
Campbell Clinic, Memphis, Tennessee

MONIQUE C. CHAMBERS, MD, MSL
Clinical and Translational Research Fellow,
Division of Orthopaedics and Rehabilitation,
Southern Illinois University School of
Medicine, Springfield, Illinois

ARISTIDES I. CRUZ Jr, MD
Assistant Professor of Orthopaedic Surgery,
The Warren Alpert Medical School of Brown
University, Hasbro Children's Hospital,
Providence, Rhode Island

ERIC W. EDMONDS, MD
Staff Pediatric Orthopaedic Surgeon, Rady
Children's Hospital, San Diego, California

MOUHANAD M. EL-OTHMANI, MD
Clinical Research Associate, Division of
Orthopaedics and Rehabilitation, Southern
Illinois University School of Medicine,
Springfield, Illinois

MATTHEW D. ELLINGTON, MD
Pediatric Orthopaedic Surgery Fellow, Rady
Children's Hospital, San Diego, California

PETER D. FABRICANT, MD, MPH
Pediatric Orthopaedic Surgery Service,
Hospital for Special Surgery; Instructor in
Orthopaedic Surgery, Weill Cornell Medical
College, New York, New York

JOHN J. FELDMAN, MD
Resident, Department of Orthopaedics,
University of Tennessee-Campbell Clinic,
Memphis, Tennessee

THEODORE J. GANLEY, MD
Associate Professor of Orthopaedic Surgery,
The Children's Hospital of Philadelphia,
Philadelphia, Pennsylvania

MICHAEL C. GREASER, MD
Assistant Professor, Department of
Orthopedic Surgery, University of Texas
Health Science Center at Houston, McGovern
Medical School, Houston, Texas

DANIEL HATZ, MD
Senior Resident, Division of Orthopaedics and
Rehabilitation, Southern Illinois University
School of Medicine, Springfield, Illinois

CHANCE J. HENDERSON, MD, LTC USAF
Chief, Hand Surgery, USAF Academy, USAFA,
Colorado

KY M. KOBAYASHI, MD
Orthopaedic Center of Excellence, Colorado
Springs, CO

MININDER S. KOCHER, MD, MPH
Associate Director, Division of Sports
Medicine, Department of Orthopedic Surgery,
Boston Children's Hospital; Professor of
Orthopedic Surgery, Harvard Medical School,
Boston, Massachusetts

BENJAMIN M. MAUCK, MD
Department of Orthopaedic Surgery and
Biomechanical Engineering, University of
Tennessee-Campbell Clinic, Memphis,
Tennessee

JAMES E. MOYER, MD
Non-operative Pediatric Orthopedics, Kosair
Children's Hospital, Children's Orthopaedics
of Louisville, Louisville, Kentucky

F. PATTERSON OWINGS, MD
Department of Orthopaedic Surgery and
Biomechanical Engineering, University of
Tennessee-Campbell Clinic, Memphis,
Tennessee

JASON PATTON, MD
Senior Resident, Division of Orthopaedics and
Rehabilitation, Southern Illinois University
School of Medicine, Springfield, Illinois

BARRY B. PHILLIPS, MD
Associate Professor, Department of
Orthopaedics, Campbell Clinic Orthopaedics,
University of Tennessee-Campbell Clinic,
Germantown, Tennessee

**KHALED J. SALEH, MD, MSc, FRCS (C),
MIICM, CPE**
Executive-in-Chief, Department of
Orthopaedic and Sports Medicine, Detroit
Medical Center, Detroit, Michigan

ZAIN SAYEED, MSc, MHA
Clinical and Translational Research Fellow,
Division of Orthopaedics and Rehabilitation,
Southern Illinois University School of
Medicine, Springfield, Illinois

STEVEN H. SHAHA, PhD, DBA
Professor, Center for Public Policy and
Administration, University of Utah, Salt Lake
City, UT

KEVIN G. SHEA, MD
St. Luke's Children's Hospital, Boise, Idaho

RICHARD B. SIEGRIST, MBA, MS, CPA
Director of Innovation and Entrepreneurship,
Harvard T.H. Chan School of Public Health,
Harvard University, Boston, Massachusetts

MEGAN WALTERS, MD
Senior Resident, Division of Orthopaedics and
Rehabilitation, Southern Illinois University
School of Medicine, Springfield, Illinois

JOHN C. WEINLEIN, MD
Assistant Professor, Department
of Orthopaedics, University of
Tennessee-Campbell Clinic, Memphis,
Tennessee

PETER K. WONG, PhD, MSc, MBA, RPh
VP and Chief Performance Improvement
Officer, Illinois Divisions, HSHS Medical
Group, Hospital Sisters Health System (HSHS),
Springfield, Illinois

HUSSEIN A. ZEINEDDINE, MD
Department of Surgery, University of Chicago,
Chicago, Illinois

CONTENTS

The Future of Arthroplasty
Patrick C. Toy

> The US health care system has been fragmented for more than 40 years; this model created a need for modification. Sociopoliticomedical system-related factors led to the Affordable Care Act (ACA) and a restructuring of health care provision/delivery. The ACA increases access to high-quality "affordable care" under cost-effective measures. This article provides a comprehensive review of health reform and the motivating factors that drive policy to empower arthroplasty providers to effectively advocate for the field of orthopedics as a whole, and the patients served.

> As health care reforms continue to improve quality of care, significant emphasis will be placed on evaluation of orthopedic patient outcomes. Total joint arthroplasty (TJA) has a proven track record of enhancing patient quality of life and are easily replicable. The outcomes of these procedures serve as a measure of health care initiative success. Specifically, length of stay, will be targeted as a marker of quality of surgical care delivered to TJA patients. Within this review, we will discuss preoperative and postoperative methods by which orthopedic surgeons may enhance TJA outcomes and effectively reduce length of stay.

> Surgical site infection in total joint arthroplasty is a challenging complication that warrants discussion with regard to prevention and management. Limiting postoperative infection rate is a paramount quest in the orthopedic community. Several preoperative risk factors have been identified in orthopedic literature with regards to likelihood of developing postoperative infection. This article evaluates several factors that predispose total joint arthroplasty patients to infection. Methods of patient surgical preparation designed to decrease postoperative infection, decreasing intraoperative traffic during procedural settings, and elaborate intraoperative prophylactic advancements are assessed. Approaches to decrease postoperative infection by discussing means of lowering rates of postoperative transfusion, wound drainage, and hematoma formation are analyzed.

Hospital readmission is a focus of quality measures used by the Center for Medicare and Medicaid (CMS) to evaluate quality of care. Policy changes provide incentives and enforce penalties to decrease 30-day hospital readmissions. CMS implemented the Readmission Penalty Program. Readmission rates are being used to determine reimbursement rates for physicians. The need for readmission is deemed an indication for inadequate quality of care subjected to financial penalties. This reviews identifies risk factors that have been significantly associated with higher readmission rates, addresses approaches to minimize 30-day readmission, and discusses the potential future direction within this area as regulations evolve.

Within the past 3 decades, a recent trend in the growth of musculoskeletal service lines has been seen nationally. Orthopedics offers an appealing concourse for implementation of service-line care. Within this review, the authors address the components involved in planning and building a musculoskeletal service line. The authors also address methods by which orthopedic surgeons can maintain the efficacy of their service lines by examining how orthopedic surgeons can navigate their service line through recent advents in health care reform. Finally, the authors review successful examples of musculoskeletal service lines currently in practice within the orthopedic community.

As health care reimbursement models shift from volume-based to value-based models, orthopedic surgeons must provide patients with highly reliable care, while consciously minimizing cost, maintaining quality, and providing timely interventions. An established means of achieving these goals is by implementing a highly reliable care model; however, before such a model can be initiated, a safety culture, robust improvement strategies, and committed leadership are needed. This article discusses interdependent and critical changes required to implement a highly reliable care system. Specific operative protocols now mandated are discussed as they pertain to high reliability of orthopedic care and elimination of wrong-site procedures.

Patient-centered care (PCC) is gaining considerable momentum among health care professionals and policy-making authorities. The need for PCC stems from the innumerable benefits of adopting such a system. The practice of PCC in orthopedic surgery in general, and in total joint replacement in particular, is still in its youth. However, present literature already establishes the need for applying PCC in total joint replacement. Extensive research and effort should be invested to better grasp and define the dimensions of PCC as they relate to total joint replacement.

Under the Patient Protection and Affordable Care Act (ACA), the Centers for Medicare and Medicaid Services' Innovation was chartered to develop new models of health care delivery. The changes meant a drastic need to restructure the health care system. To minimize costs and optimize quality, new laws encourage continuity in health care delivery within an integrated system. Affordable care organizations provided a model of high-quality care while reducing costs. Bundled payments can have a substantial effect on the national expenditures. This article examines new developments in bundle payments, affordable care organizations, and gainsharing agreements as they pertain to arthroplasty.

Recent trends in clinical research have moved attention toward reporting clinical outcomes and resource consumption associated with various care processes. This change is the result of technological advancement and a national effort to critically assess health care delivery. As orthopedic surgeons traverse an unchartered health care environment, a more complete understanding of how clinical research is conducted using large data sets is necessary. The purpose of this article is to review various advantages and disadvantages of large data sets available for orthopaedic use, examine their ideal use, and report how they are being implemented nationwide.

This article explores how integration of data from clinical registries and electronic health records produces a quality impact within orthopedic practices. Data are differentiated from information, and several types of data that are collected and used in orthopedic outcome measurement are defined. Furthermore, the concept of comparative effectiveness and its impact on orthopedic clinical research are assessed. This article places emphasis on how the concept of big data produces health care challenges balanced with benefits that may be faced by patients and orthopedic surgeons. Finally, essential characteristics of an electronic health record that interlinks musculoskeletal care and big data initiatives are reviewed.

Trauma
John C. Weinlein

Tibial stress fractures are common in the athlete. There are various causes of these fractures, the most common being a sudden increase in training intensity. Most of these injuries are treated conservatively; however, some may require operative intervention. Intervention is mostly dictated by location of the fracture and failure of conservative treatment. There are several surgical options available to the treating surgeon, each with advantages and disadvantages. The physician must understand the nature of the fracture and the likelihood for it to heal in a timely manner in order to best treat these fractures in this patient subset.

Pediatrics
Jeffrey R. Sawyer

Pediatric overuse injuries are becoming more prevalent in today's society with more children competitively playing year-round sports at a younger age. The importance of prompt diagnosis and treatment is paramount to the treatment for these injuries, second only to rest and activity modification. This article will focus on overuse injuries of the upper extremity, specifically: little league elbow, elbow osteochondritis dissecans, and gymnast wrist. It will also discuss the pathophysiology, diagnosis, imaging, and treatment of each of these entities.

Shoulder injuries in pediatric athletes are typically caused by acute or overuse injuries. The developing structures of the shoulder lead to injury patterns that are distinct from those of adult athletes. Overuse injuries often affect the physeal structures of the proximal humerus and can lead to pain and loss of sports participation. Shoulder instability is common in pediatric athletes, and recurrence is also a concern in this population. Fractures of the proximal humerus and clavicle are typically treated with conservative management, but there is a trend toward surgical intervention.

Osteochondritis dissecans (OCD) can cause knee pain and dysfunction in children. The etiology of OCD remains unclear; theories on causes include inflammation, ischemia, ossification abnormalities, genetic factors, and repetitive microtrauma. Most OCD lesions in skeletally immature patients will heal with nonoperative treatment. The success of nonoperative treatment decreases once patients reach skeletal maturity. The goals of surgical treatment include maintenance of articular cartilage congruity, rigid fixation of unstable fragments, and repair of osteochondral defects with cells or tissues that can adequately replace lost or deficient cartilage. Unsalvageable OCD lesions can be treated with various surgical techniques.

Dramatic increases in youth competitive athletic activity, early sport specialization, and year-round training and competition, along with increased awareness of anterior cruciate ligament (ACL) injuries in children, have led to a commensurate increase in the frequency of ACL tears in the skeletally immature. Recent understanding of the risks of nonoperative treatment and surgical delay have supported a trend toward early operative treatment. This article discusses treatment strategies for ACL injuries in children and adolescents, and offers our preferred treatment strategy for skeletally immature youth athletes with ACL tears.

Upper Extremity
Benjamin M. Mauck and James H. Calandruccio

Ulnar-sided wrist pain can be a challenging entity for the hand surgeon and even more so in the athletic population. The authors present 8 causes of ulnar-sided wrist pain in an athlete (hook of hamate fracture, pisiform fracture, hypothenar hammer syndrome, triangular fibrocartilage complex injuries, ulnocarpal impaction syndrome, lunotriquetral ligament tears, extensor carpi ulnaris tendinitis, subluxation of extensor carpi ulnaris) and their associated imaging and treatment options.

Hand injuries account for up to 15% of sports injuries and are common in contact sports and in sports with a high risk of falling. Appropriate management requires knowledge of the type of injury, demands of the sport and position, competitive level of the athlete, future athletic demands and expectations, and the role of rehabilitation and protective splints for return to play. Management of the athlete requires aggressive and expedient diagnostic intervention and treatment. This article describes ligamentous injuries to the thumb, including thumb carpometacarpal dislocations, thumb metacarpophalangeal dislocations, collateral ligament injuries and interphalangeal dislocations, their evaluation, treatment and outcomes.

Foot and Ankle
Benjamin J. Grear

The incidence of stress fractures in the general athletic population is less than 1%, but may be as high as 15% in runners. Stress fractures of the foot and ankle account for almost half of bone stress injuries in athletes. These injuries occur because of repetitive submaximal stresses on the bone resulting in microfractures, which may coalesce to form complete fractures. Advanced imaging such as MRI and triple-phase bone scans is used to evaluate patients with suspected stress fracture. Low-risk stress fractures are typically treated with rest and protected weight bearing. High-stress fractures more often require surgical treatment.

SPORTS-RELATED INJURIES

THE CLINICS ARE AVAILABLE ONLINE!

Access your subscription at:
www.theclinics.com

PREFACE

Sports-Related Injuries

"Sports injuries" are injuries that happen when playing sports or exercising. The severity of these injuries can range from minor to very serious, with some injuries requiring surgery to fully heal. There are many reasons for these injuries, such as poor training practices, improper equipment, or may just be an accident. Injuries can also occur when a person is not in proper condition to play the sport. Youth athletes often begin their competitive sports careers as early as age seven, if not sooner. With so many youth programs in the United States, the opportunity for injury in children and adolescents is enormous. Sports injuries are one of the leading causes of emergency room visits for children and adolescents.

The authors of these sections have done an excellent job of including types of sports injuries that they see in their patients, and treat. In lieu of an Adult Reconstruction Section, we are including a Special Section, The Future of Arthroplasty, that we feel is relative to this issue and very informative. All of these articles are written by experienced surgeons in orthopedics, and we thank them for providing their wisdom.

Articles in The Future of Arthroplasty Section will focus on the following: Healthcare Reform: Impact on Total Joint Replacement, Reducing Length of Stay in Total Joint Arthroplasty Care, Approach to Decrease Infection Following Total Joint Arthroplasty, Reducing 30-day Readmission After Joint Replacement, Planning, Building, and Maintaining a Successful Musculoskeletal Service Line, High Reliability of Care in Orthopedic Surgery—Are We There Yet?, Patient Centeredness in Total Joint Replacement – Beyond the Slogan, Affordable Care Organizations and Bundled Pricing: A New Philosophy of Care, Big Data, Big Research: Implementing Population Health-based Research Models and Integrating Care to Reduce Cost and Improve Outcomes, and Big Data, Big Problems: Incorporating Mission, Values, and Culture in Provider Affiliations.

Articles in the Trauma Section will focus on the following: Tibial Stress Fractures in Athletes.

Articles in the Pediatric Section will focus on the following: Pediatric Elbow and Wrist Pathology Related to Sports Participation, Shoulder Injuries in Pediatric Athletes, Pediatric Knee Osteochondritis Dissecans Lesions, and Anterior Cruciate Ligament Injuries in Children and Adolescents.

Articles in the Upper Extremity Section will focus on the following: Ulnar-Sided Wrist Pain in the Athlete and Thumb Ligament Injuries in the Athlete.

Articles in the Foot and Ankle Section will focus on the following: Foot and Ankle Stress Fractures in Athletes.

I hope that our readers will be engaged in this exciting issue and find the material useful.

Jennifer Flynn-Briggs
Senior Clinics Editor, Elsevier
E-mail address:
j.flynn-briggs@elsevier.com

Orthop Clin N Am 47 (2016) xv
http://dx.doi.org/10.1016/j.ocl.2016.07.001
0030-5898/16/© 2016 Published by Elsevier Inc.

The Future of Arthroplasty

Health Care Reform
Impact on Total Joint Replacement

Monique C. Chambers, MD, MSL[a],
Mouhanad M. El-Othmani, MD[a],
Khaled J. Saleh, MD, MSc, FRCS (C), MHCM, CPE[b],*

KEYWORDS
• Health care reform • ACA • Quality care • TJA • MIPS • MACRA • CMS

KEY POINTS
• The implementation of the Affordable Care Act changed the traditional approaches to payment reform and delivery of care, with an emphasis on integrated delivery systems.
• Quality care and reimbursements that drive efficiency, when implemented properly, can be a motivating factor toward improving the health of the nation.
• Understanding health reform and policy will empower arthroplasty providers to effectively advocate for the field of orthopedics as a whole, and the patients we serve.

INTRODUCTION

The US health care system has existed in a fragmented nature for more than 40 years. In his book "The Healing of America," T.J. Reid clearly outlines the 4 models of care in his search for a health care system that would provide the highest quality of care in the most cost-efficient way.[1] Under the Bismarck system, private insurers pay private physicians; the system is funded through the employer and payroll deductions, but the profits that private insurance companies are allowed to make are highly regulated.[1] In the United States, this system is applied to most workers under the age of 65 years.[2] In contrast, the universal care Beveridge model is reflected in the care provided for groups such as the US military, veterans, and Native Americans.[1] These more recognized models, such as the Bismarck system of Germany or the Beveridge model of the United Kingdoms, have been morphed into a complex array of systems that separate access to health care services based on socioeconomic factors. Many politicians, insurance companies, and providers have resisted policies that reflect the type of "socialized" medicine that is provided in models like Canada's National Health Insurance. Nonetheless, this model that uses private sector providers who are paid by government insurance agencies is seen in the 50-year-old American Medicare/Medicaid programs.[2] Ultimately, the American model has included all 3 of these models, and for the 17% of Americans who do not neatly fall into one of these categories, they are forced to pay out of pocket for medical services like the citizens of India.[1] This structure has created vast disparities in access and quality of health care provided to different social classes based on the payment that health professionals accept for medical services provided.

The disjointed model of medical access and payment created a great need for modification in the US health care system. The combination of increasing health care costs with inconsistent

Disclosures: The authors have no conflicts of interest to disclose. No funding sources were used for this article.
[a] Division of Orthopaedics and Rehabilitation, Southern Illinois University School of Medicine, 701 North First Street, Springfield, IL 62781, USA; [b] Department of Orthopaedic and Sports Medicine, Detroit Medical Center, 311 Mack Avenue, 5th Floor, Detroit, MI 48201, USA
* Corresponding author.
E-mail address: kjsaleh@gmail.com

Orthop Clin N Am 47 (2016) 645–652
http://dx.doi.org/10.1016/j.ocl.2016.05.005

and suboptimal quality of care that fared poorly in comparison with other nations meant that wide-scale structural changes were warranted.[3] The inconsistency of care has been observed in the approach providers take to manage back pain, osteoarthritis, and other musculoskeletal conditions.[4] The geographic region in the United States has been correlated with determining the options of intervention, whether it is more likely to be surgical or conservative medical treatment with physical therapy, in orthopedic surgery.[5] Additionally, the geographic location has been shown to be an independent variable affecting cost of delivered care. The recent increase in the proportion of Americans covered by Medicare and Medicaid has been governed by the increase in the elderly population, the low-income population, and greater patient complexity. This change will shift a greater proportion of health care expenditures and costs toward the federal and state governments. In an attempt to provide more sustainable methods for health care coverage, the development of a system that increased access, improved quality, and curtailed costs was presumed to be the best option for the American population.

There have been several unsuccessful attempts to revamp the America health care system. The unique combination of sociopoliticomedical system-related factors led to the passage of the Affordable Care Act (ACA) and a complete restructure of health care provision and delivery. Socially, the recession just before the 2008 election led to the highest unemployment rate in several decades and to an increased awareness of the magnitude of health care costs and their impact on the unemployed population. Several constituents were now denied access to care that was provided through their relationship with an employer. The topic of health care reform quickly became a national focal point of the 2008 presidential debates and the newly elected administration of President Obama had become very familiar with the process of remodeling the system. Politically, it was the first time in several years that the party of the executive branch also held the majority in the legislative branch. This meant there were fewer barriers needed to successfully align political goals and pass a bill through Congress that would also be supported by the president. Finally, the new health care model was shaped largely after ideas developed and implemented in Massachusetts, a progressive state in all health care advances. These factors greatly increased the chances of passage and success for revitalizing the health care system.

The 2010 implementation of the ACA changed the traditional approaches to payment reform and delivery of care, with an emphasis on integrated delivery systems.[6] One of the first areas in medicine, and the first area of orthopedics to be impacted by these alterations, were in total joint arthroplasty (TJA). These changes include payment reform through value-based purchasing or bundled payments, and a shift toward multidisciplinary care provided by accountable care organizations and patient-centered medical homes.[7,8] A closer look at the legislative provisions of the ACA allow the orthopedic provider to better understand how these changes can impact their practice, and subsequently the care and outcomes of patients undergoing TJA.

The Three Prongs of the Affordable Care Act: Increase Access, Reduce Cost, Improve Quality

The prongs of the ACA were implemented to increase access to "affordable care" of the highest possible quality under cost-effective measures (Fig. 1). However, most policy provisions have addressed primarily access to care. Currently, there are 14 million more patients insured through Medicaid than there were 3 years ago, with more than 4.2 million insured through the health care marketplace insurance exchanges.[9] It is projected that the number of total hip arthroplasty procedures will increase to 520,000 and the number of total knee arthroplasty (TKA) will be approximately 3.48 million by 2030.[10] Growth rates of upper extremity arthroplasty have been shown to be comparable with or greater than rates of total knee or hip procedures.[11] Procedure volume of shoulder arthroplasty increased at annual rates of up to 13% between 1993 to 2007, with an estimated total increase of 322% since 2007.[11] The Medicaid expansion means even more of the population will qualify for elective procedures, such as TJA, because these projections do not account for the increased access to care brought about through the ACA.

Assessing Quality in Care Delivery

The other 2 prongs have become the focus of reimbursement models in which payments are linked to the assessment of quality of care provided. There have been several regulatory responses to help improve quality in arthroplasty care. Approaches to standardize optimal medical practice that would decrease the rate of medical errors and complications have become more commonplace. Organizations, such as the American Academy of Orthopaedic Surgeons

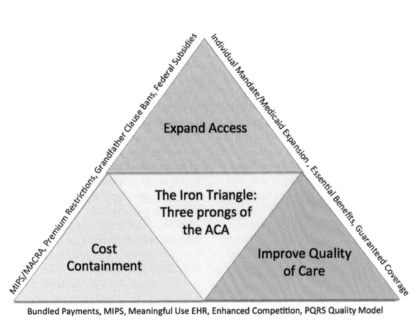

Fig. 1. The 3 prongs of the Affordable Care Act (ACA). EHR, electronic health record; MIPS/MACRA, Merit-Based Incentive Payment Systems/Medicare Access and Children's Health Insurance Program Reauthorization Act; PQRS, Physician Quality Reporting System.

or the American Association of Hip and Knee Surgeons, are updating guidelines continuously to reflect proficient evidence-based care recommendations. For example, orthopedic societies becoming more involved in driving policy has led to the widespread use of surgical hoods during arthroplasty procedures and the first guidelines concerning deep vein thrombosis prophylaxis in the arthroplasty perioperative period.[12,13] An effort to encourage providers to report and learn from medical errors occurs in forums where surgeons can discuss openly patient morbidity and mortality, without the fear of legal ramifications for mistakes made. This avenue allows providers to collaborate and analyze system-related causes to medical error. If regulatory agencies employed policies that encourage transparency of medical errors, the health care system could experience improved delivery of care and patient outcomes.[14] Other efforts to improve quality have focused on accountability in care delivery. The growing body of arthroplasty literature highlights the importance of using medical resources to minimize risk of adverse outcomes.[15–17] Although orthopedic surgeons bound by ethical considerations are unable to pick their patients, the unique opportunity exists to optimize patients medically before scheduling an elective arthroplasty procedure. This approach defies the historic view that specialists are isolated providers who only care for the system in which

they have expertise. It further places more weight on the responsibility of the provider to care for the patient and not solely the condition of degenerative joint disease. This has also fostered more collaboration surrounding the perioperative care of arthroplasty patients. Hospitals have adopted the use of hospitalists or specialized orthopedic surgery units to provide integrated and efficient care to patients after surgical intervention. When specialized orthopedic surgery units are prioritized in patients after TKA, there is a reduction in hospital duration of stay and hospital costs.[18] Hospitals directing patient flow to units dedicated to providing expert care specifically for arthroplasty patients can better improve resource use and patient outcomes.[18]

As the number and costs of arthroplasty procedures continue to increase, institutions are required to examine their existing practices for financial sustainability.[18] Various influences are placed on the physician through quality assessment from the patient, the employer, and federal agencies. These internal forces have also been placed on health care organizations since the US Institute of Medicine's report on medical errors and health care quality published in 1999.[19,20] The effort to minimize error occurrence and establish transparency in error reporting led to heightened focus on improving the quality of care provided to patients in the face of reports of nearly 100,000 deaths per year from medical mistakes and failure to provide evidence-based care.[3] Modern-day assessment of arthroplasty quality care address measures such as 30-day readmission rates and hospital-acquired conditions (ie, infection, deep vein thrombosis, pulmonary embolism). Hospitals are resorting to innovative and alternative approaches to optimize the perioperative and postdischarge course stemming from studies that identify factors that may reduce 30-day readmissions after TJA.[21] These initiatives include predischarge interventions through appropriate patient education, adequate discharge planning, accurate medication reconciliation, and prescheduling follow-up appointments. Postdischarge interventions are equally vital and include timely follow-up, communication with the primary care provider, implementing patient hotlines, and providing home visits. Some institutions have also implemented intervention programs designed to bridge the gap between the surgical care team and the patient. Known as transition programs, the team consists of a transition coach who provides individualized patient-centered discharge instructions and allows for continuity with the provider.[22,23] Finally, the implementation of electronic patient chart tracking allows patients up-to-date access to their electronic health records and constant communication with their providers. All of these measures collectively provide a closer follow-up and contact with patients, and aim to improve postoperative functional outcomes and patient satisfaction. The impact of these changes is reflected in platforms like the Consumer Assessment of Healthcare Providers.

Cost Containment Under Health Care Reform

Measures to improve the quality of delivered care center around the fact that the United States spends 17.6% of the gross domestic product on health care expenditures, but remains 37th in terms of quality of care.[24,25] The US spends more per capita on medical services than any other industrialized nation and spending under the old system was projected to reach $5.4 trillion, 20% of the gross domestic product by 2024.[26] Therefore, an equal or greater focus must be placed on containing where the US dollar is spent. Cost containment models are guided by a simple philosophy: reward those who practice medicine best. However, this simple idea is complicated by the vast array of contributors to our health care budget and expenses. Appropriately addressing this problem means an understanding of why Americans spend so much on health care. As a country of great wealth and capitalism, the

United States has a foundation of creating market structures that drive competition. However, there has been little regulation to control costs and the interplay between those who receive, provide, and finance care. Therefore, competition has not controlled costs, but instead has created an environment that allows for price increases to ensure profits and structural market sustainability. The elderly population has grown at a rate of 7% annually, leading to a greater number of patients that qualify for Medicare and increased access to necessary medical interventions, such as TJA.[27] The increase in the Baby Boomer population has meant more patients with chronic degenerative disease. Waste, fraud, and abuse also contribute to cost, although it only accounts for 20% of US expenses.[27] Other trivial contributors to costs include malpractice payments and professionals that feel trapped into practicing defensive medicine. To curtail these costs, orthopedists and leaders within the orthopedic community have been very active in successful advances of tort reform. Additionally, administrative fees associated with maintaining the fragmented insurance and private payer systems play a major role in driving up costs. Finally, efforts to advance health information technology hoped to decrease the need for administrative personnel and improve exchange of health information. However, the initial startup costs and maintenance is reflected by an increase of total expenditures for many organizations that are supported by federal trust funds under the American Reinvest and Recovery Act. The complex interaction of these factors has continued to drive the downward spiral of economic resources that are intended to sustain the US health care model.

To address this, in addition to its expansion and reform of health insurance coverage, the ACA contains numerous provisions intended to resolve underlying problems in how health care is paid in the United States. These reforms have motivated progressive contributions to the momentum across the United States to improve the value obtained for our health care dollar.[28] The Merit-Based Incentive Payment Systems (MIPS) was established through the Medicare Access and Children's Health Insurance Program Reauthorization Act to provide an avenue to report quality care for Medicare patients.[29] Because Medicare patients are the primary recipients of arthroplasty procedures, a thorough understanding of MIPS program phases should be explored by the orthopedic surgeon. The MIPS program shifts the basis for Medicare payments from volume to value by improving on current measures in 3 broad areas: the Physician Quality Reporting System, the Value-Based Modifier (VBM), and meaningful use of electronic health records. Although all 3 of these components will be combined into 1 MIPS composite score starting in 2019, each is individually reported and used as a measure to calculate payments until the end of 2018.[29]

The Physician Quality Reporting System allows organizations to elect to participate in various areas of performance. Providers are evaluated based on their ability to provide timely care that includes a patient's ability to obtain an appointment in a timely manner and receive accurate information in a timely fashion to address their medical concerns. Continuous progress in the medical field has led to an emphasis on shared decision making and less of a paternalistic approach to the doctor–patient relationship. This is a vital part of the process when patients are making decisions concerning an elective procedure, such as arthroplasty. Therefore, reporting also assesses how well providers communicate and participate in the shared decision making process with their patients. The orthopedic surgeon is also held accountable for promoting healthy habits and educating patients on factors that can impact their postoperative recovery, such as smoking cessation, weight loss related to obesity, or adequate glucose level control. When the medical management is out of the scope of the orthopedist, evaluations will include their effort to coordinate with other specialists and help the patient obtain necessary resources. Finally, Consumer Assessments of Healthcare Providers are used to get an accurate reflection of how patients rate their provider and how this interaction impacts the patient's functional health status and use of medical resources. Aspects of this system will continue to guide the MIPS model, but incentive payments within the Physician Quality Reporting System model were phased out at the end of 2015.[29]

During this transition, the VBM will be used to monitor volume, quality, and cost of services provided.[30] In line with the goals of the ACA, the characteristics of the VBM are improved health, better care, and lower costs through value-based purchasing.[31,32] The VBM establishes a value modifier that allows for differential reimbursements under the Medicare physician fee schedule. VBP programs create incentives for physicians to pursue these aims and to reward value over volume.[31] Medicare reimbursement will be tied directly to the achievement of certain cost and quality benchmarks,

including those related to patient satisfaction. Medicare will also cut reimbursement for hospital services related to preventable readmissions and hospital-acquired conditions. Many arthroplasty surgeons reasonably want to know how the VBM will impact their practice and reimbursements. The Centers for Medicare and Medicaid Services will use the quality and cost scores to determine the upward, downward, or neutral penalties a group or solo practitioner can receive according to their quality tier and practice size. These payments are based on a hospitals ability to meet performance measurements in 6 care domains: (1) patient safety, (2) care coordination, (3) clinical processes and outcomes, (4) population or community health, (5) efficiency and cost reduction, and (6) patient- and caregiver-centered experiences.[31] The measures are standardized to allow for a universal system to implement payment models, but will also adjusted for risk based on the local standards of the region and hospital for adaptability. Exceptions will apply to arthroplasty providers in rural areas, orthopedic surgeons working in critical access hospitals or federally qualified health centers, and group practices that are part of the Medicare Shared Savings Program or involved in an accountable care organization under the ACA pioneer allowances.

Finally, MIPS will evaluate an institution's Meaningful Use of electronic health records. The main components of Meaningful use are specified in the 2009 American Reinvest and Recovery Act.[33] The American Reinvest and Recovery Act articulates that meaningful use providers should be able to use certified electronic health records technology in ways that can be measured significantly in quality and quantity, and allow for the exchange of health information to improve the quality of health care.[34] After complete transition to MIPS, all Medicare-eligible professionals and hospitals must meet meaningful use or be subject to a financial penalty.[29]

Cost containment under MIPS will be largely contributed to by the concept of budget neutrality. Composite scores applied to hospitals will be weighed between providers that score above the threshold and balanced with those scoring below. Unlike the current VBM model, there is no requirement for "penalties" and "rewards" to be equal or balanced. If all providers score above the performance threshold, then rewards will be appropriated for all high-performing providers. Additionally, performance assessments will be on a sliding scale so that credit will be given for those who meet part of the performance metrics.[29] In other words, it is possible for all providers to be rewarded if their performance meets threshold standards. The shift in calculating reimbursements is designed to strengthen, incorporate, and consolidate financial impacts of the current models that have continually resulted in lags in payment reimbursements compared with inflation in costs for providing care to arthroplasty patients. For example, the national Medicare reimbursement in 1992 for a TKA was $2102. Despite an increase in the costs of running an orthopedic practice, reimbursement for joint procedure had decreased 30% with TKA reimbursement rate being $1470.[35]

Physicians have long desired an adjustment to the old sustainable growth rate formula that guided reimbursements and have pushed for reform that included predictable Medicare payments.[36] However, some argue that the structure of the reimbursements handicap the provider from being able to provide the highest level of care available, especially with the vast procedural volume projected for arthroplasty patients.[37] Concerns of orthopedic surgeons center around ideas of standardized care that cannot be individualized.[38] Surgeons have also expressed reservations that pay for performance models will not ensure protection of at-risk populations that are more likely to suffer worse outcomes, and may have their operations delayed by apprehensive providers.[39] Economically, the mandates on reporting quality data can potentially be more challenging and costly for private practice and smaller groups, and eventually force them to collaborate or merge with larger groups.[5] From 2004 to 2010, the percentage of respondents to the biannual American Academy of Orthopaedic Surgeons member survey who were in private practice dropped 28%, whereas the percentage of respondents who are hospital employed increased by more than 300%.[40] This trend is expected to worsen owing to practices attempting to survive the costs of the reporting requirements.

Sustainability of the Affordable Care Act: Will It Last in Orthopaedics?

For those who criticize the ability of this new system to provide effective care, efforts have been made to thwart the new health care system's sustainability. Arguments against the individual mandate were denied when the Supreme Court upheld the constitutionality of the individual mandate provision in NFIB v Sebelius in 2012.[41] For the field of arthroplasty, this decision implied increased access to elective orthopedic procedures for the higher percent of insured

American population that would otherwise be subjected to chronic disability and loss of function. The ACA was again challenged in 2014 regarding health care subsidies obtained through the federal government, rather than through the state marketplace exchanges. In King v Burwell, the Supreme court upheld the interpretation that federal tax credits coverage purchased in federal exchanges were consistent with the intent of the provision in the ACA to cover subsidies and encourage accessible care for all that could obtain insurance through the exchange system.[42] This decision preserved the Medicaid expansion and financial assistance for up to 6.4 million low- and middle-income individuals.[42] The impact of the ACA has expanded beyond Medicare reimbursement programs. For private insurers, a number of plans have begun to adopt ACA-type measures. Blue Cross Blue Shield of Massachusetts and other large national plans are engaging actively in various accountable care organization–like arrangements with providers.[43] Additionally, insurers are required to provide coverage that abides by major underwriting reforms, bans old grandfather clauses, and expands coverage access.

The development of diagnosis-related groups, changes in resource distribution, and the sustainable growth rate are 3 defining policies that were designed to control costs. Health care policy has changed drastically, and with the 50-year anniversary of the passage of Medicare in 2015, the relationship between the current health care system and impacts to various subspecialties has become increasingly important. These policies had an unpredictable impact on those caring for the orthopedic trauma population.[44] Legislation continues to be directed by the study of patient outcomes, providing an opportunity for orthopedists to contribute to future changes in policy. Although the ACA has currently withstood 2 major battles, it has yet to be proven if the system itself will stand the test of time. For the orthopedic surgeon, this uncertainty should motivate providers to become more active in helping to shape policy that will benefit their patients, optimize care delivery, and maximize the opportunity to address disparities that exist in patient outcomes and access to care.

SUMMARY

Degenerative joint disease is a major contributor to disability in Americans and impacts their daily activities. Decreased function and immobility is associated with an increase in medical comorbidities and early mortality. As a result, this will be reflected in a decrease in quality-adjusted life years, the measure by which the national health status is rated and compared with other nations. Therefore, any hindrance to providing the necessary relief associated with addressing poor quality of life through TJA means a hindrance to the health status of our nation. Quality care and reimbursements that drive efficiency, when implemented properly, can be a motivating factor toward improving the health of the nation. With more changes in health care policy forthcoming, it is increasingly important for the orthopedic surgeon to understand how changes in policy will affect practice. A thorough comprehension of health reform and the motivating factors that drive policy will empower arthroplasty providers to effectively advocate for the field of orthopedics as a whole, and the patients we serve.

ACKNOWLEDGMENTS

The authors thank Dr Jerry Kruse for presenting this topic during the *Central Illinois Healthcare Management Summit* chaired by Dr K.J. Saleh.

REFERENCES

1. Reid TJ. The Healing of America: a global quest for better, cheaper, and fairer health care. New York: Penguin Press; 2010.
2. Wallace LS. A view of health care around the world. Ann Fam Med 2013;11(1):84.
3. McGlynn EA, Asch SM, Adams J, et al. The quality of health care delivered to adults in the United States. N Engl J Med 2003;348(26):2635–45.
4. Fisher ES, Wennberg JE. Health care quality, geographic variations, and the challenge of supply-sensitive care. Perspect Biol Med 2003; 46(1):69–79.
5. Jayadev C, Khan T, Coulter A, et al. Patient decision aids in knee replacement surgery. Knee 2012; 19(6):746–50.
6. Maeda JL, Lee KM, Horberg M. Comparative health systems research among Kaiser Permanente and other integrated delivery systems: a systematic literature review. Perm J 2014;18(3):66–77.
7. Guterman S, Davis K, Schoenbaum S, et al. Using Medicare payment policy to transform the health system: a framework for improving performance. Health Aff (Millwood) 2009;28(2):w238–50.
8. Rittenhouse DR, Shortell SM. The patient-centered medical home: will it stand the test of health reform? JAMA 2009;301(19):2038–40.
9. Obamacare Medicaid Expansion Overview. Available at: http://obamacarefacts.com/obamacares-medicaid-expansion/. Accessed November 2, 2015.
10. Kurtz S, Ong K, Lau E, et al. Projections of primary and revision hip and knee arthroplasty in the United States from 2005 to 2030. J Bone Jt Surg Am 2007; 89(4):780–5.
11. Day JS, Lau E, Ong KL, et al. Prevalence and projections of total shoulder and elbow arthroplasty in the United States to 2015. J Shoulder Elbow Surg 2010;19(8):1115–20.
12. Hirpara KM, O'Halloran E, O'Sullivan M. A quantitative assessment of facial protection systems in elective hip arthroplasty. Acta Orthop Belg 2011;77(3):375–80.
13. Lewis CG, Inneh IA, Schutzer SF, et al. Evaluation of the first-generation AAOS clinical guidelines on the prophylaxis of venous thromboembolic events in patients undergoing total joint arthroplasty: experience with 3289 patients from a single institution. J Bone Jt Surg Am 2014;96(16):1327–32.
14. Twigg D, Duffield C, Thompson PL, et al. The impact of nurses on patient morbidity and mortality - the need for a policy change in response to the nursing shortage. Aust Health Rev 2010;34(3):312–6.
15. Froimson M. Perioperative management strategies to improve outcomes and reduce cost during an episode of care. J Arthroplasty 2015;30(3):346–8.
16. Illingworth KD, Mihalko WM, Parvizi J, et al. How to minimize infection and thereby maximize patient outcomes in total joint arthroplasty: a multicenter approach: AAOS exhibit selection. J Bone Jt Surg Am 2013;95(8):e50.
17. Layton JL, Rubin LE, Sweeney JD. Advanced blood management strategies for elective joint arthroplasty. R I Med J 2013;96(3):23–5.
18. Batsis JA, Naessens JM, Keegan MT, et al. Resource utilization of total knee arthroplasty patients cared for on specialty orthopedic surgery units. J Hosp Med 2008;3(3):218–27.
19. Corrigan DM. To Err Is Human: Building a Safer Health System. Washington, DC: National Academy Press; 1999.
20. Committee on Quality of health Care in America, Institute of Medicine. Crossing the quality chasm: a new health system for the 21st century. Washington, DC: National Academy Press; 2001.
21. Avram V, Petruccelli D, Winemaker M, et al. Total joint arthroplasty readmission rates and reasons for 30-day hospital readmission. J Arthroplasty 2014;29(3):465–8.
22. Ashton CM, Wray NP. A conceptual framework for the study of early readmission as an indicator of quality of care. Soc Sci Med 1996;43(11):1533–41.
23. Coleman EA, Min SJ, Chomiak A, et al. Posthospital care transitions: patterns, complications, and risk identification. Health Serv Res 2004;39(5):1449–65.
24. Murray CJ, Frenk J. Ranking 37th—measuring the performance of the U.S. health care system. N Engl J Med 2010;362(2):98–9.

25. Moses H 3rd, Matheson DH, Dorsey ER, et al. The anatomy of health care in the United States. JAMA 2013;310(18):1947–63.

26. McCarthy M. US healthcare spending will reach 20% of GDP by 2024, says report. BMJ 2015;351: h4204.

27. Furrow BA, Greaney TL, Johnon SH, et al. Health law: cases, materials and problems. 7th edition. St Paul (MN): West; 2013. p. 530–7.

28. Abrams M, Nuzum R, Zezza M, et al. The Affordable Care Act's payment and delivery system reforms: a progress report at five years. Issue Brief (Commonw Fund) 2015;12:1–16.

29. Delivery System Reform, Medicare Payment Reform, & the MACRA. Available at: www.cms.gov/Medicare/Quality-Initiatives-Patient-Assessment-Instruments/Value-Based-Programs/MACRA-MIPS-and-APMs/MACRA-MIPS-and-APMs.html. Accessed November 2, 2015.

30. Patient Protection and Affordable Care Act, Note 1. Section 3007. 2010.

31. VanLare JM, Conway PH. Value-based purchasing–national programs to move from volume to value. N Engl J Med 2012;367(4):292–5.

32. Centers for Medicare and Medicaid Services (CMS) website - Hospital Value Based Purchasing. Available at: www.cms.gov/Medicare/Quality-initiatives-patient-assessment-instruments/hospital-value-based-purchasing/index.html. Accessed October 4, 2015.

33. Burchill KR. ARRA and meaningful use: is your organization ready? J Healthc Manag 2010;55(4):232–5.

34. Baker DB, Perlin JB, Halamka J. Evaluating and classifying the readiness of technology specifications for national standardization. J Am Med Inform Assoc 2015;22(3):738–43.

35. Nordt JC, Connair MP, Gregorian JA. Esq. as Medicare costs rise, reimbursements drop.

Rosemont (IL): AAOS; 2012. Available at: www.aaos.org/news/aaosnow/dec12/cover1.asp. Accessed October 10, 2015.

36. Eisner W. Goodbye SGR, Hello MIPS and APR. 2015. Available at: https://ryortho.com/2015/04/goodbye-sgr-hello-mips-and-aps/. Accessed October 5, 2015.

37. Schwarzkopf R, Phan DL, Hoang M, et al. Do patients with income-based insurance have access to total joint arthroplasty? J Arthroplasty. 2014;29(6):1083–6.e1.

38. Cassel CK, Jain SH. Assessing individual physician performance: does measurement suppress motivation? JAMA 2012;307(24):2595–6.

39. Wharam JF, Frank MB, Rosland AM, et al. Pay-for-performance" as a quality improvement tool: perceptions and policy recommendations of physicians and program leaders. Qual Manag Health Care 2011;20(3):234–45.

40. Tongue JR. Orthopaedic economics 1017. Rosemont (IL): AAOS; 2013. Available at: www.aaos.org/news/aaosnow/feb13/youraaos1.asp. Accessed October 4, 2015.

41. National Federation of Independent Business v. Sebelius, 132 S.Ct. 2566 (2012). Benefits Q 2013; 29(1):64–6.

42. Gostin LO, DeBartolo MC, Hougendobler DA. King v Burwell: subsidizing US health insurance for low- and middle-income individuals. JAMA 2015;314(4): 333–4.

43. Chernew ME, Mechanic RE, Landon BE, et al. Private-payer innovation in Massachusetts: the 'alternative quality contract'. Health Aff (Millwood). 2011;30(1):51–61.

44. Mitchell PM, Thakore R, Obremskey A, et al. Orthopaedic trauma and the evolution of healthcare policy in America. J Orthop Trauma 2014;28(Suppl 10):S2–4.

Reducing Length of Stay in Total Joint Arthroplasty Care

Megan Walters, MD[a], Monique C. Chambers, MD, MSL[a],
Zain Sayeed, MSc, MHA[a], Afshin A. Anoushiravani, MD[a],
Mouhanad M. El-Othmani, MD[a],
Khaled J. Saleh, MD, MSc, FRCS (C), MHCM, CPE[b],*

KEYWORDS

- Length of stay • Total joint arthroplasty • Improved care pathways • Surgical optimization
- Fast track

KEY POINTS

- Preoperative, intraoperative, and postoperative factors should be optimized to decrease hospital length of stay.
- Risk factors—age over 64 years, operating time, American Society of Anesthesiologists score of 2 or greater, and comorbid conditions—may result in prolonged duration of stay.
- Many fast track protocols have been adopted to improve postoperative outcomes and decrease length of stay.
- Patient education and activation remain important measures that optimize overall outcomes.

INTRODUCTION

The United States consistently ranks as the leader of developed nations in per capita health care expenditures. Approximately 19.6% of the economy's spending share will be health care driven, resulting in US$5.4 trillion projected to be spent per year by 2024.[1] Recent policy changes and impending future modifications, such as bundle payments and outcome-based reimbursement, are aimed at reducing costs by improving the efficiency of the provided care. Amid methods to alleviate such spending projections, orthopedic surgeons continue to strive to develop practices that provide evidence-based care that is both individualized, as well as standardized for an aging population.

In 2009, 284,000 primary total hip arthroplasties (THAs) and 619,000 total knee arthroplasties (TKAs) were performed.[2] In only 5 years, these figures are projected to increase to 610,583 THAs and 1,557,975 TKAs.[2] With substantial numbers of procedures being performed annually, optimizing patients' outcomes while maximizing efficiency remains an overarching goal in total joint arthroplasty (TJA) care. For several decades, literature references that 30% of hospital expenses associated with TJA were allocated toward the patient's hospital room.[3] Notably, a shorter length of stay (LOS) has been associated with decreased hospital costs.[3] Thus, minimizing the time spent in hospital after TJA has the potential to limit the future financial burden.

There is substantial economic benefit of decreasing LOS in arthroplasty patients.[4] However, few studies directly link reduced LOS with patient satisfaction. An evaluation of 445 TJA

Funding Sources: No additional funding sources were used for this article.

Conflicts of Interest: No conflicts of interest are evident for authors of this article.

[a] Division of Orthopaedics and Rehabilitation, Southern Illinois University School of Medicine, 701 North First Street, Springfield, IL 62781, USA; [b] Department of Orthopaedic and Sports Medicine, Detroit Medical Center, 311 Mack Avenue, 5th Floor, Detroit, MI 48201, USA

* Corresponding author.

E-mail address: kjsaleh@gmail.com

http://dx.doi.org/10.1016/j.ocl.2016.05.006
0030-5898/16/$ – see front matter

patients who underwent "fast track" procedures, aimed toward maximizing efficiency and reducing in-hospital time, reported a 90% patient satisfaction with shorter LOS.[5] Furthermore, the risk of surgical site infection has been shown to be correlated with LOS in TJA patients.[6] Reducing LOS is a realistic target for health care institutions and has the potential to maximize economic efficiency, while simultaneously improving quality and postoperative outcomes. The aim of this review is to explore strategies that have proven effective in reducing LOS, and thereby improving quality of care delivered to TJA patients.

FACTORS THAT AFFECT HOSPITAL STAY

At the most basic level, to decrease LOS, the time required for patients to meet discharge criteria must be minimized. The final decision to discharge a patient is multifactorial and takes into consideration the patient's level of independence, pain control, mental status, control of other medical conditions, gastrointestinal and genitourinary function, and dietary intake, among others. Husted and colleagues[7] reported that "age, sex, marital status, co-morbidity, preoperative use of walking aids, pre- and postoperative hemoglobin levels, the need for blood transfusion, ASA [American Society of Anesthesiologists] score, and time between surgery and mobilization, were all found to influence postoperative outcome in general, and LOS and patient satisfaction in particular." A retrospective study assessing 10,000 TJAs examined primary reasons for delayed discharge from the hospital.[8] In almost 6000 THA patients, the leading causes of prolonged LOS were wound drainage (41.5%), slow physical therapy (22%), discharge issues (17%), and previous health conditions.[8] In the TKA cohort, hospital-acquired conditions (22.5%) was also frequently noted.[8] In a recent study, Inneh concluded that age over 64 years, operating room time, American Society of Anesthesiologists score greater than or equal to 2, and comorbid conditions were risk factors for prolonged LOS after primary TJA, and general anesthesia increased LOS in THA patients specifically.[9,10]

FAST TRACK PATHWAYS

In recognition of the interplay affecting the in-hospital stay duration, "fast track" protocols have been developed. The underlying premise is to devise a multimodal, evidence-based treatment plan that aims to improve efficiency and clinical outcomes.[11] Areas of focus for these pathways include preoperative education and assessment, anesthesia, fluid therapy, pain therapy, and early postoperative mobilization.[7,11,12] Pour and colleagues[13] reported that patients in the fast track had shorter hospital stays, increased walking distance at discharge, and an higher probability of discharge to home versus an extended care facility. Similarly, a recent study noted a significant reduction in LOS from 8.1 days to 3.1 days after implementing a fast track treatment plan for TJA patients.[11]

Owing to its multidisciplinary nature, it is unlikely that a single intervention will decrease LOS in TJA patients across institutions. A further reaching protocol that incorporates and addresses preoperative, intraoperative, and postoperative variables to maximize efficiency at each stage of the patient's experience will likely produce more preemptive improvements. However, this requires the collaboration of the orthopedic surgeon with various providers in other specialties as well as ancillary staff to develop a well-rounded care-plan. The implementation of a multidisciplinary horizontal hierarchal structure of multidisciplinary teams that approaches patient care through the learning cycle of diagnosis, design, action, and reflection, has been proposed as an effective way to promote the necessary cooperative environment. This system of repeated reevaluation and reflection has demonstrated improved quality of care and patient outcomes in preliminary implementation.[14]

PREOPERATIVE EDUCATION

The process of maximizing efficiency of care to reduce LOS for TJA patients begins in the preoperative period. Preparing the patient both mentally and physically for the upcoming surgical experience has been shown to have positive effects on clinical outcomes. A randomized controlled trial conducted by Giraudet-Le Quintrec and colleagues,[15] reported a decrease in preoperative anxiety and pain in THA patients who received preoperative education. Conversely, a systematic review by Panteli and colleagues[16] did not report reduction in LOS in TJA patients who received preoperative education when compared with those who did not. Importantly, one of the limitations of this review was the lack of consistency in the type of preoperative education provided or the delivery method chosen among the included studies.

In contrast, Yoon and colleagues[17] reported a decrease in LOS and increased probability of home discharge among their TJA patients who received preoperative education. Furthermore, joint classes, during which TJA candidates receive education specific to the procedure, achieved shorter hospital stays among participating patients.[18] Many fast track protocols have adopted a preoperative patient education component.[4,7,9,11,14,19,20] These programs range from telephone question-and-answer sessions to multiple physical therapy and informative classes. The most cost-effective form of preoperative education has yet to be determined.[13] Nevertheless, it is an important component of any arthroplasty care plan aimed at optimizing outcomes and efficiency.

ASSESSING NUTRITIONAL STATUS

The effect of a patient's nutritional status also aids in determining the length of hospital stay. Malnutrition is defined by a total lymphocyte count of less than 1500 cells/mm^3 and/or serum albumin concentration of less than 3.5 g/dL. Multiple studies reported an association between malnutrition and impaired wound healing in TJA patients.[21–23] A prospective evaluation of preoperative nutritional status in 213 TKA patients found a significant increase in both superficial and deep wound infections in malnourished patients by anthropometric means.[24] In particular, obese patients with a body mass index of greater than 39 kg/m^2 were noted to have a 9-fold increase in periprosthetic knee infection.[25] Among THA patients, obesity was reported to be a significant risk factor for hospital stay greater than 3 days.[11] Furthermore, malnourished patients often display impaired wound healing with prolonged drainage, which has been shown to be a source for prolonged hospital stay after TJA.[26] Therefore, patients must be optimized before undergoing TJA procedures to decrease the risk of such postoperative complications.[23]

Optimization of medical conditions and comorbidities is imperative for proceeding with surgery. Preoperative evaluation by an internist is recommended as an important step toward maximizing rate of postoperative recovery.[4,7,11,19,20] Comorbidities pertaining to the circulatory, respiratory, and genitourinary systems are especially associated with prolonged hospitalization.[27] Specifically, poorly controlled diabetes mellitus has been associated with increased local and systemic complications, mortality, and LOS in arthroplasty patients.[28] Diabetes diagnosed at time of surgery has been shown to increase the likelihood of postoperative prosthetic joint infection, and as such, glycemic control in the perioperative period remains crucial.[29]

MINIMIZING RISK OF POSTOPERATIVE INFECTION

Multiple studies have examined ways to decrease the rate of infections after TJA.[30–33] Decolonization protocols are supported; however, the wide variation in protocols makes it difficult to recommend any one regimen over the other.[34] These include intranasal mupirocin, clorhexidine baths, and clorhexidine mouth wash in combination or alone for up to 5 days preoperatively.[30–33] Perioperative antibiotics are used as a prophylactic measure to eliminate microorganisms that might gain access to the surgical site during the procedure. Antibiotic dosages and timing of administration should exceed the minimum inhibitory concentration of organisms likely to be encountered for the duration of the operation.[35] The use of antibiotics has been well-documented to decrease the risk of infection, and thereby decrease the likelihood of delayed discharge.

ANESTHESIA MODALITY AND BLOOD MANAGEMENT

In addition to prophylactic antibiotics, modality of anesthesia administration has been assessed as a factor that contributes to postoperative LOS. A systematic review identified a large body of randomized, controlled trials that reported lower pain scores and morphine consumption postoperatively with the use of regional anesthesia in comparison with general anesthesia in TKA patients.[36] Another randomized control trial evaluated the use of peripheral femoral nerve block in TJA, and the authors reported improved pain control and a 24-hour shorter LOS among this cohort.[37] Regional anesthesia may lead to shorter operative times in THA candidates correlating with reduced LOS.[9,10,38,39] Helwani and colleagues[40] recently examined 13,000 THAs and noted a decrease in deep surgical site infection and LOS in patients who had received regional anesthesia—spinal or epidural—versus those who received general anesthesia. General anesthesia has also been shown to increase risk of cerebrovascular events and cardiac arrest in comparison with spinal anesthesia, despite its tendency to be used in younger patients with lower Charlson Comorbidity Indexes.[38]

Furthermore, anesthesia modality has an impact on blood loss, further affecting the hospital LOS.[37] A recent study reported an overall blood transfusion rate of approximately 17% after THA.[41] Intuitively, LOS and hospital cost are both increased in patients that receive an allogenic transfusion in comparison to those who do not.[41–43] This same patient population also experiences increased infection rate, pulmonary compromise, thromboembolic events, and mortality rate.[41–43] Reported risk factors for allogenic transfusion are age, race, payer status, and medical comorbidities.[41,42] Protocols that can decrease the rate of blood transfusion among arthroplasty patients have significant potential to improve postoperative outcomes and reduce hospital stay. Limiting allogenic transfusions to patients whose hemoglobin is less than 8 g/dL or exhibiting symptoms of anemia, and transfusing 1 unit at a time has displayed a 10% reduction in rate of transfusion.[21] Furthermore, orthopedic surgeons must be cognizant that patients who receive transfusion remain in the hospital on average 1 day longer.[21] Nonetheless, the initial step in achieving this goal is to educate staff and other providers, including anesthesiologists, on transfusion guidelines for the patient.

In efforts to minimize the amount of blood loss, surgeons have turned to hypotensive epidural anesthesia (HEA). HEA is achieved by using a continuous infusion epidural catheter to achieve total sympathetic blockade with a target mean arterial pressure of 45 to 50.[44] A randomized, controlled trial of 30 TKAs demonstrated that HEA reduced transfusion rate compared with spinal anesthesia.[45] Interestingly, it does not seem that the hypotension alone is the driving force in this difference. Hypotensive total intravenous anesthesia has not been shown to be as effective in decreasing intraoperative blood loss or total number of units transfused when compared with HEA, despite having no difference in mean arterial pressure, heart rate, or partial pressure of oxygen.[46]

URINARY CATHETERIZATION

Postoperative urinary retention, a potential factor that contributes to longer LOS, is not uncommon, and the incidence has been reported to be as high as 84% after arthroplasty procedures.[47] It was historically reported that short-term catheterization after arthroplasty decreases the incidence of urinary retention without increasing the rate of urinary tract infections.[48,49] Conversely, recent studies have demonstrated that postoperative patients who are not catheterized experience better outcomes. In a retrospective study that evaluated 6154 TKA patients, patients who were not managed with postoperative catheterization were noted to have shorter hospital stay, lower cost, decreased complications, and lower rates of 30-day readmission.[50] Routine catheter use should be avoided, but intermittent catheterization may be required for a select group of patients.

USE OF TRANEXAMIC ACID

Another intervention that has recently demonstrated promising effects on hemodynamic stability after arthroplasty is the use of tranexamic acid (TXA). TXA is a lysine derivate that competitively inhibits plasmin resulting in impaired fibrinolysis.[51] Reduction in postoperative hemoglobin was significantly lower in patients who received an intraarticular TXA injection at the conclusion of THA versus those who did not.[52] Several studies have demonstrated decreased blood loss and lower transfusion rates among TJA patients who received TXA perioperatively; either periarticularly or intravenously.[52–55] Additionally, increased risk of venous thromboembolism and pulmonary embolism has not been reported after TXA administration.[43,56] Studies comparing single to double administration of TXA have shown promising improvement in overall blood loss and transfusion rate in double administration cohorts.[53,54] Thus, TXA use is a reasonable consideration in TJA patients, so long as contraindications such as prior stroke, venous thromboembolism, allergy, and severe coronary artery disease are absent.[43]

POSTOPERATIVE MANAGEMENT

Efficient postoperative management is critical for reducing hospital stay. Infection is one of the most common complication within 3 postoperative days after TJA. Efforts to minimize infection largely rely on proper wound management. Traditional dressings require frequent changes, which may expose the wound to external sources of contamination as well as skin breakdown and blistering.[57] Modern dressings are specifically designed for the demands of TJA patients. One comparative study approximates that 75% of patients who receive the modern dressings are discharged by postoperative day 4 compared with day 6 in the traditional group.[57] Advances in wound care management have also included the use of negative-pressure wound therapy. Negative-pressure wound therapy has been used more and more as a means to assist in closing primary surgical wounds. However, a randomized, controlled trial reported no difference in the rate of surgical site infection over a 6-week period, compared with patients with standard absorbent dressings.[58] Future research is needed to determine if the use of negative-pressure wound therapy may in fact reduce wound infections. Recently, there have also been advances in occlusive dressings that maintain a sterile environment and minimize risk of bacterial entry to the surgical incision.[59]

Finally, the application of cryotherapy has been used as standard care for decades to minimize inflammation and the extent of trauma to the surrounding soft tissues after TJA. However, the efficacy of the practice has not been established. Studies demonstrate that use of cryotherapy serves benefit in terms of blood loss and range of motion at discharge.[60] Cryotherapy did not provide a benefit in transfusion and analgesia requirements, pain, swelling, or LOS.[60] The use of cryotherapy remains a common practice after TJA, but may not provide any substantial benefit to discharging patients earlier. Nonetheless, the clinical benefits of decreased blood loss and increase in range of motion at discharge may allow patients to mobilize sooner and provide welfare to the patients' overall health status.

Managing medical comorbidities is vital to reducing LOS. Comanagement by multidisciplinary teams demonstrates ability to reduce minor postoperative complication rates and is the preferred model for midlevel staff and surgeons.[61] Additionally, care pathways implementation often results in shorter LOS, decreased costs, and a lesser rate of complications.[50] One of the major complications that the care delivery teams attempt to prevent is a thromboembolic event. Without prophylactic measures, the risk of deep venous thrombosis (DVT) can be as high as 46%, with the highest likelihood of occurrence being within the first 3 postoperative days.[62] There is variation in the type of mechanical device that is best suited for patients after TJA. Above-the-knee compression devices and compression stockings have not been shown to be efficacious, possibly increase risk of DVT owing to a reverse gradient flow.[63] Below-the-knee devices provide intermittent compression and have been shown to be beneficial in reducing rates of pulmonary embolism and DVT.[63]

In tandem with mechanical compressive devices, pharmacotherapy minimizes the formation of DVT by treating hematologic etiology. Thromboprophylaxis trends have moved away from aggressive anticoagulation to reduce intraoperative bleeding and rates of transfusion.[64,65] Recent studies have shown that patients receiving prophylactic aspirin have significantly fewer symptomatic DVTs and pulmonary embolisms compared with patients receiving a standard dose of warfarin.[65] This was followed by American Academy of Orthopaedic Surgeons' guidelines recommending the use of aspirin and has led to a greater trend of aspirin use as thromboprophylaxis after TJA. A systematic review of the literature found that varying specialty organizations provide inconsistent guidelines on the use of mechanical and/or chemoprophylaxis.[66] Future studies are needed to determine optimal thromboprophylactic regimens that are cost effective and therapeutically sound for TJA patients.

Early postoperative mobilization may increase patient morale and satisfaction, and prepare the patient for an earlier discharge. Postoperative care pathways have focused on earlier rehabilitation for TJA patients.[67,68] Patients who experience rapid rehabilitation with physiotherapy while in the recovery room report reduced LOS than patients who began therapy on postoperative day 1.[67,68] This has been supported by similar enhanced recovery after surgery programs in other countries.[69] Enhanced recovery after surgery programs include a combination of evidence-based interventions used in a multimodal, integrated clinical care approach to achieve improved functional outcomes and rapid recovery. Patients in enhanced programs experienced shorter hospital stays and were more likely to be ready to be discharged on day 3 after surgery.[69]

PATIENT ACTIVATION

Many TJA patients are elderly with limited support systems. Providing patients with tools that increase outpatient support may lead to earlier hospital discharge. Poor patient compliance and repetitive postoperative visits to the hospital may result in limited range of motion, infection at the surgical site, pressure sores, and possibly scar tissue contractures.[70] Factors that can motivate patients to take shared responsibility in their health care, a concept known as patient activation, should be sought to maximize patient outcomes. Postoperative orthopedic education combines verbal and written information that is valuable to offer patients methods of relieving postoperative pain.[71] As such, the use of digital technology that combines such information for specific patient populations may be associated with effective behavioral changes.[72]

SUMMARY

Health care reform will place greater emphasis on hospitals and orthopedists to minimize hospital LOS associated with TJA procedures. As replicable procedures that demonstrate high patient satisfaction, the effects of such reform on TJA will serve as a model for other procedures throughout the nation. Thus, the preoperative period should focus on optimizing patients for the demands of a surgical intervention. In the postoperative period, the patient should be given the necessary support to have a successful discharge, without increasing the risk of a hospital readmission. Decreasing LOS increases patient satisfaction, reduces economic burden, and minimizes risks to nosocomial complications. To provide the highest quality of care delivery, orthopedic surgeons should understand the various factors that contribute to these postoperative outcomes.

ACKNOWLEDGMENTS

The authors thank Dr Javad Parvizi for presenting this topic during the Central Illinois Healthcare Management Summit chaired by Dr K.J. Saleh.

REFERENCES

1. Keehan SP, Cuckler GA, Sisko AM, et al. National health expenditure projections, 2014-24: spending growth faster than recent trends. Health Aff (Project Hope) 2015;34(8):1407–17.
2. Kurtz SM, Ong KL, Lau E, et al. Impact of the economic downturn on total joint replacement demand in the United States: updated projections to 2021. J Bone Joint Surg Am 2014;96(8):624–30.
3. Healy WL, Rana AJ, Iorio R. Hospital economics of primary total knee arthroplasty at a teaching hospital. Clin Orthop Relat Res 2011;469(1):87–94.
4. Lovald ST, Ong KL, Malkani AL, et al. Complications, mortality, and costs for outpatient and short-stay total knee arthroplasty patients in comparison to standard-stay patients. J Arthroplasty 2014;29(3):510–5.
5. Specht K, Kjaersgaard-Andersen P, Kehlet H, et al. High patient satisfaction in 445 patients who underwent fast-track hip or knee replacement. Acta Orthopaedica 2015;86(6):702–7.
6. Pulido L, Ghanem E, Joshi A, et al. Periprosthetic joint infection: the incidence, timing, and predisposing factors. Clin Orthop Relat Res 2008;466(7): 1710–5.
7. Husted H, Gromov K, Malchau H, et al. Traditions and myths in hip and knee arthroplasty. Acta Orthopaedica 2014;85(6):548–55.
8. Lyman S, Fields KG, Nocon AA, et al. Prolonged length of stay is not an acceptable alternative to coded complications in assessing hospital quality in elective joint arthroplasty. J Arthroplasty 2015; 30(11):1863–7.
9. Inneh IA. The Combined Influence of Sociodemographic, Preoperative Comorbid and Intraoperative Factors on Longer Length of Stay After Elective Primary Total Knee Arthroplasty. J Arthroplasty 2015;30(11):1883–6.
10. Inneh IA, Iorio R, Slover JD, et al. Role of sociodemographic, co-morbid and intraoperative factors in length of stay following primary total hip arthroplasty. J Arthroplasty 2015;30(12):2092–7.
11. Winther SB, Foss OA, Wik TS, et al. 1-year follow-up of 920 hip and knee arthroplasty patients after implementing fast-track. Acta Orthopaedica 2015; 86(1):78–85.
12. Khan SK, Malviya A, Muller SD, et al. Reduced short-term complications and mortality following Enhanced Recovery primary hip and knee arthroplasty: results from 6,000 consecutive procedures. Acta Orthopaedica 2014;85(1):26–31.
13. Pour AE, Parvizi J, Sharkey PF, et al. Minimally invasive hip arthroplasty: what role does patient preconditioning play? J Bone Joint Surg Am 2007; 89(9):1920–7.
14. Nawaz H, Edmondson AC, Tzeng TH, et al. Teaming: an approach to the growing complexities in health care: AOA critical issues. J Bone Joint Surg Am 2014;96(21):e184.
15. Giraudet-Le Quintrec JS, Coste J, Vastel L, et al. Positive effect of patient education for hip surgery: a randomized trial. Clin Orthop Relat Res 2003;(414):112–20.
16. Panteli M, Habeeb S, McRoberts J, et al. Enhanced care for primary hip arthroplasty: factors affecting length of hospital stay. Eur J Orthop Surg Traumatol 2014;24(3):353–8.
17. Yoon RS, Nellans KW, Geller JA, et al. Patient education before hip or knee arthroplasty lowers length of stay. J Arthroplasty 2010;25(4):547–51.
18. Huang SW, Chen PH, Chou YH. Effects of a preoperative simplified home rehabilitation education program on length of stay of total knee arthroplasty patients. Orthop Traumatol Surg Res 2012;98(3): 259–64.
19. Kolisek FR, McGrath MS, Jessup NM, et al. Comparison of outpatient versus inpatient total knee arthroplasty. Clin Orthop Relat Res 2009;467(6): 1438–42.
20. Berger RA, Sanders SA, Thill ES, et al. Newer anesthesia and rehabilitation protocols enable outpatient hip replacement in selected patients. Clin Orthop Relat Res 2009;467(6):1424–30.
21. Markel DC, Allen MW, Zappa NM. Can an arthroplasty registry help decrease transfusions in

primary total joint replacement? A quality initiative. Clin Orthop Relat Res 2016;474(1):126–31.

22. Jaberi FM, Parvizi J, Haytmanek CT, et al. Procrastination of wound drainage and malnutrition affect the outcome of joint arthroplasty. Clin Orthop Relat Res 2008;466(6):1368–71.

23. Cross MB, Yi PH, Thomas CF, et al. Evaluation of malnutrition in orthopaedic surgery. J Am Acad Orthop Surg 2014;22(3):193–9.

24. Font-Vizcarra L, Lozano L, Rios J, et al. Preoperative nutritional status and post-operative infection in total knee replacements: a prospective study of 213 patients. Int J Artif Organs 2011;34(9):876–81.

25. Dowsey MM, Choong PF. Obese diabetic patients are at substantial risk for deep infection after primary TKA. Clin Orthop Relat Res 2009;467(6):1577–81.

26. Ibrahim MS, Khan MA, Nizam I, et al. Peri-operative interventions producing better functional outcomes and enhanced recovery following total hip and knee arthroplasty: an evidence-based review. BMC Med 2013;11:37.

27. Kurtz S, Ong K, Lau E, et al. Projections of primary and revision hip and knee arthroplasty in the United States from 2005 to 2030. J Bone Joint Surg Am 2007;89(4):780–5.

28. Marchant MH Jr, Viens NA, Cook C, et al. The impact of glycemic control and diabetes mellitus on perioperative outcomes after total joint arthroplasty. J Bone Joint Surg Am 2009;91(7):1621–9.

29. Jamsen E, Nevalainen P, Eskelinen A, et al. Obesity, diabetes, and preoperative hyperglycemia as predictors of periprosthetic joint infection: a single-center analysis of 7181 primary hip and knee replacements for osteoarthritis. J Bone Joint Surg Am 2012;94(14):e101.

30. Buehlmann M, Frei R, Fenner L, et al. Highly effective regimen for decolonization of methicillin-resistant Staphylococcus aureus carriers. Infect Control Hosp Epidemiol 2008;29(6):510–6.

31. Kim DH, Spencer M, Davidson SM, et al. Institutional prescreening for detection and eradication of methicillin-resistant Staphylococcus aureus in patients undergoing elective orthopaedic surgery. J Bone Joint Surg Am 2010;92(9):1820–6.

32. Rao N, Cannella BA, Crossett LS, et al. Preoperative screening/decolonization for Staphylococcus aureus to prevent orthopedic surgical site infection: prospective cohort study with 2-year follow-up. J Arthroplasty 2011;26(8):1501–7.

33. Wendt C, Schinke S, Wurttemberger M, et al. Value of whole-body washing with chlorhexidine for the eradication of methicillin-resistant Staphylococcus aureus: a randomized, placebo-controlled, double-blind clinical trial. Infect Control Hosp Epidemiol 2007;28(9):1036–43.

34. Illingworth KD, Mihalko WM, Parvizi J, et al. How to minimize infection and thereby maximize patient outcomes in total joint arthroplasty: a multicenter approach: AAOS exhibit selection. J Bone Joint Surg Am 2013;95(8):e50.

35. Hansen E, Belden K, Silibovsky R, et al. Perioperative antibiotics. J Arthroplasty 2014;29(2 Suppl):29–48.

36. Macfarlane AJ, Prasad GA, Chan VW, et al. Does regional anesthesia improve outcome after total knee arthroplasty? Clin Orthop Relat Res 2009;467(9):2379–402.

37. Macfarlane AJ, Prasad GA, Chan VW, et al. Does regional anaesthesia improve outcome after total hip arthroplasty? A systematic review. Br J Anaesth 2009;103(3):335–45.

38. Basques BA, Toy JO, Bohl DD, et al. General compared with spinal anesthesia for total hip arthroplasty. J Bone Joint Surg Am 2015;97(6):455–61.

39. Hu S, Zhang ZY, Hua YQ, et al. A comparison of regional and general anaesthesia for total replacement of the hip or knee: a meta-analysis. J Bone Joint Surg Br 2009;91(7):935–42.

40. Helwani MA, Avidan MS, Ben Abdallah A, et al. Effects of regional versus general anesthesia on outcomes after total hip arthroplasty: a retrospective propensity-matched cohort study. J Bone Joint Surg Am 2015;97(3):186–93.

41. Saleh A, Small T, Chandran Pillai AL, et al. Allogenic blood transfusion following total hip arthroplasty: results from the nationwide inpatient sample, 2000 to 2009. J Bone Joint Surg Am 2014;96(18):e155.

42. Browne JA, Adib F, Brown TE, et al. Transfusion rates are increasing following total hip arthroplasty: risk factors and outcomes. J Arthroplasty 2013;28(8 Suppl):34–7.

43. Levine BR, Haughom B, Strong B, et al. Blood management strategies for total knee arthroplasty. J Am Acad Orthop Surg 2014;22(6):361–71.

44. Sharrock NE, Mineo R, Urquhart B. Hemodynamic response to low-dose epinephrine infusion during hypotensive epidural anesthesia for total hip replacement. Reg Anesth 1990;15(6):295–9.

45. Juelsgaard P, Larsen UT, Sorensen JV, et al. Hypotensive epidural anesthesia in total knee replacement without tourniquet: reduced blood loss and transfusion. Reg Anesth Pain Med 2001;26(2):105–10.

46. Eroglu A, Uzunlar H, Erciyes N. Comparison of hypotensive epidural anesthesia and hypotensive total intravenous anesthesia on intraoperative blood loss during total hip replacement. J Clin Anesth 2005;17(6):420–5.

47. Hollman F, Wolterbeek N, Veen R. Risk factors for postoperative urinary retention in men undergoing

total hip arthroplasty. Orthopedics 2015;38(6): e507–11.

48. Michelson JD, Lotke PA, Steinberg ME. Urinary-bladder management after total joint-replacement surgery. N Engl J Med 1988;319(6): 321–6.

49. Oishi CS, Williams VJ, Hanson PB, et al. Perioperative bladder management after primary total hip arthroplasty. J Arthroplasty 1995;10(6):732–6.

50. Loftus T, Agee C, Jaffe R, et al. A simplified pathway for total knee arthroplasty improves outcomes. J Knee Surg 2014;27(3):221–8.

51. Astedt B. Clinical pharmacology of tranexamic acid. Scand J Gastroenterol Suppl 1987;137:22–5.

52. Ralley FE, Berta D, Binns V, et al. One intraoperative dose of tranexamic Acid for patients having primary hip or knee arthroplasty. Clin Orthop Relat Res 2010;468(7):1905–11.

53. Iwai T, Tsuji S, Tomita T, et al. Repeat-dose intravenous tranexamic acid further decreases blood loss in total knee arthroplasty. Int Orthop 2013;37(3): 441–5.

54. Lee SH, Cho KY, Khurana S, et al. Less blood loss under concomitant administration of tranexamic acid and indirect factor Xa inhibitor following total knee arthroplasty: a prospective randomized controlled trial. Knee Surg Sports Traumatol Arthrosc 2013;21(11):2611–7.

55. Seo JG, Moon YW, Park SH, et al. The comparative efficacies of intra-articular and IV tranexamic acid for reducing blood loss during total knee arthroplasty. Knee Surg Sports Traumatol Arthrosc 2013; 21(8):1869–74.

56. Yang ZG, Chen WP, Wu LD. Effectiveness and safety of tranexamic acid in reducing blood loss in total knee arthroplasty: a meta-analysis. J Bone Joint Surg Am 2012;94(13):1153–9.

57. Hopper GP, Deakin AH, Crane EO, et al. Enhancing patient recovery following lower limb arthroplasty with a modern wound dressing: a prospective, comparative audit. J Wound Care 2012;21(4):200–3.

58. Gillespie BM, Rickard CM, Thalib L, et al. Use of negative-pressure wound dressings to prevent surgical site complications after primary hip arthroplasty: a pilot RCT. Surg Innov 2015;22(5):488–95.

59. Shetty VD. Drywounds matter: the use of occlusive sterile sanitary napkin dressing in hip and knee replacement wounds. Int Wound J 2010;7(5):428–9.

60. Adie S, Naylor JM, Harris IA. Cryotherapy after total knee arthroplasty a systematic review and meta-analysis of randomized controlled trials. J Arthroplasty 2010;25(5):709–15.

61. Huddleston JM, Long KH, Naessens JM, et al. Medical and surgical comanagement after elective hip and knee arthroplasty: a randomized, controlled trial. Ann Intern Med 2004;141(1):28–38.

62. Cordell-Smith JA, Williams SC, Harper WM, et al. Lower limb arthroplasty complicated by deep venous thrombosis. Prevalence and subjective outcome. J Bone Joint Surg Br 2004;86(1):99–101.

63. Best AJ, Williams S, Crozier A, et al. Graded compression stockings in elective orthopaedic surgery. An assessment of the in vivo performance of commercially available stockings in patients having hip and knee arthroplasty. J Bone Joint Surg Br 2000;82(1):116–8.

64. Castillo Monsegur J, Bisbe Vives E, Santiveri Papiol X, et al. Low-dose aspirin doesn't increase surgical bleeding nor transfusion rate in total knee arthroplasty. Rev Esp Anestesiol Reanim 2012;59(4):180–6 [in Spanish].

65. Raphael IJ, Tischler EH, Huang R, et al. Aspirin: an alternative for pulmonary embolism prophylaxis after arthroplasty? Clin Orthop Relat Res 2014;472(2): 482–8.

66. Sharma V, Morgan PM, Cheng EY. Factors influencing early rehabilitation after THA: a systematic review. Clin Orthop Relat Res 2009;467(6):1400–11.

67. Stewart SP. Joint replacement and rapid mobilization: a clinical perspective on rapid arthroplasty mobilization protocol. Orthop Nurs 2012;31(4): 224–9 [quiz: 30–1].

68. Tayrose G, Newman D, Slover J, et al. Rapid mobilization decreases length-of-stay in joint replacement patients. Bull Hosp Jt Dis (2013) 2013;71(3): 222–6.

69. Christelis N, Wallace S, Sage CE, et al. An enhanced recovery after surgery program for hip and knee arthroplasty. Med J Aust 2015;202(7): 363–8.

70. Robbins CE, Casey D, Bono JV, et al. A multidisciplinary total hip arthroplasty protocol with accelerated postoperative rehabilitation: does the patient benefit? Am J Orthopedics (Belle Mead, NJ) 2014;43(4):178–81.

71. Derman PB, Fabricant PD, David G. The role of overweight and obesity in relation to the more rapid growth of total knee arthroplasty volume compared with total hip arthroplasty volume. J Bone Joint Surg Am 2014;96(11):922–8.

72. Abroms LC, Ahuja M, Kodl Y, et al. Text2Quit: results from a pilot test of a personalized, interactive mobile health smoking cessation program. J Health Commun 2012;17(Suppl 1):44–53.

Approach to Decrease Infection Following Total Joint Arthroplasty

Daniel Hatz, MD[a], Afshin A. Anoushiravani, MD[a],
Monique C. Chambers, MD, MSL[a], Mouhanad M. El-Othmani, MD[a],
Khaled J. Saleh, MD, MSc, FRCS (C), MHCM, CPE[b,*]

KEYWORDS

- Surgical site infection • Prevention • Total joint arthroplasty • Prosthetic joint infection
- Total knee infection • Total hip infection

KEY POINTS

- Surgical site infections are a debilitating and costly adverse outcome following total joint replacement that is minimized with proper preoperative, intraoperative, and postoperative screening.
- The most effective means of preventing surgical site infections is through the preoperative optimization of all total joint surgical candidates.
- New pharmacologic and intraoperative technologies are allowing orthopedic surgeons to better prevent and if needed combat surgical site infections.

INTRODUCTION

Degenerative joint osteoarthritis is a debilitating disease, profoundly altering a patient's functional capacity and quality of life. Advancements in total joint arthroplasty (TJA) have allowed for excellent pain relief and restoration of biomechanical function. By the year 2030, demand for TJA in the United States is expected to exceed 4 million TJA procedures a year.[1] One of the most concerning and serious complications of any TJA is deep infection. However, periprosthetic joint infections (PJI) have a reasonably low reported incidence at 0.5% to 3%.[1,2] As such, PJIs remain one of the most challenging orthopedic complications in terms of prevention and treatment. Unsuccessful treatment can result in devastating morbidity including several reoperations; overall loss of function; and significant cost to patient,

caregivers, and the health care system. Estimated cost of a single PJI has been reported at approximately $50,000, increasing to greater than $100,000 for resistant organisms.[1] Reported cost of revisions because of infection in 2009 was $566 million and projected to reach up to $4 billion by 2030.[1] A better understanding of successful approaches to prevent periprosthetic infections will allow orthopedic surgeons to better optimize their patients preoperatively, intraoperatively, and postoperatively, improving patient outcomes.

Although eradicating periprosthetic infection may seem daunting, a methodical approach minimizes operative risks while improving outcomes. The development of PJI can result from several perioperative factors. Preoperative patient selection and optimization, intraoperative emphasis on sterility, and postoperative

Funding Sources: No additional funding sources were used for this article.
Conflicts of Interest: No conflicts of interest are evident for authors of this article.
[a] Division of Orthopaedics and Rehabilitation, Southern Illinois University School of Medicine, 701 North First Street, Springfield, IL 62781, USA; [b] Department of Orthopaedic and Sports Medicine, Detroit Medical Center, 311 Mack Avenue, 5th Floor, Detroit, MI 48201, USA
* Corresponding author.
E-mail address: kjsaleh@gmail.com

antibiotics and wound care play a pivotal role in avoiding the dreaded complications of infection. This article discusses current measures and concepts to decrease risks for deep infections in TJA.

PREOPERATIVE MEASURES
Optimizing the Patient
Assessment of the general medical health of each patient with a thorough history and physical examination is an important precursor for infection prevention. Several medical comorbidities have been shown to generate a significant propensity for infection, most notably diabetes, rheumatoid arthritis, obesity, and immunosuppression (including chronic steroid use).[3,4] The combination of these comorbidities is demonstrated to significantly increase the overall risk for infection.[5] Special care should be taken in selecting patients with manageable medical comorbidities and optimizing all current medical issues before proceeding with TJA.

Diabetes
Several studies have reported diabetes as an integral contributor to the development of infections. Diabetes combined with any other comorbidity has been shown to significantly increase infection rates.[2,6] Hemoglobin A_{1C} is a frequently ordered outpatient blood test representative of glucose control over the past 3 months. Marchant and colleagues[7] reported that patients with moderately elevated hemoglobin A_{1C} are two to four times as likely to develop PJI. However, other studies have suggested that the risk for PJI is more closely associated with the patient's current glycemic status rather than the patient's long-term glycemic control.[7] Mraovic and colleagues[8] reported patients with blood glucose levels greater than 200 mg/dL on postoperative Day 1 are twice as likely to have a PJI, compared with patients with well-controlled glucose levels. Surgical procedures, such as TJA, can result in stress-induced hyperglycemia postoperatively.[9] Patients with diabetes have increased variability in perioperative glycemic levels, increasing the propensity for PJI. Thus, orthopedic surgeons must be cognizant of the long-term and perioperative effects of poor glycemic control in all TJA candidates, but particularly those with diabetes mellitus.[2,4]

Obesity
Although an area of controversy, recent literature supports the correlation between obesity and morbid obesity with PJI.[3,10–14] Dowsey and

Choong[11] prospectively examined 1214 consecutive primary total knee arthroplasties (TKA) comparing deep infection rates of morbidly obese and obese patients with nonobese control subjects. The results indicated morbidly obese patients (body mass index >40) were nearly at nine times higher risk of developing deep infection.[11] No infections were recorded in nonobese patients. Furthermore, obese patients (body mass index <40) did not demonstrate an increased risk for periprosthetic knee infections when compared with the nonobese control subjects.[3,4,10,15] A similar study in total hip arthroplasty (THA) patients evaluating obese and morbidly obese patients indicated increased risk for PJI in both cohorts.[16] Namba and colleagues[14] evaluated deep infections in obese patients with THA and TKA, concluding that obese patients had a 6.7- and 4.2-fold increased risk of developing deep infection following TKA and THA, respectively. In addition, the combination of obesity with diabetes revealed a nearly seven-fold increase in periprosthetic knee infections when compared with obese patients without diabetes.[3,4,10,15]

Other comorbidities
Comorbidities, such as cardiovascular disease, chronic anemia, rheumatoid arthritis, and chronic immunosuppression, have demonstrated increased rates of PJI.[3,4,10,15] In a study evaluating greater than 56,000 TKAs, patients with an American Society of Anesthesiologists score greater than three demonstrated a statistically significant increased infection rate of 53.3% compared with 38.2%.[17] Males are twice as likely to have PJI, than their female counterparts.[18] Patients with the human immunodeficiency virus, hemophilia, and those with CD4 counts of less than or equal to 200/mm^3 are at increased risk for PJI because of their immunocompromised status.[18,19] Hence, patients with high-risk comorbidities should be counseled extensively and medically optimized before elective surgical intervention.

Nutritional status
Nutritional status is predictive of infection and postoperative wound healing.[4,20–22] Malnutrition is most commonly delineated with a series of serologic tests including serum transferrin less than 200 mg/dL, serum albumin less than 3.5 g/dL, and a total lymphocyte count less than 1500/mm^3.[23] Poor nutritional status is most frequently cited in the elderly, bariatric patients, and the morbidly obese. Jaberi and colleagues[24] prospectively examined 10,325

patients following TJA with 300 developing persistent wound drainage greater than 48 hours. In their study, they concluded that malnourished patients had a higher rate of PJI.[24] Greene and colleagues[21] similarly assessed the impact of surgery on the nutritional status of 217 patients with TJA. Postoperatively, patients' total lymphocyte counts had dropped 57% and serum albumin had dropped 72% from preoperative values.[21] By postoperative Day 10, no patient had returned to preoperative levels.[21] Lavernia and colleagues[25] reported the effect of poor nutrition on length of stay following TKA. They prospectively examined 119 and found that patients with albumin levels less than 3.4 g/dL had a 32.7% higher hospital charge and longer length of stay (3.4 days).[25] Zorilla and colleagues[26] examined serum zinc levels as a predictor of postoperative outcomes. They prospectively examined 97 patients who underwent hemiarthroplasty for acute hip fracture and found an 11.8-fold increased risk for delayed wound healing.[26] Prolonged wound healing greater than 5 days has been shown to increase the likelihood of PJI by 12.5-fold.[27,28] Because of its prevalence among patients with TJA, it is crucial to optimize the nutritional status before surgical intervention.

Smoking

The detrimental effects of smoking tobacco on wound healing and all-cause complications are well documented in patients with TJA.[4,29–31] In one large retrospective study smokers were 32% more likely to suffer from postoperative complications including mortality.[29] Furthermore, there was an association between the number and severity of systemic complications and the number of pack-years smoked.[29,30] Peersman and colleagues[4] study demonstrated smokers were at a statistically significant risk for PJI when compared with nonsmokers. Clinicians should inform their patients about the various medical risks associated with smoking tobacco, and encourage them to quit smoking at least 6 to 8 weeks before surgery.[32]

Infection Starts with the Host

Surgical site infection (SSI) and wound drainage greater than 48 hours has been correlated to the development of PJI.[24] In addition to optimizing the patient's ability to heal postoperatively, prevention of SSI involves minimizing risk from superficial bacterial sources. A study by von Eiff and colleagues[33] used the bacterial genotype to demonstrate that 80% of nosocomial SSIs originated from native endogenous

Staphylococcus aureus. The prevalence of colonization with *S aureus* has been dropped from 32.4% to 28.6% of infections, whereas the prevalence of methicillin-resistance *S aureus* (MRSA) has increased from 0.8% to 1.5%.[34,35] Both *S aureus* and MRSA colonization have been associated with a significant increase in risk for SSI.[2,33,36–38] In a study by Yano and colleagues[36] preoperative screening for nasal colonization of MRSA in orthopedic patients revealed that 4% of patients had MRSA-positive nasal cultures of which 26% developed MRSA wound infections. Conversely, of the patients with negative nasal colonization, only 1.3% developed SSI.[36]

However, whether SSIs result from exogenous bacterial contamination or endogenous self-inoculation and colonization is still controversial. Although intranasal *S aureus* colonization is a risk factor for orthopedic SSI, most postoperative bacterial strains recovered from the surgical suites were different strains than those identified in preoperative nasal samples. Despite the uncertainty of the origin, several studies have shown the effectiveness of implementation of prehospital screening and decolonization protocols in decreasing SSI.[39,40] Decolonization protocols started 5 days before surgery include combination of nasal mupirocin ointment, chlorhexidine total body wash, and chlorhexidine mouth rinse and have been demonstrated to reduce postoperative infections.[2,33,36–38] Buehlmann and colleagues[41] revealed that such preadmission protocols were 98% effective in preventing PJI and decolonizing the nares and groin. In contrast, Wendt and colleagues[42] compared decolonization protocols with a placebo group in various regions of the body and reported that preadmission decolonization protocols were only successful in eradicating MRSA from the groin, but not the nares, throat, or perineum.

INTRAOPERATIVE MEASURES

The surgeon has control over several factors within the operating room that may decrease the risk of PJI. Intraoperative considerations include use of effective skin preparations, control over sterile operative and facility environments, perioperative prophylactic antibiotics, and wound management. It is also important for the surgeon to have a team that is cohesive and aware of TJA protocols designed to increase sterility, and maximize operating room efficiency.

Skin Preparation

It is beneficial to thoroughly examine the patient's skin in the office and in the preoperative area. Detection of abrasions, bruising, ulcers, pet scratches, psoriatic patches, or cellulitis should be routine practice and may reduce the risk for wound infections.[3,4,10,15] It is important to appreciate existing incisional scars. Incorporating previous incisions into the new incision decreases the risk for devascularized skin bridges, postoperative skin necrosis, and subsequent wound infection.[3,4,10,15] Removal of hair around the incision site has become a routine part of the preoperative preparation. There are limited data to support hair removal in prevention of SSI. A Cochrane review article showed no statistical difference between hair removal and decrease in SSI.[43] In fact, SSI statistically increased when hair was removed with a razor as compared with clippers.[2,43] Alcohol or aqueous skin preparations have been shown to have a skin penetration of only 300 μm.[44] This leaves viable bacteria deep inside hair follicles and skin recolonization may occur in 30 minutes.[3,4,10,15] Although, hair removal does not reduce the risk for SSI, it does improve surgical site visibility. When implemented, it is recommended that hair be removed immediately before surgery with an electric clipper, minimizing bacterial recolonization and epidermal abrasions.

Several preoperative skin preparations are currently available; however, no one agent has superiority over the other.[2] Investigators have compared the use of preparation regimens containing DuraPrep (3M Company, St. Paul MN) solution and a povidone-iodine scrub before TJA.[45–47] Both methods were found to be equivalent in reducing the frequency of SSIs and PJIs.[45–47] The addition of alcohol to aqueous skin preparations, such as chlorhexidine, has been shown to be beneficial, but has the disadvantage of drying out the skin's top layer. Disruption of the most superficial skin layers aids bacterial proliferation. The use of skin preparation agents, such as Avagard (3M Company), moisturizes the skin preventing its drying.[46]

Draping out the prepared surgical area is an important step in conserving sterility and decreasing the risk for infection. Care must be taken to only isolate skin that has been adequately sterilized. Plastic adhesive drapes have shown decreased rates of contamination when compared with traditional cloth drapes.[2,48] Use of an iodine-impregnated drape, such as Ioban (3M Company), may theoretically decrease PJI. A Cochrane article reviewed more than 3000 patients in five different studies and found no significant decrease in PJI with antimicrobial-incorporated adhesive drapes.[2,49] Appropriate draping including a water-tight seal around non-sterilized skin and use of adhesive drapes over the incision site is imperative to maintain sterility and decrease infection rates.[48,49]

Prophylactic Antibiotics

Systemic prophylactic antibiotic use before TJA has been shown in several studies to reduce the rate of infection.[1,2,50] In a recent meta-analysis of seven studies, antibiotic prophylaxis reduced the absolute risk of SSI in TJA by 8% and the relative risk by 81% compared with no antibiotic prophylaxis.[51] Antibiotics need to be effective against organisms responsible for postoperative infections, such as S aureus, Staphylococcus epidermidis, Escherichia coli, and Proteus. Currently, the American Academy of Orthopedic Surgeons recommends antibiotics for prophylaxis with a first- or second-line cephalosporin, most commonly cefazolin and cefuroxime, in the absence of a β-lactam allergy.[37,50,52] Clindamycin, vancomycin, or teicoplanin can be used in the presence of a documented cephalosporin allergy or known antibiotic-resistant organism, such as MRSA.[37] Given the increasing prevalence of MRSA, it is important to recognize patients who are at higher risk of being colonized. Risk factors for MRSA include recent antibiotic use, hospitalization, female sex, diabetes, age greater than 65 years, human immunodeficiency virus, or health care workers. Those patients should have their prophylactic antibiotics adjusted accordingly.[18,50]

Fulkerson and colleagues[50] examined bacterial cultures from infected TJA and susceptibilities to prophylactic antibiotics. They found that only 61% of bacterial isolates were sensitive to cefazolin. In patients previously treated with antibiotics, the vancomycin sensitivity was only 78%, and cefazolin sensitivity was 0%.[50] Sewick and colleagues[53] examined the use of a dual antibiotic prophylaxis with preoperative cefazolin and vancomycin on 1828 TJAs. They found no statistical difference in SSI when compared with cefazolin alone.[53] The use of vancomycin as a primary prophylactic antibiotic is controversial and current literature supports primary prophylaxis with a first- or second-line cephalosporin when applicable.

To reach minimal inhibitory concentration, prophylactic antibiotics should be initiated within 1 hour of start of the procedure.[2,52] Several studies confirm that 24 hours of antibiotics is as effective as 48 or 72 hours.[4,54] Current recommendations include one intraoperative dose of antibiotics followed by one or two additional perioperative doses.[2,35,52] A second additional dose of antibiotics may be administered during prolonged surgical duration beyond the half-life of the antibiotic (typically 4 hours) or when blood loss exceeds 1000 mL.

Our Own Worst Enemy

A potential source for intraoperative wound contamination includes airborne bacteria. These bacteria almost commonly originate from operating room staff. Bacterial shedding from one operating room staff member can be 10,000 bacteria per minute.[55] When compared with a completely empty operating room, the addition of five personnel increases the airborne microbial count 15-fold.[56–59] This source of contamination has been well documented over the years. In fact, Charnley[58] is credited with saying, "The living body of personnel in an operating room is by far the most important source of pathogenic organisms." Several techniques have been implemented to minimize the circulating airborne bacterial load and promote a "clean air" environment.

Traffic Control

Ambient airborne particulate and bacteria counts increase because of bacterial shedding from operating room personnel and air exchange between the sterile operating room and nonsterile hallways.[57,60] The repeated opening and closing of operating room doors has been shown to be a predictor of the number of airborne particulates in an operating room.[57,60] In the modern operating room, restricting presence to only scrubbed sterile personnel is not practical because most operating room staff must regularly travel between operating rooms. To combat airborne contamination, clean air enclosures have been established within the operating room. This allows anesthesia and other unscrubbed personnel to remain physically separate from the sterile surgical field. Currently, there are little data to support the use of clean air enclosures within the operating room. Although some amount of foot traffic within the operating room is to be expected, excessive use of the operating room doors and increased number of personnel should be discouraged.

Space Suits and Laminar Flow Systems

Lidwell and colleagues[61] first examined the use of ultraclean laminar air flow (LAF) systems in the operating room for control of airborne contamination compared with typical turbulent flow rooms. They examined greater than 8000 operating rooms and found a 75% decrease in SSI with LAF compared with a control room.[61,62] Historically, use of LAF without the use of preoperative antibiotics was shown to decrease the prevalence of SSI from 3.4% to 1.2%.[1–3] Vertical LAF units have demonstrated 80% to 93% reduction in environmental and surface contamination.[63] The accepted airborne bacterial counts for ultraclean LAF is less than or equal to 10 cfu/m^3.[62] When combined with the use of body exhaust systems (BES), operating room bacterial counts decrease to 1 cfu/m^3.[59,64] Ritter and colleagues[56] showed that BESs reduce airborne contamination by 38% when compared with sterile gowns and up to 69% when compared with plain surgical scrubs.[57] Despite several studies showing the significant decrease in airborne contamination with the combination of LAF and BES, the efficacy of these methods at decreasing infection rates is still controversial. Hooper and colleagues[65] analyzed greater than 51,000 primary THAs and greater than 36,000 TKAs assessing LAF and BES use and the rate of revision for early deep infection. Their data failed to demonstrate any decrease in the rate of infection in either modality.[65] Similarly, Ahl and colleagues[66] showed no statistical difference in deep infection rate when examining greater than 8000 TKAs with laminar flow rooms and body suits. Whyte and colleagues[67] revealed that air contamination does not significantly reflect surface contamination, and proposed surface bacteria as a more substantial risk factor for SSI. Ultraclean laminar flow systems and BES remain extremely popular in TJA despite debate over their efficacy.[63,65,66]

An alternative to using LAF systems to reduce the number of airborne bacterial and particulate load in addition to decreasing surface contaminates involves directly killing bacteria using ultraviolet lighting (UVL).[68] UVL at 290 µW/cm^2 has been shown to decrease surface bacterial counts more than with LAF alone.[68] Ritter and colleagues[68] prospectively examined 5890 TJA with and without UVL and revealed a 3.1 times decrease in SSI, solely by using UVL. Although effective in preventing SSI, there exist safety concerns for patient and personnel because of the carcinogenic properties of UVL. Currently, the Centers for Disease Control and Prevention and National Institutes of Health recommend against the use of UVL, citing significant safety hazards.[68–70] The use of UVL seems to be an effective adjunct to ultraclean air operating room environment and with proper operating room staff and patient protective equipment, could be a cost-effective addition or alternative to LAF.

Intraoperative Anesthesia Measures

The anesthesia team plays an important intraoperative role in the prevention of postoperative wound complications and deep infections. During the procedure, the anesthesia team is responsible for implementing protocols to optimize postoperative healing. This includes an appropriate timing of perioperative antibiotics, intraoperative monitoring of blood glucose, and temperature controls.

Because of the increase in physiologic stress during the operation, insulin requirements are typically elevated. This is especially important with patients with decreased insulin response, such as type 1 and 2 diabetes. An estimated 8% of all TJAs are performed on patients with diabetes.[71] Frequent intraoperative blood glucose monitoring is also encouraged and is of particular importance in patients with type 1 diabetes. Continual postoperative glycemic checks are required because insulin requirements may fluctuate as the patients metabolic needs readjust.

Mild hypothermia during a major operation is a common event. This has been shown to trigger thermoregulatory vasoconstriction and decrease subcutaneous perfusion and oxygen tension and promote postoperative wound infection.[72] Reduction of oxygen tension may also impair the oxidative mechanism of neutrophils, decreasing the tissues ability to immunogenic and anabolic activity. Hypothermia also directly impairs function of the patient's natural overall immune function.[31] A multicenter, randomized controlled trial assessing intraoperative warming in colorectal patients demonstrated that patients with normothermia had a significantly lower risk of developing postoperative infections than their hypothermic counterparts (6% vs 19%, respectively).[31] Hence, intraoperative normothermia is likely to decrease SSI in patients undergoing major TJA and should be implemented by the anesthesia team.

Antibiotic Bone Cement

Prevention of infection in TJA may be augmented with the use of antibiotic-impregnated cement. The addition of heat-resistant antibiotics to bone cement allows for the direct delivery of antimicrobials to the area with the greatest concern. Antibiotic-impregnated cement has been demonstrated to have bactericidal activity for at least 7 to 10 days following implantation and up to 10 years in some studies.[73–77] Antibiotic-loaded bone cement (ALBC) allows for the delivery of high antibiotic concentrations at the operative site, reducing the adverse systemic effects while increasing antibiotic concentration at the surgical site.[78] The use of ALBC in conjunction with systemic antibiotics has been shown to decrease wound infection and PJI revision rates.[79,80] A randomized prospective study by Chiang and Chiu[81] examined the prophylactic use of ALBC in primary TKAs and compared their outcomes with standard polymethyl methacrylate bone cement. In the cohort receiving ALBC, no infections were reported, whereas the standard polymethyl methacrylate cohort had a 3.1% infection rate.[81]

Despite the promising data, the use of ALBC continues to be controversial. Concerns regarding routine use of ALBC in primary TJA include decreasing bone cement strength, development of antibiotic resistance, hypersensitivity reactions, and increased cost. Although the addition of large amounts of antibiotics to bone cement can alter cement properties, the use of lower doses has been shown to have negligible mechanical effects.[77,78] The increased cost associated with the use of ALBC can adversely affect the use of TJA. To offset increased cost of approximately $60,000 per 100 patients undergoing TJA, the decrease in infection incidence needs to be greater than 1.2%.[78] However, the use of prophylactic ALBC in high-risk patients with a history of bacterial infections or immunocompromised status is generally well accepted.[78] Although still controversial, the use of prophylactic ALBC has been demonstrated to be effective and beneficial in properly selected patients with TJA.

POSTOPERATIVE MEASURES

Postoperative Blood Transfusions

Perioperative hemoglobin levels can adversely affect the patients' risk for postoperative infection. Patients receiving allogeneic blood transfusions may be up to 2.1 times more likely to develop postoperative infections than those not receiving blood products.[82] This correlation is possibly caused by the generalized immunomodulatory effect of allogeneic blood, compounded by the impaired microcirculation of oxygen and nutrients to the surgical wound site.[10] Furthermore, the unfavorable effects of allogeneic blood transfusions increase directly with the number of units transfused.[82] To minimize the detrimental effects of postoperative transfusions, preoperative preventative measures, such as screening and correction of anemia, optimization of other comorbidities, and meticulous intraoperative hemostasis, must be used.

Several intraoperative practices may also be implemented to reduce blood loss and the need for postoperative transfusions. The application of above-knee pneumatic tourniquets has been a well-used technique at minimizing intraoperative blood loss. However, this method has been shown to result in considerable soft tissue damage, ultimately delaying the recovery process. Furthermore, use of a tourniquet for greater than 1 hour has been shown to increase the risk for arterial and venous thrombi.[83] Application of tranexamic acid (TXA), a fibrinolytic agent, has been shown to be a cost-effective method of decreasing postoperative transfusions and the incidence of postoperative hematomas. A prospective randomized controlled trial evaluated intravenous TXA versus placebo in patients with TKA without the use of a tourniquet.[83] This study demonstrated no transfusions in the group receiving two perioperative doses of 15 g/kg of TXA, whereas 32% of the placebo group required transfusion.[83] Intravenous administration of TXA has been accepted in patients without significant cardiovascular comorbidities or history of intracranial bleed. Although considered as a safe practice, intravenous TXA carries a small risk of thromboembolic complications.[84] Only a small concentration of TXA injected intravenously eventually reaches the target area.[85] To decrease systemic effects of TXA, topical or intra-articular administration of TXA has been advocated. In a study by Digas and colleagues[85] intra-articular TXA was comparatively assessed with intravenous TXA and a placebo cohort. Patients in the placebo group had a significant increase in blood loss and transfusion requirements (43%), whereas the intravenous TXA and intra-articular cohorts demonstrated significantly reduced transfusion requirements, 23% and 17% respectively.[85] Furthermore, Digas and colleagues[85] noted that intra-articular injections were the preferred means of TXA administration, because it may be associated with reduced postoperative bleeding and transfusion requirements.

Wound Drainage and Hematoma
Postoperative hematomas are a nidus for bacteria to propagate and subsequently result in infection. Use of an intraoperative closed suction drain has the theoretic benefit of evacuating any residual blood; however, its use continues to be an area of debate. A meta-analysis of closed suction drains following TKAs has shown no benefit in decreasing infection.[86] A randomized

controlled trial evaluating the efficacy of closed suction drains following THA demonstrated no benefit in terms of infection, complication rates, or early functional outcomes.[87]

Excessive wound drainage, defined by persistent drainage for greater than 5 days, may lead to a persistent communicating tract reaching to the joint space and facilitating transition of epidermal flora. In a study by Jaberi and colleagues,[24] persistently draining wounds were 12.5 times more likely to result in PJI. Similar studies have reported that the incidence of PJI in patients with persistent wound drainage is near 50%.[24,27,88,89] Moreover, each additional day of prolonged wound drainage increases the chance for deep infection by approximately 42% in THA and 29% in TKA.[89]

Thromboprophylaxis is essential in patients with TJA because they are at an increased risk of developing deep venous thrombi and pulmonary emboli. Although prevention of deep venous thrombi and pulmonary emboli is paramount, the administration of prophylactic pharmacologic regimens complicates the management of postoperative hematoma and wound drainage. Some advocate decreasing thromboprophylactic doses, until the drainage ceases.[90] Other interventions, such as initiating prophylactic antibiotics, are discouraged because they can mask the underlying infection.[90] Persistent wound drainage (5–7 days) secondary to aggressive thromboprophylaxis is unlikely to subside without surgical intervention.[24] Several studies have reported positive outcomes after surgical debridement within the first 7 days following the onset of wound drainage.[24,27,88–90] Surgical intervention with irrigation and debridement, in combination with polyethylene exchange, and the addition of prophylactic antibiotics should be promptly initiated after a hematoma is identified if persistent wound drainage is present.

Management of postoperative wounds is essential for the prevention of wound infections. Sterile dressings should be appropriately applied in the operating room. Dressings should be permeable, waterproof, transparent, and flexible enough to withstand joint movement. Wounds should be tended to at postoperative visits, with special attention given to wound maceration, drainage, and signs of infection.[91]

Dental Procedures
In certain circumstances prophylactic measures are indicated in patients with TJA undergoing dental procedures. Historically, antibiotic prophylaxis has been indicated for this population.

However, few studies have demonstrated a correlation between dental procedures and an increased risk for infection.[15] Although no clear association exists, the American Academy of Orthopedic Surgeons continues to recommend prophylactic antibiotics in patients with TJA undergoing dental or other invasive procedures, without specifying the duration.[92]

SUMMARY

Prevention is always preferred to surgical management, particularly in the setting of infection. Although TJAs are considered one of the most successful surgical procedures, a rare but devastating complication is the PJI. Several evidence-based preoperative, intraoperative, and postoperative practices may help reduce the risk for postoperative infections, further reducing the morbidity and mortality associated with TJA.

ACKNOWLEDGMENTS

The authors thank Dr Javad Parvizi for presenting this topic during the Central Illinois Healthcare Management Summit chaired by Dr K.J. Saleh.

REFERENCES

1. Bozic KJ, Katz P, Cisternas M, et al. Hospital resource utilization for primary and revision total hip arthroplasty. J Bone Joint Surg Am 2005;87(3): 570–6.
2. Parvizi J, Bender B, Saleh KJ, et al. Resistant organisms in infected total knee arthroplasty: occurrence, prevention, and treatment regimens. Instr Course Lect 2009;58:271–8.
3. Bozic KJ, Chiu V. Emerging ideas: shared decision making in patients with osteoarthritis of the hip and knee. Clin Orthop Relat Res 2011;469(7): 2081–5.
4. Peersman G, Laskin R, Davis J, et al. Infection in total knee replacement: a retrospective review of 6489 total knee replacements. Clin Orthop Relat Res 2001;(392):15–23.
5. Ong KL, Kurtz SM, Lau E, et al. Prosthetic joint infection risk after total hip arthroplasty in the Medicare population. J Arthroplasty 2009;24(6 Suppl):105–9.
6. Malinzak RA, Ritter MA, Berend ME, et al. Morbidly obese, diabetic, younger, and unilateral joint arthroplasty patients have elevated total joint arthroplasty infection rates. J Arthroplasty 2009; 24(6 Suppl):84–8.
7. Marchant MH Jr, Viens NA, Cook C, et al. The impact of glycemic control and diabetes mellitus on perioperative outcomes after total joint arthroplasty. J Bone Joint Surg Am 2009;91(7):1621–9.
8. Mraovic B, Suh D, Jacovides C, et al. Perioperative hyperglycemia and postoperative infection after lower limb arthroplasty. J Diabetes Sci Technol 2011;5(2):412–8.
9. Ramos M, Khalpey Z, Lipsitz S, et al. Relationship of perioperative hyperglycemia and postoperative infections in patients who undergo general and vascular surgery. Ann Surg 2008;248(4):585–91.
10. Pulido L, Ghanem E, Joshi A, et al. Periprosthetic joint infection: the incidence, timing, and predisposing factors. Clin Orthop Relat Res 2008;466(7): 1710–5.
11. Dowsey MM, Choong PF. Obese diabetic patients are at substantial risk for deep infection after primary TKA. Clin Orthop Relat Res 2009;467(6): 1577–81.
12. Dowsey MM, Choong PF. Early outcomes and complications following joint arthroplasty in obese patients: a review of the published reports. ANZ J Surg 2008;78(6):439–44.
13. Dowsey MM, Choong PF. Obesity is a major risk factor for prosthetic infection after primary hip arthroplasty. Clin Orthop Relat Res 2008;466(1): 153–8.
14. Namba RS, Paxton L, Fithian DC, et al. Obesity and perioperative morbidity in total hip and total knee arthroplasty patients. J Arthroplasty 2005;20(7 Suppl 3):46–50.
15. Berbari EF, Hanssen AD, Duffy MC, et al. Risk factors for prosthetic joint infection: case-control study. Clin Infect Dis 1998;27(5):1247–54.
16. Hayakawa K, Nakagawa K. Treatment of infected total knee arthroplasty in patients with rheumatoid arthritis. Mod Rheumatol 2004;14(5):376–82.
17. Namba RS, Inacio MC, Paxton EW. Risk factors associated with deep surgical site infections after primary total knee arthroplasty: an analysis of 56,216 knees. J Bone Joint Surg Am 2013;95(9): 775–82.
18. Parvizi J, Sullivan TA, Pagnano MW, et al. Total joint arthroplasty in human immunodeficiency virus-positive patients: an alarming rate of early failure. J Arthroplasty 2003;18(3):259–64.
19. Ragni MV, Crossett LS, Herndon JH. Postoperative infection following orthopaedic surgery in human immunodeficiency virus-infected hemophiliacs with CD4 counts < or = 200/mm3. J Arthroplasty 1995;10(6):716–21.
20. Jensen JE, Jensen TG, Smith TK, et al. Nutrition in orthopaedic surgery. J Bone Joint Surg Am 1982; 64(9):1263–72.
21. Greene KA, Wilde AH, Stulberg BN. Preoperative nutritional status of total joint patients. Relationship to postoperative wound complications. J Arthroplasty 1991;6(4):321–5.

22. Marin LA, Salido JA, Lopez A, et al. Preoperative nutritional evaluation as a prognostic tool for wound healing. Acta Orthop Scand 2002;73(1):2–5.

23. Cross MB, Yi PH, Thomas CF, et al. Evaluation of malnutrition in orthopaedic surgery. J Am Acad Orthop Surg 2014;22(3):193–9.

24. Jaberi FM, Parvizi J, Haytmanek CT, et al. Procrastination of wound drainage and malnutrition affect the outcome of joint arthroplasty. Clin Orthop Relat Res 2008;466(6):1368–71.

25. Lavernia CJ, Sierra RJ, Baerga L. Nutritional parameters and short term outcome in arthroplasty. J Am Coll Nutr 1999;18(3):274–8.

26. Zorrilla P, Salido JA, Lopez-Alonso A, et al. Serum zinc as a prognostic tool for wound healing in hip hemiarthroplasty. Clin Orthop Relat Res 2004;(420):304–8.

27. Saleh K, Olson M, Resig S, et al. Predictors of wound infection in hip and knee joint replacement: results from a 20 year surveillance program. J Orthop Res 2002;20(3):506–15.

28. Dennis DA. Wound complications in TKA. Orthopedics 2002;25(9):973–4.

29. Singh JA. Smoking and outcomes after knee and hip arthroplasty: a systematic review. J Rheumatol 2011;38(9):1824–34.

30. Lavernia CJ, Sierra RJ, Gomez-Marin O. Smoking and joint replacement: resource consumption and short-term outcome. Clin Orthop Relat Res 1999;(367):172–80.

31. Kurz A, Sessler DI, Lenhardt R. Perioperative normothermia to reduce the incidence of surgical-wound infection and shorten hospitalization. Study of Wound Infection and Temperature Group. N Engl J Med 1996;334(19):1209–15.

32. Canale ST, Daugherty K. Smoking threatens orthopaedic outcomes. Available at: http://www.aaos.org/news/aaosnow/jun12/cover2.asp. Accessed October 6, 2015.

33. von Eiff C, Becker K, Machka K, et al. Nasal carriage as a source of Staphylococcus aureus bacteremia. Study Group. N Engl J Med 2001;344(1):11–6.

34. Gorwitz RJ, Kruszon-Moran D, McAllister SK, et al. Changes in the prevalence of nasal colonization with Staphylococcus aureus in the United States, 2001-2004. J Infect Dis 2008;197(9):1226–34.

35. Illingworth KD, Mihalko WM, Parvizi J, et al. How to minimize infection and thereby maximize patient outcomes in total joint arthroplasty: a multicenter approach: AAOS exhibit selection. J Bone Joint Surg Am 2013;95(8):e50.

36. Yano K, Minoda Y, Sakawa A, et al. Positive nasal culture of methicillin-resistant Staphylococcus aureus (MRSA) is a risk factor for surgical site infection in orthopedics. Acta Orthop 2009;80(4):486–90.

37. Parvizi J, Matar WY, Saleh KJ, et al. Decolonization of drug-resistant organisms before total joint arthroplasty. Instr Course Lect 2010;59:131–7.

38. Davis KA, Stewart JJ, Crouch HK, et al. Methicillin-resistant Staphylococcus aureus (MRSA) nares colonization at hospital admission and its effect on subsequent MRSA infection. Clin Infect Dis 2004;39(6):776–82.

39. Rao N, Cannella BA, Crossett LS, et al. Preoperative screening/decolonization for Staphylococcus aureus to prevent orthopedic surgical site infection: prospective cohort study with 2-year follow-up. J Arthroplasty 2011;26(8):1501–7.

40. Gernaat-van der Sluis AJ, Hoogenboom-Verdegaal AM, Edixhoven PJ, et al. Prophylactic mupirocin could reduce orthopedic wound infections. 1,044 patients treated with mupirocin compared with 1,260 historical controls. Acta Orthop Scand 1998;69(4):412–4.

41. Buehlmann M, Frei R, Fenner L, et al. Highly effective regimen for decolonization of methicillin-resistant Staphylococcus aureus carriers. Infect Control Hosp Epidemiol 2008;29(6):510–6.

42. Wendt C, Schinke S, Wurttemberger M, et al. Value of whole-body washing with chlorhexidine for the eradication of methicillin-resistant Staphylococcus aureus: a randomized, placebo-controlled, double-blind clinical trial. Infect Control Hosp Epidemiol 2007;28(9):1036–43.

43. Tanner J, Norrie P, Melen K. Preoperative hair removal to reduce surgical site infection. Cochrane Database Syst Rev 2011;(11):CD004122.

44. Karpanen TJ, Conway BR, Worthington T, et al. Enhanced chlorhexidine skin penetration with eucalyptus oil. BMC Infect Dis 2010;10:278.

45. Jacobson C, Osmon DR, Hanssen A, et al. Prevention of wound contamination using DuraPrep solution plus Ioban 2 drapes. Clin Orthop Relat Res 2005;439:32–7.

46. Birnbach DJ, Meadows W, Stein DJ, et al. Comparison of povidone iodine and DuraPrep, an iodophor-in-isopropyl alcohol solution, for skin disinfection prior to epidural catheter insertion in parturients. Anesthesiology 2003;98(1):164–9.

47. Brown AR, Taylor GJ, Gregg PJ. Air contamination during skin preparation and draping in joint replacement surgery. J Bone Joint Surg Br 1996;78(1):92–4.

48. French ML, Eitzen HE, Ritter MA. The plastic surgical adhesive drape: an evaluation of its efficacy as a microbial barrier. Ann Surg 1976;184(1):46–50.

49. Webster J, Alghamdi A. Use of plastic adhesive drapes during surgery for preventing surgical site infection. Cochrane Database Syst Rev 2015;(4):CD006353.

50. Fulkerson E, Valle CJ, Wise B, et al. Antibiotic susceptibility of bacteria infecting total joint

arthroplasty sites. J Bone Joint Surg Am 2006;88(6): 1231–7.

51. AlBuhairan B, Hind D, Hutchinson A. Antibiotic prophylaxis for wound infections in total joint arthroplasty: a systematic review. J Bone Joint Surg Br 2008;90(7):915–9.

52. Watters W 3rd, Rethman MP, Hanson NB, et al. Prevention of orthopaedic implant infection in patients undergoing dental procedures. J Am Acad Orthop Surg 2013;21(3):180–9.

53. Sewick A, Makani A, Wu C, et al. Does dual antibiotic prophylaxis better prevent surgical site infections in total joint arthroplasty? Clin Orthop Relat Res 2012;470(10):2702–7.

54. Prokuski L. Prophylactic antibiotics in orthopaedic surgery. J Am Acad Orthop Surg 2008;16(5):283–93.

55. Sadrizadeh S, Holmberg S. Surgical clothing systems in laminar airflow operating room: a numerical assessment. J Infect Public Health 2014;7(6):508–16.

56. Ritter MA, Eitzen H, French ML, et al. The operating room environment as affected by people and the surgical face mask. Clin Orthop Relat Res 1975;(111):147–50.

57. Ritter MA. Operating room environment. Clin Orthop Relat Res 1999;(369):103–9.

58. Charnley J. Postoperative infection after total hip replacement with special reference to air contamination in the operating room. Clin Orthop Relat Res 1972;87:167–87.

59. Lidwell OM. Air, antibiotics and sepsis in replacement joints. J Hosp Infect 1988;11(Suppl C):18–40.

60. Scaltriti S, Cencetti S, Rovesti S, et al. Risk factors for particulate and microbial contamination of air in operating theatres. J Hosp Infect 2007;66(4): 320–6.

61. Lidwell OM, Lowbury EJ, Whyte W, et al. Effect of ultraclean air in operating rooms on deep sepsis in the joint after total hip or knee replacement: a randomised study. Br Med J 1982; 285(6334):10–4.

62. Nilsson KG, Lundholm R, Friberg S. Assessment of horizontal laminar air flow instrument table for additional ultraclean space during surgery. J Hosp Infect 2010;76(3):243–6.

63. Miner AL, Losina E, Katz JN, et al. Deep infection after total knee replacement: impact of laminar airflow systems and body exhaust suits in the modern operating room. Infect Control Hosp Epidemiol 2007;28(2):222–6.

64. Der Tavitian J, Ong SM, Taub NA, et al. Body-exhaust suit versus occlusive clothing. A randomised, prospective trial using air and wound bacterial counts. J Bone Joint Surg Br 2003;85(4): 490–4.

65. Hooper GJ, Rothwell AG, Frampton C, et al. Does the use of laminar flow and space suits reduce early deep infection after total hip and knee replacement?: the ten-year results of the New Zealand Joint Registry. J Bone Joint Surg Br 2011;93(1): 85–90.

66. Ahl T, Dalen N, Jorbeck H, et al. Air contamination during hip and knee arthroplasties. Horizontal laminar flow randomized vs. conventional ventilation. Acta Orthop Scand 1995; 66(1):17–20.

67. Whyte W, Hambraeus A, Laurell G, et al. The relative importance of routes and sources of wound contamination during general surgery. I. Non-airborne. J Hosp Infect 1991;18(2):93–107.

68. Ritter MA, Olberding EM, Malinzak RA. Ultraviolet lighting during orthopaedic surgery and the rate of infection. J Bone Joint Surg Am 2007;89(9): 1935–40.

69. Evans RP. Current concepts for clean air and total joint arthroplasty: laminar airflow and ultraviolet radiation: a systematic review. Clin Orthop Relat Res 2011;469(4):945–53.

70. Carlsson AS, Nilsson B, Walder MH, et al. Ultraviolet radiation and air contamination during total hip replacement. J Hosp Infect 1986;7(2):176–84.

71. Bolognesi MP, Marchant MH Jr, Viens NA, et al. The impact of diabetes on perioperative patient outcomes after total hip and total knee arthroplasty in the United States. J Arthroplasty 2008;23(6 Suppl 1):92–8.

72. Davis TR, Wood MB, Vanhoutte PM. The effect of hypothermic ischemia on the alpha-adrenergic mechanisms of the canine tibia vascular bed. J Orthop Res 1992;10(1):149–55.

73. Davies JP, O'Connor DO, Burke DW, et al. Influence of antibiotic impregnation on the fatigue life of Simplex P and Palacos R acrylic bone cements, with and without centrifugation. J Biomed Mater Res 1989;23(4):379–97.

74. Buchholz HW, Elson RA, Engelbrecht E, et al. Management of deep infection of total hip replacement. J Bone Joint Surg Br 1981;63-B(3): 342–53.

75. Carlsson AS, Josefsson G, Lindberg L. Revision with gentamicin-impregnated cement for deep infections in total hip arthroplasties. J Bone Joint Surg Am 1978;60(8):1059–64.

76. Masri BA, Duncan CP, Beauchamp CP. Long-term elution of antibiotics from bone-cement: an in vivo study using the prosthesis of antibiotic-loaded acrylic cement (PROSTALAC) system. J Arthroplasty 1998;13(3):331–8.

77. Joseph TN, Chen AL, Di Cesare PE. Use of antibiotic-impregnated cement in total joint arthroplasty. J Am Acad Orthop Surg 2003;11(1):38–47.

78. Jiranek WA, Hanssen AD, Greenwald AS. Antibiotic-loaded bone cement for infection prophylaxis in total joint replacement. J Bone Joint Surg Am 2006;88(11):2487–500.

79. Chiu FY, Chen CM, Lin CF, et al. Cefuroxime-impregnated cement in primary total knee arthroplasty: a prospective, randomized study of three hundred and forty knees. J Bone Joint Surg Am 2002;84-A(5):759–62.

80. Espehaug B, Engesaeter LB, Vollset SE, et al. Antibiotic prophylaxis in total hip arthroplasty. Review of 10,905 primary cemented total hip replacements reported to the Norwegian arthroplasty register, 1987 to 1995. J Bone Joint Surg Br 1997;79(4): 590–5.

81. Chiang CC, Chiu FY. Cefuroxime-impregnated cement and systemic cefazolin for 1 week in primary total knee arthroplasty: an evaluation of 2700 knees. J Chin Med Assoc 2012;75(4):167–70.

82. Garvin KL, Konigsberg BS. Infection following total knee arthroplasty: prevention and management. J Bone Joint Surg Am 2011;93(12):1167–75.

83. Bidolegui F, Arce G, Lugones A, et al. Tranexamic acid reduces blood loss and transfusion in patients undergoing total knee arthroplasty without tourniquet: a prospective randomized controlled trial. Open Orthop J 2014;8:250–4.

84. Wingerter SA, Keith AD, Schoenecker PL, et al. Does tranexamic acid reduce blood loss and transfusion requirements associated with the periacetabular osteotomy? Clin Orthop Relat Res 2015; 473(8):2639–43.

85. Digas G, Koutsogiannis I, Meletiadis G, et al. Intra-articular injection of tranexamic acid reduce blood loss in cemented total knee arthroplasty. Eur J Orthop Surg Traumatol 2015;25(7):1181–8.

86. Zhang XN, Wu G, Xu RZ, et al. Closed suction drainage or non-drainage for total knee arthroplasty: a meta-analysis. Zhonghua wai ke Za Zhi 2012;50(12):1119–25 [in Chinese].

87. Fichman SG, Makinen TJ, Lozano B, et al. Closed suction drainage has no benefits in revision total hip arthroplasty: a randomized controlled trial. Int Orthop 2015;40(3):453–7.

88. Weiss AP, Krackow KA. Persistent wound drainage after primary total knee arthroplasty. J Arthroplasty 1993;8(3):285–9.

89. Patel VP, Walsh M, Sehgal B, et al. Factors associated with prolonged wound drainage after primary total hip and knee arthroplasty. J Bone Joint Surg Am 2007;89(1):33–8.

90. Proceedings of the International Consensus Meeting on Periprosthetic Joint Infection. Available at: https://www.efort.org/wp-content/uploads/2013/10/Philadelphia_Consensus.pdf. Accessed October 7, 2015.

91. Tustanowski J. Effect of dressing choice on outcomes after hip and knee arthroplasty: a literature review. J Wound Care 2009;18(11):449–50, 452, 454, passim.

92. Matar WY, Jafari SM, Restrepo C, et al. Preventing infection in total joint arthroplasty. J Bone Joint Surg Am 2010;92(Suppl 2):36–46.

Reducing 30-day Readmission After Joint Replacement

Monique C. Chambers, MD, MSL[a], Mouhanad M. El-Othmani, MD[a],
Afshin A. Anoushiravani, MD[a], Zain Sayeed, MSc, MHA[a],
Khaled J. Saleh, MD, MSc, FRCS (C), MHCM, CPE[b],*

KEYWORDS

• Readmission • Complications • TJA • Quality measures • 30-day readmissions

KEY POINTS

- Hospital readmission rate contributes a practically avoidable source of waste and financial burden; the topic is a focus in the surgical literature and a target for quality improvement.
- Unplanned readmissions bring about severe ramifications for the patient, patient families, the institution, and the health care system.
- The implications of readmission within 30 days of discharge should drive providers, administrators, and policymakers to turn more attention to system-based procedures.
- These system-based procedures can help to decrease readmission, and ultimately improve quality of care while decreasing health care–associated costs.

INTRODUCTION

Total joint arthroplasty (TJA) is one of the most effective and efficient interventional procedures in medicine, because it offers a successful option to address chronic pain and functional disability of the associated joint.[1] Although it was developed initially to address degenerative changes seen in the elderly population, TJA indications have continued to expand to include conditions that affect younger, more active patients.[2,3]

It is projected that there will be as many as 610,582 primary and 99,898 revision total hip arthroplasty (THA) procedures annually by 2020.[4] For total knee arthroplasty (TKA), as many as 1.5 million primary TKA procedures and 161,405 revision TKAs are anticipated in the same year.[5] Based on current trends, 5.6% of those THAs and 3.3% of TKAs are followed by a readmission within 30 days of discharge.[6] Hospital readmission has become a focus of quality measures used by the Centers for Medicare and Medicaid (CMS) to evaluate quality of care. Recent policy changes provide incentives and enforce penalties to decrease 30-day hospital readmissions, with the hopes of improving the quality of health care delivery.

In 2013, the CMS rolled out the implementation of the Readmission Penalty Program. Hospitals are no longer reimbursed for necessary care of patients that are readmitted within 30 days of discharge, with few exceptions to the primary diagnosis for readmission.[7] As more provisions within the Patient Protection and Affordable Care Act are developed, readmission rates, as part of a bigger set of quality metrics, are being used to determine reimbursement rates for physicians. Further, the need for readmission is

Funding Sources: No additional funding sources were used for this article.

Conflicts of Interest: No conflicts of interest are evident for authors of this article.

[a] Division of Orthopaedics and Rehabilitation, Southern Illinois University School of Medicine, 701 North First Street, Springfield, IL 62781, USA; [b] Department of Orthopaedic and Sports Medicine, Detroit Medical Center, 311 Mack Avenue, 5th Floor, Detroit, MI 48201, USA

* Corresponding author.

E-mail address: kjsaleh@gmail.com

deemed as an indication for inadequate quality of care, and is therefore subjected to financial penalties.[7] However, readmissions may often be a result of an independent incident, unrelated to the surgical arthroplasty procedure. As such, surgeons and administrators are pressed with the challenge to accommodate the growing number of patients who qualify for arthroplasty procedures, while also improving quality of care and decreasing the costs to the system. With this daunting task before total joint surgeons, the purpose of this review is to identify risk factors that have been significantly associated with higher readmission rates, address approaches to minimize 30-day readmission, and discuss the potential future direction within this area as new government regulations arise.

UNDERSTANDING THE ECONOMIC SCOPE OF 30-DAY READMISSIONS

The rate of THA being performed in the United States is 4 times higher than it was in 2005, with associated economic burden of $13.43 billion. Following a similar trend, TKAs have increased by up to 5 times with a total cost of $40.8 billion, further straining financial resources and expenditures.[5,8] Unplanned readmissions carry a cost burden of $17.5 billion for Medicare patients alone.[9,10] However, the etiology and the cost associated with the event of readmission after arthroplasty vary greatly. As such, understanding the various factors and variables that lead to readmission after TJA is a principal goal for both policymakers and hospital administrators.

The high efficiency and impact of TJA has led to further resource allocation, as TJA expenditure constitutes the greatest share of Medicare funds.[11] Because the hospital readmission rate contributes a practically avoidable source of waste and financial burden, the topic became a central focus in the surgical literature and a target for multiple quality improvement approaches. The average cost of readmissions for THA is $17,103 and readmissions after TKA are $13,008.[9] The financial costs for revision operations are even greater, with the average revision owing to a surgical complication being $29,893.[9] Considering the substantial costs of an additional hospital admission, the goal of reducing 30-day readmission rates has become a primary focus of the CMS.

Risk and gain sharing strategies will continue to evolve as more provisions within the Patient Protection and Affordable Care Act are implemented. It is important that such changes do not negatively impact quality of care or the sustainability of hospitals and providers to ensure access to high-quality care. Shared responsibility for the gains and risks associated with care delivery will be bundled into a single payment for an entire episode of care. As such, physicians should be equipped with the tools to negotiate bundle payments, taking into account the costly reality of a possible readmission. More emphasis should be placed on quality improvement, and as such, understanding factors that increase the risk of readmissions is vital to adequately mitigate poor patient outcomes and financial waste.

RISK FACTORS ASSOCIATED WITH INCREASED 30-DAY READMISSION RATES

Orthopedic readmissions are owing to a number of variables, both nonmodifiable and modifiable. A multitude of factors have been analyzed in the literature. These range from hospital-related factors, such as hospital and surgeon volume; to patient-associated elements, including demographics, age, and comorbidities; to orthopedic/surgical-specific facets like surgical time.[12–15] Determining patients at risk for readmission requires identification of a number of variables beyond merely the patients' background and comorbidities. In fact, establishing a predictive model for readmissions requires thorough consideration of a broad category of variables such as social history, family support, economic status, and the interplay between these factors.

Patient-Specific Factors

Patient demographics, such as age, race, and gender have been shown to be associated significantly with an increased risk in readmission rates.[9,14,16–19] Patients over the age of 40 have a steady increase in hospital readmission risk until over the age of 75, and then there is a decreased risk of unrelated readmission.[20,21] African American race and male gender have also been identified as independent predictors of readmission, with an odds ratio of 1.5 for males compared with females.[22] The higher readmission risk noted in these populations might be partly explained by the association of these variables with an increased risk for other medical comorbidities. Although patient demographics are nonmodifiable factors, they can be used to establish patient expectations and to better guide preoperative optimization for TJA candidates.

Additional patient-specific variables, such as comorbid conditions independent of the index surgery, have also been studied to determine their impact on 30-day readmission.[23] Among the most common comorbidities in the aging US population is obesity. Obesity has been associated with an increased risk of surgical complications, compounded comorbid illness, and increased readmission after TJA.[24] The rest of the identified comorbidities represent serious medical conditions and poor health status before the index procedure. Among those, the strongest correlation with higher readmission rates is reported in pulmonary circulation disease, chronic pulmonary disease, hypothyroidism, bleeding disorder, history of cancer, and psychoses.[13,24] Several studies also assessed the burden of comorbidity with standardized scoring systems such as the Charlson comorbidity index and have shown that worse preoperative scores are predictive of worse outcomes, higher postoperative complications, and higher rates of readmission.[23]

Care Delivery Factors

Other modifiable factors associated with an increased likelihood of 30-day readmission are related to the care delivery process. Studies demonstrate that the level of expertise has an impact on the postoperative course and readmission. THA patients who were operated on in a high-volume surgical center have lower readmission rates, although greater surgeon volume was associated with greater readmission rates.[24] However, in patients who underwent TKA, there is a lower rate of complications and readmission with higher provider volume.[25] This finding is consistent when accounting for all TJA patients.[26] Patients undergoing surgical intervention in public hospitals had higher readmission rates compared with those receiving the procedure at private or teaching institutions.[27]

Identifying and addressing these factors will allow institutions to develop guidelines around perioperative surgical management of TJA patients. Also, all arthroplasty procedures do not carry equal risk for hospital readmission. TKA procedures tend to result in greater readmission rates than unilateral knee arthroplasty procedures, which is likely related to the longer surgical time, older patient population, and complication rate.[28] In total elbow arthroplasty, osteoarthritis and infectious arthritis posed a greater risk for reoperation and readmission than posttraumatic arthroplasty.[29] Additionally, the type of anesthesia might impact complication rates. Patients who had epidural anesthesia were 56% more likely to have a minor systemic complication and 2.6 times more likely to have a major systemic complication than patients

who had spinal anesthesia, which can lead to readmission in the geriatric patient population undergoing joint arthroplasty.[30] The use of a multidisciplinary care team in the management of operative patients as well as process standardization in the care of TJA patients reduced readmission, revision operation, and mortality.[26,31]

Health system factors related to care, such as insurance type and discharge destination, are reported consistently to be associated with readmission risk. When the cost of the index admission is greater, there is an increased risk of readmission.[25] Rather than this being identified as an independent factor, it may suggest a longer index admission that was the result of complications, putting the patient at greater risk for subsequent readmissions. Interestingly, payer status has been suggested as a factor that can be incorporated in a predictive model for 30-day readmission. Medicare and Medicaid patients are more likely to return to the hospital within the 30-day readmission observation period.[25,27,32] Also, TJA patients discharged to skilled nursing facilities or homes with home health care are also at a greater risk for readmission.[33,34] Although poorer health status upon discharge might be assumed as a confounding variable in this population, more recent studies have adjusted for preoperative comorbidities and postoperative complications that suggest place of discharge may independently have an impact on readmission outcomes.[33]

Complications

Several studies have identified postoperative complications as the leading cause for all-cause surgical readmission.[35] Complications associated with higher readmission include wound infections, sepsis, thromboembolic and cardiac events, and respiratory issues.[13] Within arthroplasty, deep or superficial surgical site infection is the leading cause of 30-day readmission after TKA and accounts for 12.1% of unplanned readmissions.[6] Other complications are broken down into broad categories that may be joint specific, such as dislocation, prosthetic misalignment, ligamentous laxity, periprosthetic fracture, a septic joint, or systemic complications including cardiac, pulmonary, and circulatory issues. The postoperative course, including inadequate pain control, inability to mobilize, falling episodes, anemia, or hematoma, account for the second leading cause for 30-day readmission rates particularly among THA patients.[6] Thromboembolic disease (deep vein thrombosis or pulmonary embolism) accounts for the third most common reason for hospital readmission after both THA and TKA procedures.[6] All of these factors have an impact on the length of in-hospital stay after the index admission. Although still accounting for the various factors that determine hospital length of stay, patients should be discharged as soon as possible. This is primarily pertinent in the elderly population, where increased duration of primary hospitalization has been associated with increased readmission rates.[22]

In addition to the aforementioned factors, it should also be noted that as many as 50% of THA readmissions are not related to the index surgery.[23] This suggests that they may have been planned readmissions or were unpreventable. Understanding this dynamic allows administrators to address the modifiable factors that predict readmission, while also realizing that completely eliminating readmissions may not be feasible. This should also empower physicians to advocate for appropriate reimbursement models that provide adequate compensation for the care provided, without penalizing providers or patients for unpredictable circumstances.

APPROACHES TO REDUCE 30-DAY READMISSIONS

With the increase in access and indications, federal regulations attempt to encourage a higher emphasis on adequate care during the primary hospital admission. Proper patient selection and optimization is a vital aspect to reducing readmission after elective procedures. Patients must have access to an internist or primary care physician who manages their medical comorbidities. In the past, there has been a disconnect between the primary provider and secondary or multispecialty physicians. The orthopedic surgeon must have an invested relationship with all physicians and stakeholders involved in the care of their patients to ensure appropriate preoperative expectations and continuity of care. Optimizing the patient with preoperative medical clearance and communication with all providers and family members involved in the perioperative course are steps that should be included. The medical comorbidities that have been associated with higher readmission rates (pulmonary circulation disease, chronic pulmonary disease, hypothyroidism, bleeding disorder, history of cancer and psychoses) should be optimized to ensure the patient has the lowest possible risk for postoperative complications. Malnutrition can be an easily overlooked factor affecting the postoperative period, with the stress of responding to a surgical intervention. Albumin levels, zinc, and nitric oxide are all predictors of outcomes in terms of the body's ability to heal and the immune system competency, and these levels should be obtained and brought within normal limits. Finally, because thromboembolic disease is one of the leading causes of readmission, following proper anticoagulation guidelines is pivotal to improve outcomes and decrease readmission rates in candidates for TJA.

Appropriate intraoperative processes can also help to reduce the risk of readmission. Management of the patient immediately before the surgical procedure and during all aspects of care in the operating room can have an impact on patient satisfaction and postoperative outcomes. Care efficiency and standardized protocols have an impact on quality of care and can improve readmission rates. Institutions that perform a higher volume of TJAs have lower rates of mortality, complications, and readmissions compared with those that perform lower volumes.[36] Surgeons and hospitals must commit to providing resources and implementing processes that can improve their TJA volume. The implementation of dedicated arthroplasty operating rooms or running parallel rooms, increases procedural volume, and decreases surgical time and the duration of hospitalization.[36,37]

In addition to establishing a surgical team/ vision centered around quality care goals, heightened focus should be allocated to compliance with standardized surgical protocols. Preventing surgical wound infection, the primary cause of readmissions after TJA, starts before the operation, with perioperative measures that include proper skin preparation and prophylactic antibiotics. Intraoperatively, meticulous care is crucial to ensure the maintenance of the sterility of the operating field. Minimizing particle count in the operating room will also decrease risk of postoperative infection by using body exhaust suits, laminar flow, ultraviolet light, controlling operating room traffic, and antibiotic-loaded bone cement.[38] Finally, the use of tourniquets can minimize blood loss and the need for transfusions, which may contribute to longer duration of stay and impact risk for readmission.[39]

After surgical intervention, efforts should be directed towards minimizing risk of complications during in-hospital care and in the postdischarge period. Keeney and colleagues[40] advocate for the multimodal treatment approach, which had a great impact on reducing surgically related complications after TKA. Appropriate anticoagulation and use of compression stockings are prophylactic measures for patients who suffer from thromboembolic disease, a common cause of readmission in the THA population.[41] Appropriate antibiotic prophylaxis regimens are aimed at decreasing the risk of potential infection.[38] Routine monitoring will also allow timely recognition of hematoma development, copious wound drainage, or need for early blood transfusion.[38]

Several readmission reduction initiatives reported in the literature, focus on minimizing hospital length of stay and influencing discharge destination.[42,43] Decreasing the duration of hospital stay became an approach to continuing managed care in patients when the diagnosis related group payment system was coming into play.[44] This shifted care from the inpatient setting to an outpatient rehabilitation facility and lowered costs related to the hospitalization.[44] However, discharging patients to home has been shown to decrease readmissions.[45,46] In an attempt to achieve both of these goals, the use of patient management support systems have been implemented to provide rapid recovery after discharge, while minimizing patients' risk to hospital acquired conditions.[44] Edwards and colleagues[44] used support teams by engaging with the patient at all phases of care and in collaboration with a "navigator" team member in the immediate postdischarge period. This system resulted in an increased home discharge rate of all TJA patients to 94%, decreased length of stay to less than 2 days, and decreasing readmission rate from 16% to 9.2%.[44]

Postoperative care can consume up to 50% of the overall cost of the perioperative care cycle.[11] The use of perioperative care teams and home monitoring systems, through mobile devices or electronic systems, can lead to better transition from the time of discharge to the first follow-up visit.[47,48] Providing quality care requires the surgeon to become invested and equipped with the resources needed to empower patients to play an active role in their health care and optimize their outcomes. Patient activation is vital in the postoperative period, but starts from the initial preoperative appointment. An "activated" patient has improved quality of life, lower health-related costs, fewer complications, and greater satisfaction.[49] Surgical outcome is the result of many components within the system and failure, at any 1 step, may result in an adverse outcome mitigating the risk for an unplanned readmission. As such, the optimization of the postoperative course and the decrease

in 30-day readmission rates could be achieved by the improvement and perfection of every step in the surgical process.

Future Directions

Recent studies reported in the orthopedic surgery literature have delved into components of readmissions ranging from cost burden, risk factors, as well as proper coding and assessments.[9,14,16–19] Although some success has been achieved in reducing the duration of stay through rapid recovery protocols without compromising readmission rates, gaps in our understanding of readmissions still exist. One study suggested that one-half of readmissions are not associated with a complication or the index admission.[33,50]

Studies to bridge the gap in the literature would aid in providing a model to predict hospital readmission founded on evidence-based factors and guide medical management to minimize such risks. This review further highlights the disparities in our understanding of readmission factors, the dearth of studies in certain domains of risk factors, and the limited number of prospective studies. Also, the variation in criteria of what constitutes a readmission across studies and the arbitrary 30-day quality measure used by CMS, prevents effective pooling of the data. In fact, some variables cannot be studied quantitatively because of the significant heterogeneity and the lack of consistency, especially in reporting terminology. Several current studies focus extensively on the patient and provider factors, with a clear paucity in reported data for social, procedural, and diagnostic factors that influence readmission rates. There is also a need to further explore factors such as general medical and psychiatric health conditions including, but not limited to, depression, hypertension, and abnormal blood levels of triglycerides, cholesterol, and vitamin D. Patient compliance and accountability are also crucial factors that may impact risk of readmission and remain underreported. The patient's and/or family member's ability to process and provide adequate care in the postoperative period might have a direct impact on complications and lead to early unplanned readmission.

Furthermore, it is vital to understand the implications of not just the individual procedures and risk factors, but also the effects of multilevel interventions on readmission to significantly reduce incidence.[51] For instance, factors that otherwise would not be a major cause of readmission could play a pivotal role when compounded with other factors. Unfortunately, many current readmission predictors, such as the LACE index, have poor discriminatory power as well as limited utility.[20,52] Contrastingly, the American College of Surgeons Surgical Risk Calculator presents a strong example of the importance of clinical judgment to adjust and improve predictive power of adverse events, although it does not predict readmission risk specifically.[53] Additionally, none of these predictors are sufficiently specific for orthopedics; in a surgical specialty with a variety of specialty-specific operations, a unique, specialized predictor is required. Without investigating the effects of various interventions, optimal interventions to prevent early readmission will remain a challenging task. A comprehensive and arthroplasty-specific model is needed to reduce early readmissions to prevent providers

from further straining the medical and financial resources in the system, without actually improving the quality of delivered care.[54,55]

SUMMARY

Unplanned readmissions bring about severe ramifications for the patient, patient families, the institution, and the health care system. Several studies have attempted to identify various factors to predict hospital readmissions (summarized in Table 1). The implications of readmission within 30 days of discharge should drive providers, administrators, and policymakers to turn more attention to system-based procedures that can help decrease readmission, and ultimately improve quality of care while decreasing health care–associated costs.

Table 1
Summary of readmission risk and strategies to reduce readmission rates

Factors Associated with Increased Readmission Rates	Approaches to Reduce 30-Day Readmission
Patient specific (nonmodifiable)	Proper patient selection and optimizing the patient
• Age (>40 and <75 y)	• Internist or PCP care management
• Race (African American)	• Preoperative medical clearance
• Gender (Male)	• Communication with providers and family members
• History of cancer	• Address malnutrition
Patient specific (modifiable)	• Manage comorbidities
• Obesity	• Assess preoperative laboratory tests (albumin, Zn, NO)
• Pulmonary circulation disease	Care delivery
• Chronic pulmonary disease	• Care efficiency protocols
• Hypothyroidism	• Standardized surgical protocols
• Bleeding disorder	• Dedicate arthroplasty ORs
• Psychosis	• Minimize infectious particle count
• Preoperative Charlson Index score	• Tourniquet use
Care delivery factors	Managing complications
• Low-volume surgical centers	• Compression stockings
• Lower surgeon volume	• Proper anticoagulation
• Public hospitals	• Appropriate prophylactic antibiotics
• Infectious arthritis	• Routine monitoring
• Epidural anesthesia	• Routine wound care
Health system factors	Postoperative care
• Higher cost of index admission	• Minimize hospital length of stay
• Payer type (Medicare/Medicaid)	• Discharge to home/home health
• Discharge status (SNFs)	• Postdischarge support teams
Complications	• Encourage patient activation/involvement
• Wound infection	• Engage family members
• Sepsis	
• Surgical site infection (deep)	
• Dislocation	
• Prosthetic misalignment	
• Inadequate pain control	
• Hematoma	
• Inability to mobilize	
• Falling episodes	
• Thromboembolic disease (DVT/PE)	

Abbreviations: DVT, deep venous thrombosis; NO, nitric oxide; OR, operating room; PE, pulmonary embolism; SNF, skilled nursing facility.

REFERENCES

1. Ethgen O, Bruyere O, Richy F, et al. Health-related quality of life in total hip and total knee arthroplasty. A qualitative and systematic review of the literature. J Bone Joint Surg Am 2004;86-A(5): 963–74.

2. Karam JA, Tokarski AT, Ciccotti M, et al. Revision total hip arthroplasty in younger patients: indications, reasons for failure, and survivorship. Phys Sports Med 2012;40(4):96–101.

3. Lons A, Arnould A, Pommepuy T, et al. Excellent short-term results of hip resurfacing in a selected population of young patients. Orthop Traumatol Surg Res 2015;101(6):661–5.

4. Kurtz SM, Ong KL, Lau E, et al. Impact of the economic downturn on total joint replacement demand in the United States: updated projections to 2021. J Bone Joint Surg Am 2014;96(8):624–30.

5. Kurtz S, Ong K, Lau E, et al. Projections of primary and revision hip and knee arthroplasty in the United States from 2005 to 2030. J Bone Joint Surg Am 2007;89(4):780–5.

6. Ramkumar PN, Chu CT, Harris JD, et al. Causes and rates of unplanned readmissions after elective primary total joint arthroplasty: a systematic review and meta-analysis. Am J Orthop (Belle Mead NJ) 2015;44(9):397–405.

7. Readmissions Reduction Program. Centers for Medicare & Medicaid Services website. Available at: www.cms.gov/Medicare/Medicare-Fee-for-Service-Payment/AcuteInpatientPPS/Readmissions-Reduction-Program.html. Accessed July 27, 2015.

8. Kurtz SM, Ong KL, Schmier J, et al. Future clinical and economic impact of revision total hip and knee arthroplasty. J Bone Joint Surg Am 2007; 89(Suppl 3):144–51.

9. Bosco JA 3rd, Karkenny AJ, Hutzler LH, et al. Cost burden of 30-day readmissions following Medicare total hip and knee arthroplasty. J Arthroplasty 2014;29(5):903–5.

10. The revolving door: a report on U.S. Hospital Readmissions. An analysis of Medicare data by the Dartmouth Atlas Project. Stories from patients and health care providers by PerryUndem Research & Communication. Princeton (NJ): Robert Wood Johnson Foundation; 2013. Available at: www.rwjf.org/content/dam/farm/reports/reports/2013/rwjf404178. Accessed July 27, 2015.

11. Bozic KJ, Stacey B, Berger A, et al. Resource utilization and costs before and after total joint arthroplasty. BMC Health Serv Res 2012;12:73.

12. Birkmeyer NJ, Dimick JB, Share D, et al. Hospital complication rates with bariatric surgery in Michigan. JAMA 2010;304(4):435–42.

13. Pugely AJ, Callaghan JJ, Martin CT, et al. Incidence of and risk factors for 30-day readmission following elective primary total joint arthroplasty: analysis from the ACS-NSQIP. J Arthroplasty 2013;28(9): 1499–504.

14. Tayne S, Merrill CA, Smith EL, et al. Predictive risk factors for 30-day readmissions following primary total joint arthroplasty and modification of patient management. J Arthroplasty 2014;29(10):1938–42.

15. Weller WE, Rosati C, Hannan EL. Relationship between surgeon and hospital volume and readmission after bariatric operation. J Am Coll Surg 2007;204(3):383–91.

16. Avram V, Petruccelli D, Winemaker M, et al. Total joint arthroplasty readmission rates and reasons for 30-day hospital readmission. J Arthroplasty 2014;29(3):465–8.

17. Clement RC, Kheir MM, Derman PB, et al. What are the economic consequences of unplanned readmissions after TKA? Clin Orthop Relat Res 2014; 472(10):3134–41.

18. Saucedo J, Marecek GS, Lee J, et al. How accurately are we coding readmission diagnoses after total joint arthroplasty? J Arthroplasty 2013;28(7): 1076–9.

19. Saucedo JM, Marecek GS, Wanke TR, et al. Understanding readmission after primary total hip and knee arthroplasty: who's at risk? J Arthroplasty 2014;29(2):256–60.

20. Cotter PE, Bhalla VK, Wallis SJ, et al. Predicting readmissions: poor performance of the LACE index in an older UK population. Age Ageing 2012;41(6):784–9.

21. Teixeira A, Trinquart L, Raphael M, et al. Outcomes in older patients after surgical treatment for hip fracture: a new approach to characterise the link between readmissions and the surgical stay. Age Ageing 2009;38(5):584–9.

22. Zmistowski B, Restrepo C, Hess J, et al. Unplanned readmission after total joint arthroplasty: rates, reasons, and risk factors. J Bone Joint Surg Am 2013; 95(20):1869–76.

23. Lavernia CJ, Villa JM. Readmission rates in total hip arthroplasty: a granular analysis? J Arthroplasty 2015;30(7):1127–31.

24. Paxton EW, Inacio MC, Singh JA, et al. Are there modifiable risk factors for hospital readmission after total hip arthroplasty in a US Healthcare System? Clin Orthop Relat Res 2015;473(11):3446–55.

25. Singh JA, Kwoh CK, Richardson D, et al. Sex and surgical outcomes and mortality after primary total knee arthroplasty: a risk-adjusted analysis. Arthritis Care Res (Hoboken) 2013;65(7):1095–102.

26. Bozic KJ, Maselli J, Pekow PS, et al. The influence of procedure volumes and standardization of care on quality and efficiency in total joint replacement surgery. J Bone Joint Surg Am 2010;92(16):2643–52.

27. SooHoo NF, Lieberman JR, Ko CY, et al. Factors predicting complication rates following total knee replacement. J Bone Joint Surg Am 2006;88(3):480–5.

28. Miller AG, Margules A, Raikin SM. Risk factors for wound complications after ankle fracture surgery. J Bone Joint Surg Am 2012;94(22):2047–52.

29. Gay DM, Lyman S, Do H, et al. Indications and reoperation rates for total elbow arthroplasty: an analysis of trends in New York State. J Bone Joint Surg Am 2012;94(2):110–7.

30. Higuera CA, Elsharkawy K, Klika AK, et al. 2010 Mid-America Orthopaedic Association Physician in Training Award: predictors of early adverse outcomes after knee and hip arthroplasty in geriatric patients. Clin Orthop Relat Res 2011;469(5):1391–400.

31. Dy CJ, Dossous PM, Ton QV, et al. The medical orthopaedic trauma service: an innovative multidisciplinary team model that decreases in-hospital complications in patients with hip fractures. J Orthop Trauma 2012;26(6):379–83.

32. Matsen FA 3rd, Li N, Gao H, et al. Factors affecting length of stay, readmission, and revision after shoulder arthroplasty: a population-based study. J Bone Joint Surg Am 2015;97(15):1255–63.

33. Bini SA, Fithian DC, Paxton LW, et al. Does discharge disposition after primary total joint arthroplasty affect readmission rates? J Arthroplasty 2010; 25(1):114–7.

34. Riggs RV, Roberts PS, Aronow H, et al. Joint replacement and hip fracture readmission rates: impact of discharge destination. PM R 2010;2(9): 806–10.

35. Lawson EH, Hall BL, Louie R, et al. Association between occurrence of a postoperative complication and readmission: implications for quality improvement and cost savings. Ann Surg 2013;258(1):10–8.

36. Duffy GP. Maximizing surgeon and hospital total knee arthroplasty volume using customized patient instrumentation and swing operating rooms. Am J Orthop (Belle Mead NJ) 2011;40(11 Suppl):5–8.

37. Roberts TT, Vanushkina M, Khasnavis S, et al. Dedicated orthopaedic operating rooms: beneficial to patients and providers alike. J Orthop Trauma 2015;29(1):e18–23.

38. Illingworth KD, Mihalko WM, Parvizi J, et al. How to minimize infection and thereby maximize patient outcomes in total joint arthroplasty: a multicenter approach: AAOS exhibit selection. J Bone Joint Surg Am 2013;95(8):e50.

39. Whitehead DJ, MacDonald SJ. TKA sans tourniquet: let it bleed: opposes. Orthopedics 2011; 34(9):e497–9.

40. Keeney JA, Nam D, Johnson SR, et al. The impact of risk reduction initiatives on readmission: THA and TKA readmission rates. J Arthroplasty 2015; 30(12):2057–60.

41. Lewis CG, Inneh IA, Schutzer SF, et al. Evaluation of the first-generation AAOS clinical guidelines on the prophylaxis of venous thromboembolic events in patients undergoing total joint arthroplasty:

42. Jordan CJ, Goldstein RY, Michels RF, et al. Comprehensive program reduces hospital readmission rates after total joint arthroplasty. Am J Orthop (Belle Mead NJ) 2012;41(11):E147–51.

43. Lower HL, Dale H, Eriksen HM, et al. Surgical site infections after hip arthroplasty in Norway, 2005-2011: influence of duration and intensity of postdischarge surveillance. Am J Infect Control 2015;43(4):323–8.

44. Edwards PK, Levine M, Cullinan K, et al. Avoiding readmissions-support systems required after discharge to continue rapid recovery? J Arthroplasty 2015;30(4):527–30.

45. Mabrey JD, Toohey JS, Armstrong DA, et al. Clinical pathway management of total knee arthroplasty. Clin Orthop Relat Res 1997;(345):125–33.

46. Ramos NL, Karia RJ, Hutzler LH, et al. The effect of discharge disposition on 30-day readmission rates after total joint arthroplasty. J Arthroplasty 2014; 29(4):674–7.

47. Abroms LC, Ahuja M, Kodl Y, et al. Text2Quit: results from a pilot test of a personalized, interactive mobile health smoking cessation program. J Health Commun 2012;17(Suppl 1):44–53.

48. Evans WD, Abroms LC, Poropatich R, et al. Mobile health evaluation methods: the Text4baby case study. J Health Commun 2012;17(Suppl 1):22–9.

49. Tzeng A, Tzeng TH, Vasdev S, et al. The role of patient activation in achieving better outcomes and cost-effectiveness in patient care. Journal of Bone and Joint Surgery Reviews 2013;3(1):e4. Available at: http://reviews.jbjs.org/content/3/1/e4.

50. Stambough JB, Nunley RM, Curry MC, et al. Rapid recovery protocols for primary total hip arthroplasty can safely reduce length of stay without increasing readmissions. J Arthroplasty 2015;30(4):521–6.

51. Kripalani S, Theobald CN, Anctil B, et al. Reducing hospital readmission rates: current strategies and future directions. Annu Rev Med 2014;65:471–85.

52. Inneh IA, Lewis CG, Schutzer SF. Focused risk analysis: regression model based on 5,314 total hip and knee arthroplasty patients from a single institution. J Arthroplasty 2014;29(10):2031–5.

53. Bilimoria KY, Liu Y, Paruch JL, et al. Development and evaluation of the universal ACS NSQIP surgical risk calculator: a decision aid and informed consent tool for patients and surgeons. J Am Coll Surg 2013;217(5):833–42.e1–3.

54. Leppin AL, Gionfriddo MR, Kessler M, et al. Preventing 30-day hospital readmissions: a systematic review and meta-analysis of randomized trials. JAMA Intern Med 2014;174(7):1095–107.

55. Nicholson A, Lowe MC, Parker J, et al. Systematic review and meta-analysis of enhanced recovery programmes in surgical patients. Br J Surg 2014; 101(3):172–88.

Planning, Building, and Maintaining a Successful Musculoskeletal Service Line

Zain Sayeed, MSc, MHA[a], Mouhanad M. El-Othmani, MD[a],
Afshin A. Anoushiravani, MD[a],
Monique C. Chambers, MD, MSL[a],
Khaled J. Saleh, MD, MSc, FRCS (C), MHCM, CPE[b],*

KEYWORDS

• Service lines • Musculoskeletal care • Value-based care • Comanagement • Joint ventures

KEY POINTS

• A musculoskeletal service line can be defined as a structure used in health care organizations allowing health care providers and administrators to deliver integrated patient care, track relevant data, and manage resources and expenses.
• Identification of service-line purpose, key stakeholders, registry management, and administrative principles are becoming a necessity in the management tool kit of orthopedic surgeons as they steer musculoskeletal service lines through the era hospital-physician alignment.
• Comanagement and joint ventures serve as 2 management models that orthopedic surgeons may adopt to maintain autonomy in musculoskeletal service-line initiatives.

INTRODUCTION

The concept of service lines was first introduced to the health care industry in the 1980s.[1] As health care executives noted successes from other industry leaders, such as Proctor & Gamble, Toyota, Motorola Corporation, and the Product Line Model from General Motors, speculation of how to apply such strategic principles in health care delivery gained further attention.[2] In the first installment of service-line strategies within the health care setting, the primary driving force was interhospital competition.[1,3] In the mid 1980s, a discernable prevalence of the marketing capability of service lines was seen in health care systems in which a specific service line, such as total joint replacement, may have been used to entice patients to choose one hospital over another.[1,3,4] Additionally, the establishment of fixed reimbursement payment models in the 1980s prompted managed care organizations to use this mechanism to promote their market share.[1,3,4] As the health care industry progressed into the 1990s and 2000s, interhospital competition became a secondary focus with the establishment of specialty hospitals, ambulatory surgical centers, and physician-owned medical facilities.[1,3,4] Within the past decade, there has been a resurgence in the interest of service-line management.[5–7] Moreover, hospitals have realized that they cannot depend on volume alone to maintain financial stability. Rather, delivery of health care must meet nationally recognized quality standards. Thus, service lines became a model allowing both hospital administrators and

Funding Sources: No additional funding sources were used for this article.
Conflicts of Interest: No conflicts of interest are evident for the authors of this article.
[a] Division of Orthopaedics and Rehabilitation, Southern Illinois University School of Medicine, 701 North First Street, Springfield, IL 62781, USA; [b] Department of Orthopaedic and Sports Medicine, Detroit Medical Center, 311 Mack Avenue, 5th Floor, Detroit, MI 48201, USA
* Corresponding author.
E-mail address: kjsaleh@gmail.com

physicians the ability to monitor outcomes and resource allocation while delivering optimal care.[5-7]

Within orthopedics, a notable trend has been seen in the establishment of musculoskeletal service lines that achieve high-quality care at lower costs. This review addresses the processes involved in planning and building a successful musculoskeletal service line.

DEFINING A MUSCULOSKELETAL SERVICE LINE

A musculoskeletal service line can be defined as a process used by health care organizations allowing providers to adopt an integrated patient care pathway, track relevant data, and manage resource consumption. The service may incorporate one or all procedures involved in musculoskeletal care, including but not limited to total joint arthroplasty (TJA), hip fracture management, and spinal care, among others. Regardless of procedural variation, service lines share the fundamental centralization of the organization's efforts and allocation of resources to specific patient-population requiring specialty care. Orthopedic care has consistently been viewed as low maintenance amidst hospital administrators, with surgeons requiring minimal administrative oversight despite high costs, advanced technology, and complicated patients.[8] Furthermore, orthopedic outcome measures serve to be easily marketable, allowing administrators to establish trust and proven care within their hospital infrastructure.[4,8-10]

COMPONENTS OF A MUSCULOSKELETAL SERVICE LINE

Another asset provided by a musculoskeletal service line is the establishment of a horizontal hierarchical system of care.[11] Instead of distinct departments that are separately involved in patient care, a service line establishes parallel management of patients requiring specialty service.[4] Therefore, musculoskeletal service lines have all needed personnel and required resources to streamline processes involved. Each service line has a dedicated system that allows involved stakeholders access to physician leaders (champions) or service-line administrators. As a result, necessary concerns are conveyed leading to enhanced team communication and reporting structure. Within the past 2 decades, a substantial push toward adding value to patient care has woven its trademark in the health care industry.

Identification of value is more easily discerned in orthopedic practices, as care is results driven. Consequently, value in musculoskeletal service lines is defined by clinical and economical success measures. Clinical success relates to patient care outcomes. Economic success, on the other hand, measures profitability, contribution margins, and market share. When planning a service line, it is imperative that administrators and surgeons establish common ground based on the delineated principles before investing resources and time into such practices.

Regardless of surgical procedure, defining a central purpose for a musculoskeletal service line is imperative to its success.[12] Many organizations choose a standard Diagnostic Related Group designation that corresponds to related procedures, whereas some service lines choose the International Classification of Diseases, 9th or 10th edition, code classifications for inclusion criteria. Whichever mechanism is used, a shared vision that identifies designated metrics helps determine service-line achievement. Gee[1] suggests that the success of a service line is greatly governed by its comparability to the market. In essence, a musculoskeletal service line should have the capability of being objectively evaluated by the hospital or health care system stakeholders through well-defined and established performance metrics. Such metrics may be qualitative, including patient-reported outcomes and satisfaction, hip or knee scores, and community perception of service lines. Furthermore, quantitative measures, such as net revenue, mortality rate, and postoperative complications, may help further define the effectiveness of a service line. Service line administrators and physicians often establish goals by identifying success measures based on the Agency for Healthcare Research and Quality (AHRQ) or Centers for Medicare and Medicaid services (CMS) criteria.[13,14] Measurement of any quality improvement (QI) service-line initiative has become a necessity with recent trends toward publicly reporting data and use of Hospital Compare Scores.[15]

Identification of contributions of various stakeholders involved in a musculoskeletal service line is another fundamental step in enabling greater alignment with service-line goals. Identifying physician leaders among health care providers allows clinical leaders to serve distinct roles in the process. Some champion physicians serve as service-line medical directors or official medical advisors. Leaders from various specialties involved in musculoskeletal care delivery, including anesthesiology, emergency medicine, hospitalist medicine, and surgery, may be involved in the service-line production. This interspecialty alignment encourages needed physician advocacy once the program is implemented while simultaneously supporting process transparency.[8] Furthermore, decision-making bodies and work groups may be necessary to identify approaches to optimize musculoskeletal care. Various committees' levels and structures may be required that specialize in clinical care, QI, business planning, marketing, and finance, among other focuses. Another valuable role is that of service-line chief financial officers (CFOs). A CFO is typically a senior health care finance leader that is responsible for determining the profitability of a service line. Lang and Powers[8] suggested that a health care finance leader should pair with at least one orthopedic surgeon champion, service-line administrator, and vendor to analyze and make financial decisions in establishing the service line.

BUILDING A MUSCULOSKELETAL SERVICE LINE

Perhaps one of the greatest challenges facing the establishment of a musculoskeletal service line is garnering a relationship between orthopedic surgeons and hospital administrators.[16] Service-line leadership may consist of several stakeholders, including administrators, nurse managers, and medical directors, all of whom play an integral role in developing an institutional culture embracing and supporting service lines.[17,18] Health systems implementing musculoskeletal service lines require active involvement of orthopedic surgeons at all stages of process development. Early and active involvement by stakeholders ensures service-line sustainability and allows orthopedic surgeons to make informed decisions that are clinically and financially responsible.[19] On planning the development of a musculoskeletal service line, orthopedic surgeons and administrators use various management accounting models that allow stakeholders to track resources and revenue (discussed further later). In many hospital settings, a musculoskeletal service line is primarily used as a means of tracking adverse outcomes in one or more designated metrics by the hospital administration.[19] The service-line administrator typically responds to such outcomes by developing interventions to address costly resources and sources of waste. Intuitively, orthopedic surgeons often drive utilization of resources, in an attempt to lead to patient outcome optimization. Thus, administrators face the challenge of optimizing the financial aspect of surgical practices without compromising individual surgeon preference.[19]

The ability of service-line administrators to understand surgeon's preferences extends into assessing the relationships of surgeons and operating room (OR) case representatives.[8] The working relationship between an orthopedist and a case representative may result in new and expensive product utilization. When hospitals and orthopedic surgeons are not commonly aligned with regard to surgical equipment, surgeons may be less inclined to cooperate with service-line initiatives. A case representative can play an integral role intraoperatively by offering technical assistance or advice that allows surgeons to perform difficult cases.[8] Lang and Powers[8] note that a skilled case representative can become an organization's or surgeon's right hand by filling a void that is often unaddressed by the surgical team or OR staff. Nonetheless, the OR should be a sales-free zone in which measures that control the introduction of new technology in the OR are negotiated by stakeholders vested within the process.[8] Evidence-based decision-making is necessary to guide instrument and implant selection. Several studies assessing the survivorship and patient functionality scores of various implant designs must be considered before investment of resources.[20,21] Therefore, it is critical that early in musculoskeletal service-line development, a clear and concise method to implement surgical instrument selection be available for orthopedic surgeons and various stakeholders to review.

Such resource-control and budgeting strategies permit service-line stakeholders to create an implant selection process. In order to optimize efficiency in patients' surgical care and address the needs of orthopedic surgeons, service-line administrators must harness surgeons' input and collaboration through a committee that includes representation from champion orthopedic surgeons. Hospitals pay different prices for similar implants according to the negotiated rates between institution and supplier.[8] As orthopedic implant devices comprise a considerable share of the cost for the procedure, careful selection might warrant maintenance of high-quality care while at the same time decreasing associated costs.[8] Coincidentally, the implant is also the driver of revenue for orthopedic vendors; therefore, a selected consultant should serve as a liaison for communication.[8] Oftentimes, a surgeon will advocate for a preferred vendor based on implant preference. Such claims should be recommended through peer corroboration, documentation, or other justified means. A qualified third-party member may offer helpful navigation through difficult interactions that may develop between surgeons and service-line administrators. Hospitals in which surgeons lack such managerial experience are challenged by increased operational risks, inventory control, storage issues, and ultimately higher costs. Thus, an implant selection strategy allows a service line to have limited vendor convolution, better aligning the service lines' focus on patient-centered care while improving resources utilization.

Establishing an open forum for communication is a challenging task within the setting of musculoskeletal service lines. Success depends on creating a meaningful dialogue between stakeholders invested in the process. Amidst recent legislative changes, institutions are shifting from being volume and margin driven to quality and performance metrics. Interestingly, physicians often lack administrative training in their medical education, resulting in vulnerability of their autonomy. A discussion of various management models will allow orthopedists to play an active role in the creation and implementation of a musculoskeletal service line. Involvement of all stakeholders not only addresses concerns of all vested interests but also ensures compliance.

Hospitals match revenue from services rendered with associated costs or expenses to determine profits in a given period of time. In musculoskeletal service lines, the CFO typically tracks hospital discharge volumes or surgical caseloads representing the "sale of service."[22]

The service-line CFO often determines the cost-allocation that is generally divided into the scheme provided in Table 1. Eventually these costs help calculate the financial impact of a given musculoskeletal service line to a hospital. The most robust marker to determine such impact is the contribution margin that represents the profitability of the given musculoskeletal service line (see Table 1).[19] Once indirect expenses are covered, hospitals tend to report net profit on their investment.[19,22] If indirect expenses are unable to be covered, CFOs are left to examine expense management, identify inefficiencies, and consider efforts that may add volume or harness indirect expenses.[19,22] Some financial leaders have recognized that the greatest expense to a service line is the human component. In order to track such expenses, stakeholders must assess the time and activity-driven costs in order to effectively isolate wastes within the service line. If service lines continue to be unprofitable, evaluating accounting practices may improve the financial outcomes of the musculoskeletal line. Such evaluations require comprehensive and consistent documentation of the entire patient-care spectrum within a specified service line.

On identification of deficiencies in service-line processes, data-driven management tools may be implemented to optimize musculoskeletal care pathways. Recent focus on integrating QI methodologies, such as the Lean and Six Sigma principles, among others, are becoming ever more common within the orthopedic community.[23-25] In combination, the Lean Six Sigma (LSS) methodology allows stakeholders to map

Table 1	
Understanding the costs and contribution margin of a musculoskeletal service line	
Cost Principle	**Definition and Example**
Direct costs	Cost of surgical care directly provided to patients; may be fixed or variable Example: cost of implant used in surgical procedure
Indirect costs	Expenses associated with services that are often seen as overhead; may be fixed or variable Example: facility expenses, laundry, and electrical costs
Fixed costs	Incrementally fixed within every episode of providing care Example: cost of a specific knee implant regardless of patient
Variable costs	Incrementally changes with respect to various episodes of providing care Example: duration of operating room use and associated cost, salary of operating room nurse, and anesthetic agents.
Contribution margin	Most frequently cited markers of profitability for a service line; there are 2 types: 1. Variable contribution margin: net revenue (all the revenue the hospital receives for patient care), the variable direct cost for patients 2. Direct contribution margin: net revenue (variable direct cost + fixed direct cost)

care processes in order to detect and prevent error, while reducing waste and process variation.[26] After application, orthopedic surgeons can analyze resource consumption by identifying efficient portions of the process and addressing and eliminating wasteful resources utilization. Furthermore, application of this management methodology is designed to optimize patient outcomes in a reproducible and sustainable manner.[23–25] Although each patient receiving care from service-line providers encompasses individual needs, parameters such as time to surgery, duration of surgery, and clinical wait times may improve following implementation of LSS principles. One way to accomplish this goal is to combine service-line initiatives with tracking capabilities through the use of patient registries.[27–30]

Several studies have attempted to investigate QI initiatives by assessing how registry data tracks change within an organization.[15,29,30] One study assessed the American Association of Blood Banks' transfusion protocol installment for TJA procedures comparing pre-QI and post-QI implementation cohorts.[15] The investigators reported that the use of the Michigan Arthroplasty Registry Collaborative Quality Initiative allowed for effective outcomes tracking that identified a decrease in allogeneic transfusions following TJA.[15] In North America, national and local registries are broadening their focus to include perioperative complications and patient-reported outcomes measures following surgery.[27–30] Use of service-line registries empowers surgeons to assess outcomes and resource utilization trends in an evidence-based manner resulting in improvement of postoperative outcomes.

Furthermore, recent health care reforms have disproportionally targeted orthopedic care. The Patient Protection and Affordable Care Act in combination with high volume, high costs, and well-reimbursed care requires orthopedic surgeons to foster greater transparency. The use of detailed surgical registries in musculoskeletal service lines may enhance reporting practices and identify shortcomings in care delivery. However, simply developing a service line is not enough for the musculoskeletal line to remain effective, as it must be continuously maintained, assessed, and modified to stay up-to-date with the ever-changing health care environment.

MAINTAINING A MUSCULOSKELETAL SERVICE LINE

As the health care systems transform from volume-based to a value-driven system,[31] it is critical that orthopedic surgeons vested within musculoskeletal service lines understand how to maintain a service line while navigating through newer reimbursement models. After the recent repeal of the Sustainable Growth Rate formula, one newer modality of reimbursement includes the Merit-based Incentive Payment System (MIPS).[32,33] MIPS is a quality reporting program in which physicians and hospitals will be compensated under the traditional Medicare fee-for-service plan assessed by performance within 4 weighted subcategories: clinical quality, meaningful use of health information technology, resource use, and practice improvement.[32] Such a reimbursement system is ripe for implementation via a musculoskeletal service line, which has exposure to a high-volume of elective procedures within the Medicare population as well as a wide continuum-of-care tracking practice improvement. Another reimbursement model that currently affects service lines is the bundle payment initiative. Within this model, a payer bundles the service line's episode of care into one reimbursable sum.[8,34] In essence, the amount reimbursed is fixed and includes all services rendered, including the surgical procedure, prosthesis, and hospital stay. Reimbursement is largely unaltered by in-hospital complications sustained by patients. Additionally, a hospital may choose to contract with the CMS as part of the Bundled Payment Care Initiative, allowing for more parties, such as the various payers, to be included in service-line investment.

A common theme represented by value-based care initiatives is greater accountability and shared risk taking by both hospitals and physicians. There are several management methods to consider when orthopedic surgeons consider partnering with hospitals in the implementation of a musculoskeletal service line. These methods may include, but are not limited to, medical directorships, contractual agreements for call pay, medical coverage agreements, comanagement, gain sharing, information technology strategies, joint ventures, and support for care of unions.[35] Two of the more robust models used by orthopedic surgeons that aid in physician autonomy is comanagement and joint ventures. Comanagement agreements usually involve a base compensation in addition to an incentive scheme that promotes institutional goals, such as improved patient satisfaction or reduced health care costs.[36,37] Use of comanagement in service lines may yield greater profit margins for both the institution and health care providers while providing patients with optimal care.[36,37]

This type of financial arrangement maintains the orthopedic surgeon's clinical autonomy while promoting clinical transparency and fiscal responsibility among clinicians and hospitals. Importantly, it is advised that service-line administrators and orthopedic surgeons look to a limited liability company for negotiating comanagement arrangements in line with Stark and Anti-Kickback laws.[36,37]

Another management model that is highly amenable to musculoskeletal service lines is a joint-venture. This type of management arrangement aims to create distinct freestanding centers of care that offer specialty services to patients. These centers may include specialty surgery centers, diagnostic clinics, or immediate care facilities.[35,38] Because of the large volume of minimally invasive orthopedic surgical techniques and acuteness of orthopedic trauma, joint venture arrangements offer formation of musculoskeletal enterprises that can appeal to both patients and providers. Much like comanagement, joint ventures should be advised to seek an outside independent legal entity to carefully structure a contract that is free of astringent liability. Currently, there are examples of successful musculoskeletal service lines that are in practice nationwide. Such service lines necessitate further exploration by the orthopedic community.

CURRENT MUSCULOSKELETAL SERVICE-LINE LEADERS

In the rapidly evolving health care climate, the Hospital for Special Surgery (HSS) and TRIA, a physician-run multidisciplinary orthopedic group, have developed in such a manner to meet the demands of the modern health care system.[39,40] The success of these organizations can in large part be attributed to their commitment to clinical, research, and educational excellence.[10,39] Furthermore, their ability to align physician and administrator goals in an incentive-driven manner has led to greater efficiency and improved quality of care at reduced costs.[10]

THE HOSPITAL FOR SPECIAL SURGERY SERVICE LINE

HSS has developed a strong partnership between administrators and physicians at both an organizational and policy level.[10] A robust organizational partnership has allowed for the implementation of several initiatives, as creating orthopedic service lines.[10] At the policy level, alignment has been achieved through the effective transfer of supply management and innovative programs.[10]

The HSS orthopedic department has been separated into 10 distinct orthopedic service lines each reporting to their respective chief or cochiefs.[10] The service lines consist of surgeons and health care providers with similar areas of expertise, allowing for close collaboration in regard to clinical, educational, and research-based initiatives.[10] In addition, each service line has adjunctive administrators dedicated to fostering alignment. The service-line administrators' primary focus is developing organizational structure, streamlined decision-making processes, and strategic planning needed to promote, maintain, and harness the individual strengths of each service-line member.[10] The orthopedic surgeons devote most of their efforts to clinical protocol development, research registries, fellowship management, and marketing initiatives.[10] The administrators and individual orthopedic surgeons collaborate extensively; however, high-level requests and concerns require the involvement of the service-line chief.[10] Ultimately, all 10 service lines are overseen by the surgeon-in-chief and chief executive officer (CEO). The surgeon-in-chief schedules regular meetings with all service-line chiefs discussing issues of concern.[10] The service-line chiefs should also provide the leadership and the service line members with regular updates and follow-up reports.[10] Finally, the CEO and surgeon-in-chief meet regularly to discuss systemic issues that may arise, thus, maintaining clear organizational structure, missions, and member accountability among all service-line members.[10]

THE TRIA SERVICE LINE

TRIA, a physician-run orthopedic center, is the result of a joint venture between a sports medicine practice, a multispecialty health care provider, and the Department of Orthopaedic Surgery at the University of Minnesota.[39] From its inception, the stakeholders in TRIA recognized the breakdown in communication among different care providers, insurance companies, and hospitals.[39] In response to these failures, TRIA developed service lines in order to improve the quality of care delivery and establish a patient-centered approach within orthopedics.[39] As part of this approach, clinicians were responsible for collecting and measuring patient outcomes. By tracking outcomes on all patients, TRIA is able to improve patient care as well as implement evidence-based initiatives.[39] Although outcomes data are collected on all patients, the data on the

9 most common orthopedic procedures are most frequently evaluated. Furthermore, these outcome studies ensure that individual orthopedic surgeons and the service line as a whole are maintaining institutional standards.

One successful initiative implemented at TRIA is the Hilton Recovery Program, an evidence-based approach, allowing patients to rest and recover on an outpatient basis at the hotel while cared for by TRIA nurses and physical therapists.[39,41] The incorporation of such initiatives has not only been popular among patients and physicians but also third-party payers who realized lower fixed costs. Interestingly, the Hilton Recovery Program has been such a success that other orthopedic providers are replicating the program, increasing competition and driving down costs.[41]

SUMMARY

In the changing health care climate, orthopedic surgeons must be cognizant of the outcomes and resource utilization trends within their practice. Failure to address clinical shortcomings may result in financial penalties. The establishment of service lines by key stakeholders may not only improve outcomes and reduce resource consumption but may also enable clinicians to develop patient registries. Before vesting in a musculoskeletal service line, orthopedic surgeons should investigate management mechanism by which efficient care can be administered without compromising patient needs.

ACKNOWLEDGMENTS

The authors would like to thank Dr Marc Swiontkowski for presenting this topic during the *Central Illinois Healthcare Management Summit* chaired by Dr K.J. Saleh.

REFERENCES

1. Gee EP. Divide and compete. A new look at service lines. Healthc Financ Manage 2004;58(3):60–5.
2. Parker VA, Charns MP, Young GJ. Clinical service lines in integrated delivery systems: an initial framework and exploration. J Healthc Manag 2001;46(4):261–75.
3. Longshore GF. Service-line management/bottom-line management. J Health Care Finance 1998;24(4):72–9.
4. Patterson C. Orthopaedic service lines-revisited. Orthop Nurs 2008;27(1):12–20.
5. Greenberg GA, Rosenheck RA, Charns MP. From profession-based leadership to service line management in the Veterans Health Administration: impact on mental health care. Med Care 2003;41(9):1013–23.
6. Kwon B, Tromanhauser SG, Banco RJ. The spine service line: optimizing patient-centered spine care. Spine 2007;32(11 Suppl):S44–8.
7. Turnipseed WD, Lund DP, Sollenberger D. Product line development: a strategy for clinical success in academic centers. Ann Surg 2007;246(4):585–90 [discussion: 90–2].
8. Lang S, Powers K. Strategies for achieving orthopedic service line success. Healthc Financ Manage 2013;67(12):96–100, 2.
9. Horwitz DS. Orthopaedic surgeon-hospital alignment at Geisinger Health System. Clin Orthop Relat Res 2013;471(6):1846–53.
10. Ranawat AS, Koenig JH, Thomas AJ, et al. Aligning physician and hospital incentives: the approach at hospital for special surgery. Clin Orthop Relat Res 2009;467(10):2535–41.
11. Nawaz H, Edmondson AC, Tzeng TH, et al. Teaming: an approach to the growing complexities in health care: AOA critical issues. J Bone Joint Surg Am 2014;96(21):e184.
12. Byrne MM, Charns MP, Parker VA, et al. The effects of organization on medical utilization: an analysis of service line organization. Med Care 2004;42(1):28–37.
13. Quality AfHRa. AHRQ quality indicators tool kit for hospitals. 2014. Available at: http://www.ahrq.gov/professionals/systems/hospital/qitoolkit/index.html. Accessed November 2, 2015.
14. Services CfMaM. Quality measures - Centers for Medicare and Medicaid services. 2014. Available at: https://www.cms.gov/Medicare/Quality-Initiatives-Patient-Assessment-Instruments/QualityMeasures/index.html?redirect=/QUALITYMEASURES/. Accessed October 13, 2015.
15. Medicare. website - Hospital Compare datasets. Available at: https://data.medicare.gov/data/hospital-compare. Accessed November 4, 2015.
16. Haugh R. A joint strategy for orthopedics. Hospitals team up with docs to keep a lucrative service line. Hosp Health Netw 2002;76(9):54–8, 2.
17. Williams J. A new road map for healthcare business success. Healthc Financ Manage 2011;65(5):62–9.
18. Wilson NA, Ranawat A, Nunley R, et al. Executive summary: aligning stakeholder incentives in orthopaedics. Clin Orthop Relat Res 2009;467(10):2521–4.
19. Olson SA, Mather RC 3rd. Understanding how orthopaedic surgery practices generate value for healthcare systems. Clin Orthop Relat Res 2013;471(6):1801–8.
20. Pandit H, Hamilton TW, Jenkins C, et al. The clinical outcome of minimally invasive phase 3 Oxford unicompartmental knee arthroplasty: a 15-year follow-up of 1000 UKAs. Bone Joint J 2015;97-b(11):1493–500.

21. Felli L, Coviello M, Alessio-Mazzola M, et al. The Endo-Model rotating hinge for rheumatoid knees: functional results in primary and revision surgery. Orthopade 2016;45(5):446–51.

22. DW Y. Management accounting in health care organizations. San Francisco (CA): Jossey-Bass; 2008.

23. Bender JS, Nicolescu TO, Hollingsworth SB, et al. Improving operating room efficiency via an interprofessional approach. Am J Surg 2015;209(3):447–50.

24. DelliFraine JL, Langabeer JR 2nd, Nembhard IM. Assessing the evidence of Six Sigma and Lean in the health care industry. Qual Manag Health Care 2010;19(3):211–25.

25. Wortman B, Richardson WR, Glenn G, et al. The certified Six Sigma black belt primer. West Terre Haute (IN): Quality Council of Indiana; 2012.

26. Kubiak TM, Benbow DW. The certified Six Sigma black belt handbook 2nd edition. Milwaukee (WI): ASQ Quality Press; 2009.

27. Markel DC, Allen MW, Zappa NM. Can an arthroplasty registry help decrease transfusions in primary total joint replacement? A quality initiative. Clin Orthop Relat Res 2016;474(1):126–31.

28. Clair AJ, Inneh IA, Iorio R, et al. Can administrative data be used to analyze complications following total joint arthroplasty? J Arthroplasty 2015;30(9 Suppl):17–20.

29. Ayers DC, Franklin PD. Joint replacement registries in the United States: a new paradigm. J Bone Joint Surg Am 2014;96(18):1567–9.

30. Ahn H, Court-Brown CM, McQueen MM, et al. The use of hospital registries in orthopaedic surgery. J Bone Joint Surg Am 2009;91(Suppl 3):68–72.

31. Porter ME. A strategy for health care reform—toward a value-based system. N Engl J Med 2009;361(2):109–12.

32. Doherty RB. Goodbye, sustainable growth rate-hello, merit-based incentive payment system. Ann Intern Med 2015;163(2):138–9.

33. Sorrel AL. SGR Is Gone. Now What? Tex Med 2015;111(9):57–62.

34. Bushnell BD. Developing a bundled pricing strategy. Rosemont (IL): AAOS Now; 2014.

35. Bushnell BD. Physician-hospital alignment in orthopedic surgery. Orthopedics 2015;38(9):e806–12.

36. NC. Establishing a service line co-management agreement. 2013. Available at: http://www.aaos.org/news/aaosnow/mar13/managing1.asp. Accessed November 6, 2015.

37. Sowers KW, Newman PR, Langdon JC. Evolution of physician-hospital alignment models: a case study of comanagement. Clin Orthop Relat Res 2013;471(6):1818–23.

38. TJ G. Tips for marketing your orthopedic practice. 2007. Available at: http://www.aaos.org/news/bulletin/oct07/managing7.asp. Accessed November 6, 2015.

39. TRIA 2015. Available at: http://tria.com/about/. Accessed November 2, 2015.

40. Kaissi A. Manager-physician relationships: an organizational theory perspective. Health Care Manag (Frederick) 2005;24(2):165–76.

41. Frisch S. An orthopedic group is experimenting with having surgery patients recover in a hotel. 2011. Available at: http://www.minnesotamedicine.com/Past-Issues/Past-Issues-2011/September-2011/Hotel-Management-Sept-2011. Accessed November 2, 2015.

High Reliability of Care in Orthopedic Surgery
Are We There Yet?

Afshin A. Anoushiravani, MD[a], Zain Sayeed, MSc, MHA[a],
Mouhanad M. El-Othmani, MD[a],
Peter K. Wong, PhD, MSc, MBA, RPh[b],
Khaled J. Saleh, MD, MSc, FRCS (C), MHCM, CPE[c,*]

KEYWORDS

- High reliability • Orthopedic practice • Value-based • Safety • Lean management
- Six Sigma principles

KEY POINTS

- A prerequisite for the establishment of a highly reliable organization is "collective mindlessness," otherwise described as a team attitude.
- All team members should work together to eliminate systemic failures leading to sentinel events.
- The AAOS, Joint Commission, and World Health Organization have all developed protocols and checklists designed to reduce wrong-site procedures while delivering highly reliable care.
- Lack of proper leadership, safety culture, and quality improvement strategies make the safety protocols ineffective.

INTRODUCTION

Physicians face many hurdles when delivering care to patients, which inevitably affect outcomes and patient satisfaction. These hurdles are particularly evident within the current health care climate, as volume-based reimbursement models are replaced with value-based patient-centered approaches to health care.[1] The three overarching obstacles currently affecting health care delivery are (1) cost, (2) quality, and (3) timely intervention. Clinicians are constantly faced with the challenges of providing the highest quality of care, within the shortest time frame, at the lowest possible cost. These basic principles are particularly relevant within orthopedics, because the field is responsible for an estimated 9% to 11% of all medical malpractice claims and an estimated 30% of these claims result in legal settlements costing the health care system billions of dollars annually.[2]

High reliability of care, described as consistent performance at high levels of safety over long periods of time, may be implemented within orthopedic practices.[3] If successfully integrated, the model may standardize treatment protocols, improve the quality of care, and aid in the development of clinically applicable guidelines, while minimizing resource expenditures. This article addresses three interdependent and critical changes that need to take

Funding Sources: No additional funding sources were used for this article.
Conflicts of Interest: No conflicts of interest are evident for authors of this article.
[a] Division of Orthopaedics and Rehabilitation, Southern Illinois University School of Medicine, 701 North First Street, Springfield, IL 62781, USA; [b] Illinois Divisions, HSHS Medical Group, Hospitals Sisters Health System (HSHS), 800 E Carpenter St, Springfield, IL 62707, USA; [c] Department of Orthopaedic and Sports Medicine, Detroit Medical Center, 311 Mack Avenue, 5th Floor, Detroit, MI 48201, USA
* Corresponding author.
E-mail address: kjsaleh@gmail.com

Orthop Clin N Am 47 (2016) 689–695
http://dx.doi.org/10.1016/j.ocl.2016.05.011
0030-5898/16/$ – see front matter © 2016 Elsevier Inc. All rights reserved.

place to adopt a high-reliability care model within an orthopedic practice. Also addressed are specific operative protocols that if implemented properly may reduce the risk for wrong-site surgery and improve the quality of care.

SCOPE OF THE PROBLEM

Efforts to improve the quality of health care began with Ignaz Semmelweis,[3] the nineteenth-century obstetrician who introduced hand washing, and later with Ernest Codman,[4] an early advocate for hospital standards and outcome registries. Although significant advancements have been made in the reliability and quality of health care, the Institute of Medicine reported that an estimated 44,000 to 98,000 patients die annually in US hospitals as a direct result of medical errors.[5] Incorrect surgical procedures (wrong site, wrong side, wrong procedure, or wrong patient) account for a small but significant fraction of these errors and have been estimated to occur nationally at a rate of 5 to 10 events per day.[6] Kwaan and colleagues[7] examined a malpractice insurance database and reported that wrong-site procedures occurred at a rate of 1 in 112,994 nonspine procedures. In response to the unacceptably high rate of medical errors, regulatory bodies, such as the Joint Commission on the Accreditation of Healthcare Organizations (JCAHO), and professional medical societies, such as the American Academy of Orthopaedic Surgeons (AAOS), have been charged with the task of analyzing medical errors and developing protocols that aim to prevent future errors.[8]

REQUIREMENTS FOR IMPLEMENTING HIGH RELIABILITY OF CARE

A prerequisite for highly reliable health care organizations is "collective mindfulness," or a team attitude in which all members work together and are acutely aware of small failures or processes that can lead to sentinel events.[9] The successful implementation of highly reliable care requires that three dependent factors be in place: (1) leadership must make a long-term commitment to implementing highly reliable care, (2) the organizational culture must embrace a safety culture, and (3) tools supporting a robust process improvement strategy must be adopted.[3]

Leadership
Before implementation of care initiatives, the respective organization's leadership must be fully committed to structural and cultural

changes necessary to deliver highly reliable care. This commitment must be shared by all members of the leadership including board members, senior managers, administrators, physicians, and all other stakeholders. In addition, the organization's management must recognize that it may take 10 to 15 years to fully transition to a high-reliability care model.[3] To efficaciously implement institutional-wide changes the principles of high-reliability care should be embedded in the organization's mission statement. Furthermore, measurable organization-wide standards should be established so that the execution of goals may be objectively monitored.

Safety Culture
As described by Reason and Hobbs,[10] a "safety culture" comprised of trust, communication, and improvement is essential for the successful establishment and maintenance of highly reliable care systems. If an organization is to receive continuous information regarding possible failures and unsafe conditions, orthopedic surgeons may form trust among team members by two means. First, all personnel must trust organizational policies when identifying and uncovering problems that may implicate others. Moreover, if a team member exposes a management issue the team member must be confident that the organizations leadership will promptly fix the problem. Lack of trust among involved parties and management hinders the flow of information, resulting in organizational shortcomings and unsafe patient conditions.

Second, horizontal and vertical communication between orthopedic surgeons and all team members is required for effective execution of high-reliability care. To promote communication among the various stakeholders, administrators should establish several routes of communication, including anonymous means. An organizational culture promoting high-reliability care and patient safety can only be achieved if the philosophy is first instilled in all team members; as such, trust, communication, and the process of continuous improvement are necessary in all institutions striving to improve health care reliability.

Quality Improvement Strategy
Any organization seeking to implement high reliability of care must adopt a robust mechanism of quality improvement (QI). Since the 1990s health care organizations have been experimenting with industrial QI tools to continuously improve the quality of health care. Although some early health care organizations implementing

industrial QI principles were able to appreciate improvements, most institutions implemented QI measures within nonclinical settings, limiting their effect on patient outcomes.[11]

Within the last decade, orthopedic practices have led the way in the implementation of Lean and Six Sigma philosophies that address difficult safety- and quality-related issues.[12,13] These industrial measures have standardized treatment protocols, streamlined surgical service lines, and integrated comanagement principles within patient populations undergoing elective and emergent orthopedic surgeries (total joint arthroplasty and hip fracture, respectively).[12,13] Notably, the use of these industrial ideologies lies within their systematic approach, which eliminates waste while minimizing error.[14]

OPERATING ROOM INTERVENTIONS

Over the last two decades professional medical societies (AAOS) and large multinational organizations, such as the World Health Organization (WHO) and JCAHO, have developed several protocols aimed at reducing medical errors and improving patient safety. Although these QI initiatives have been developed by various societies and organizations, the common goal remains the same: to improve the reliability of orthopedic care.

American Academy of Orthopaedic Surgeons
As a recognized leader among professional medical societies, the AAOS commissioned the Wrong Site Surgery Task Force to undertake the society's first major QI initiative.[15] In 1998, the task force recommended the implementation of the Sign Your Site initiative (SYS) to reduce the unacceptably high rate of wrong-site procedures.[16] The initiative encouraged orthopedic surgeons to routinely initial the surgical site before operative intervention.[8] Although the recommendations were primarily aimed at reducing wrong-site surgery, it was also effective at reducing wrong-patient and wrong-procedure events.[16] Since the SYS initiative 45% of orthopedic surgeons have changed their practice habits and almost all have routinely taken some action to prevent wrong-site surgery.[17] A study by Meinberg and Stern[17] evaluating 1560 active hand surgeons revealed that 21% (217) of hand surgeons reported performing wrong-site surgeries at least once in their career. A major limitation of the SYS initiative has historically been its voluntary status and lack of support among academy fellows.[18] More recently, regulatory bodies, such as JCAHO and WHO, have

implemented similar initiatives within their protocols. Hence, the SYS initiative can be credited with being the first of many steps implemented with the goal of reducing medical errors and improving the reliability of care.[18]

Joint Commission on the Accreditation of Healthcare Organizations
In 2000 a report by the Institute of Medicine titled, *To Err Is Human: Building a Safer Health System*,[5] brought widespread attention to the concept of medical errors within all specialties of care. At the same time, JCAHO, a nonprofit accreditation body originally formed by Ernest Codman on behalf of the American College of Surgeons, was already assessing medical errors through its Sentinel Events Program. Any event resulting in death, permanent harm, or severe temporary harm is considered a sentinel event, or an event requiring an immediate investigation and "root cause analysis."[19] Additionally, JCAHO also developed the Patient Safety Event Taxonomy[20] for the analysis of additional medical errors. Although, JCAHO is not a regulatory body, endorsement by JCAHO or an equivalent accreditation body is mandated by the Centers for Medicare and Medicaid Services. Thus, initiatives developed by JCAHO may have far reaching effects. Table 1 reports a series of orthopedic-related initiatives currently investigated by JCAHO.[21]

Additionally, all medical errors tabulated by JCAHO are further evaluated by the National Quality Forum,[22] a non-for-profit public-private consensus group consisting of more than 400 organizations representing consumers, medical professionals, and public health entities. The aim of the JCAHO-National Quality Forum is to develop a national strategy for health care quality measures and reporting.[23]

The Universal Protocol
In July 2004, JCAHO enacted the Universal Protocol, a checklist developed by a panel of experts reaching consensus on principles and steps required to prevent wrong-person, wrong-side, and wrong-procedure surgical complications.[24] The Universal Protocol is separated into three stages: (1) preprocedural verification, (2) marking the procedural site, and (3) a "time out."[25] The preprocedural stage consists of addressing any missing information pertaining to the patient's relevant history or surgical procedure (Table 2).[25] During this stage, it is important that any information concerning the patient's procedure, medical history, imaging, and implant specifications be made available to

Table 1
Current projects being investigated or implemented by the JCAHO

Initiative	Status	Project Aim
Hand hygiene	Investigation initiated December 2008	The Hand Hygiene Project focuses on improving and sustaining hand hygiene compliance.
Hand-off communications	Investigation initiated August 2009	Examine hand-off communication problems and isolate specific areas of failure. The goal is to then implement validated solutions targeting these barriers.
Preventing falls	Being implemented	Falls have been identified by the Centers for Medicare and Medicaid Services as an event that is preventable and should never occur.
Safety culture	Investigation initiated October 2011	Optimize behaviors and practices resulting in an improved safety culture that reinforces and supports the prevention of patient harm.
Safe surgery	Investigation initiated July 2009	Improve the safeguards to prevent patients from wrong-site, wrong-side, and wrong-patient surgical procedures.
Venous thromboembolism prevention	Investigation initiated October 2014	Reduce venous thromboembolism rates using accurate risk assessment and appropriate use of pharmacologic and/or mechanical prophylaxis.

Adapted from Joint Commission Center for Transforming Healthcare. Targeted initiatives. Available at: http://www.centerfortransforminghealthcare.org/projects/detail.aspx?Project=3. Accessed November 30, 2015.

the orthopedic surgeon and all surgical team members.[25] The next stage of the Universal Protocol is similar to the SYS initiative. Before surgical intervention JCAHO recommends that all surgeons clearly mark the surgical site.[25]

Although surgical site markings may be delegated to surgical residents and physicians assistants, it should be noted that the orthopedic surgeon is accountable for all errors and complications that may arise as a result of ancillary

Table 2
Stages and components of JCAHO Universal Protocol

Preprocedure Verification	Mark Procedure Site	Perform a "Time Out"
Address missing information or discrepancies before starting the procedure • Verify correct patient, procedure, and surgical site • Identify items required for the procedure • Use a standardized list to document the availability of items • Relevant documentation, diagnostic, and radiology results should be available • Required blood products, implants, and devices should also be made available	At a minimum, mark the site of the surgical procedure • Mark the site before the procedure • The mark should be unambiguous and used throughout the organization • The mark is made at or near the procedure site	The procedure is not started until all questions and concerns of team members have been addressed • Conduct a "time out" immediately before the procedure or making of the incision • The "time out" should be standardized • All team members should be introduced • During the "time out" the patient, surgical site, and procedure should be confirmed • In the event two or more procedures are being done on the same patient, another "time out" needs to be performed before starting the second procedure

staff.[25] The last component of the Universal Protocol is the "time out," which is initiated by the orthopedic surgeon immediately preceding the surgical incision.[25] At this time, all team members provide their undivided attention, while the surgeon introduces the entire team and their respective roles.[25] The surgeon and anesthesiologist cross-check the patient's identity, site of surgery, and procedure (see Table 2).[25] In the event two consecutive procedures are performed, each procedure requires its own "time out" at respective start times.[25]

World Health Organization

In 2008, the WHO published the *Surgical Safety Checklist and Implementation Manual*, which in many respects emulates JCAHO's Universal Protocol.[26] The *Surgical Safety Checklist* identifies three distinct phases of an operation; each phase corresponds to specific work-flow patterns unique to the operative phase. The phases identified by the *Surgical Safety Checklist* are "sign-in," "time out," and "sign out."[26] During the "sign-in" phase the WHO recommends confirming the patient's identity, procedure consented for, and surgical site. At this time the anesthesiologist should also discuss expected blood loss and the presence or absence of allergies with the orthopedic surgeon. After induction of anesthesia, but before the surgical incision, the WHO *Surgical Safety Checklist* recommends the entire surgical team take a "time out." At this time, all team members must introduce themselves and their respective role during the procedure. The orthopedic surgeon and anesthesiologist must confirm the name of the patient, the procedure taking place, and any expected critical events. The administration of prophylactic antibiotics and any intraoperative imaging should also be discussed with the team. The last phase on the WHO *Surgical Safety Checklist* is "sign out." This phase must occur before the patient leaves the operating room, and is usually led by the nursing staff. The instruments, sponges, and needle counts are checked and rechecked; laboratory specimens are appropriately labeled; and the surgeon, anesthesiologist, and nursing staff discuss intraoperative fluid losses and possible postoperative concerns.

Universal Protocol and Surgical Safety Checklist Outcomes

Because professional medical societies and Centers for Medicare and Medicaid Services mandate that health care organizations follow the recommendations made by JCAHO and WHO, investigators have begun evaluating the efficacy of these protocols and checklists.[27,28] James and colleagues[29] looked at approximately 1.3 million orthopedic cases evaluating whether the incidence of wrong-site surgery was affected by the Universal Protocol or SYS. Surprisingly, their study reported that implementation of the Universal Protocol was not linked with a decrease in wrong-site procedures; suggesting that the SYS initiative, which had been used before the implementation of Universal Protocol was equally as effective.[29] The study concluded that additional layers of precautions may yield diminishing returns; attention should instead be directed at preventing wrong-site procedures, particularly within orthopedic subspecialties with the poorest reliability scores.[17,29]

In a similar study, Mayer and colleagues[27] evaluated the impact of the WHO checklist compliance in 6712 surgical admissions and reported risk-adjusted clinical outcomes. Only 62.1% of procedures completed the entire checklist (sign-in, time-out, sign-out), whereas completion of at least one in three checklist components was reported at 96.7% of cases.[27] Although, completion of the checklist had no effect on patient mortality; calculated population-attributable fractions demonstrated that 14% of complications could be prevented with checklist completion.[27] Conversely, a study by van Klei and coworkers[28] evaluating the effect of the WHO's *Surgical Safety Checklist* on mortality rates reported a statistically significant reduction in 30-day mortality when the WHO checklist was fully implemented. Perhaps the most comprehensive study to date assessing the efficacy of surgical checklists was conducted by Urbach and colleagues.[30] Investigators comparatively examined the efficacy of surgical checklists before and after implementation of checklist protocols to report no significant reduction in operative mortality or complications.[30]

Despite the implementation of various forms of QI measures, including the AAOS SYS initiative, WHO *Surgical Safety Checklist*, and JCAHO Universal Protocol, no method has been found to be superior. A balance of surgical autonomy and operative precautions is necessary for optimal surgical outcomes and high reliability of orthopedic care. Excessive regulations may place a greater burden on the health care system and the surgical team, inevitably having a counterproductive effect on the delivery of care. The orthopedic surgeon must also be cognizant that the goal of any checklist or protocol is to ensure communication among health care providers. As such, documenting the completion of established protocols should not be the sole priority of the surgical team. Instead team members should strive to continuously improve communication, thereby preventing systemic failures and near misses, while achieving a higher reliability of orthopedic care.[29]

American Academy of Orthopaedic Surgeons Clinical Practice Guidelines and Reliability of Care

Aside from checklists and protocols the AAOS and other medical societies have invested heavily in the development of clinical practice guidelines, defined by the Institute of Medicine as "recommendations intended to optimize patient care that are informed by a systematic review of evidence and an assessment of the benefits and harms of alternative care options."[31] Although it is well recognized that when appropriately used clinical guidelines are an evidence-based approach at standardizing and improving care,[32] their recommendations are frequently limited by their methodologic design.[33] Sabharwal and colleagues[34] assessed 14 AAOS clinical guidelines and reported that the overall quality of the guidelines was high; however, the guidelines scored poorly in respect to clinical applicability as indicated by the Appraisal of Guidelines for Research and Evaluation II criteria.[35] Specifically, the Appraisal of Guidelines for Research and Evaluation II tool assesses four subdomains including (1) whether the guideline is supported by measurement tools, (2) if organizational barriers limiting the recommendations have been addressed, (3) potential cost implications of implementing recommendations, and (4) if the guideline provides a means of monitoring its clinical use.[35] To improve the clinical applicability of guidelines studies have suggested that the involvement of health economists, the implementation of pilot studies, barrier analysis studies, clinician feedback sessions, and regularly scheduled audits monitoring the efficacy of the guidelines are warranted.[34] Moreover, implementation of a highly reliable care model, combining organizational leadership, a safety culture, and robust QI strategies, is crucial for the development and sustainability of clinically applicable guidelines.

SUMMARY

Medical errors have devastating social and financial implications on the North American health care infrastructure. The orthopedic specialty is

no exception; although wrong-site surgery accounts for 2% of claims, 84% of those claims resulted in costly legal settlements.[2] As such, orthopedic surgeons must radiate an attitude of "collective mindfulness" to motivate all team members to identify possible sentinel events. Furthermore, the health care organization's leadership must establish a long-term commitment to the application, delivery, and methodologic improvement processes necessary to implement a highly reliable care model. Once an organization has implemented all necessary changes, the efficacy of surgical checklists, protocols, and clinical guidelines may be evaluated, improving the quality of care delivered.

ACKNOWLEDGMENTS

The authors thank Dr P.K. Wong for presenting this topic during the Central Illinois Healthcare Management Summit chaired by Dr K.J. Saleh.

REFERENCES

1. Porter ME, Teisberg EO. Redefining competition in health care. Harv Bus Rev 2004;82(6):64–76, 136.
2. American Academy of Orthopaedic Surgeons. Advisory statement–wrong-site surgery. Rosemont (IL): American Academy of Orthopaedic Surgeons; 2000.
3. Chassin MR, Loeb JM. The ongoing quality improvement journey: next stop, high reliability. Health Aff (Millwood) 2011;30(4):559–68.
4. Brand RA. Ernest Amory Codman, MD, 1869-1940. Clin Orthop Relat Res 2009;467(11):2763–5.
5. Kohn LT, Corrigan JM, Donaldson MS. To err is human: building a safer health system. Washington, DC: National Academy Press; 2000.
6. Seiden SC, Barach P. Wrong-side/wrong-site, wrong-procedure, and wrong-patient adverse events: are they preventable? Arch Surg 2006; 141(9):931–9.
7. Kwaan MR, Studdert DM, Zinner MJ, et al. Incidence, patterns, and prevention of wrong-site surgery. Arch Surg 2006;141(4):353–7 [discussion: 357–8].
8. American Academy of Orthopaedic Surgeons Council on Education. Report of the Task Force on Wrong-Site Surgery. Rosemont (IL): American Academy of Orthopaedic Surgeons; 1998.
9. Weick KE, Sutcliffe KM. Managing the unexpected: resilient performance in an age of uncertainty. New York: Wiley; 2007.
10. Reason J, Hobbs A. Managing maintenance error: a practical guide. Aldershot (UK): Ashgate; 2003.
11. Goldberg HI. Continuous quality improvement and controlled trials are not mutually exclusive. Health Serv Res 2000;35(3):701–5.

12. Niemeijer GC, Flikweert E, Trip A, et al. The useful-ness of Lean Six Sigma to the development of a clinical pathway for hip fractures. J Eval Clin Pract 2013;19(5):909–14.

13. Gayed B, Black S, Daggy J, et al. Redesigning a joint replacement program using Lean Six Sigma in a Veterans Affairs Hospital. JAMA Surg 2013; 148(11):1050–6.

14. Lean Six Sigma: Wastes and principles. 2015. Available at: http://www.sixsigmaonline.org/six-sigma-training-certification-information/lean-six-sigma-wastes-and-principles/. Accessed November 30, 2015.

15. Wong DA, Herndon JH, Canale ST, et al. Medical errors in orthopaedics. Results of an AAOS mem-ber survey. J Bone Joint Surg Am 2009;91(3): 547–57.

16. Schweitzer KM Jr, Brimmo O, May R, et al. Inci-dence of wrong-site surgery among foot and ankle surgeons. Foot Ankle Spec 2011;4(1):10–3.

17. Meinberg EG, Stern PJ. Incidence of wrong-site surgery among hand surgeons. J Bone Joint Surg Am 2003;85-A(2):193–7.

18. Herndon JH. One more turn of the wrench. J Bone Joint Surg Am 2003;85-A(10):2036–48.

19. Sentinel events (SE). Available at: http://www.joint commission.org/assets/1/6/CAMH_2012_Update2_ 24_SE.pdf. Accessed November 30, 2015.

20. Chang A, Schyve PM, Croteau RJ, et al. The JCAHO patient safety event taxonomy: a standard-ized terminology and classification schema for near misses and adverse events. Int J Qual Health Care 2005;17(2):95–105.

21. Project detail. Available at: http://www.center fortransforminghealthcare.org/projects/detail.aspx? Project=3. Accessed November 30, 2015.

22. Kizer KW, Cushing TS, Nishimi RY. The Department of Veterans Affairs' role in federal emergency man-agement. Ann Emerg Med 2000;36(3):255–61.

23. Restrepo C, Parvizi J, Kurtz SM, et al. The noisy ceramic hip: is component malpositioning the cause? J Arthroplasty 2008;23(5):643–9.

24. Kelly B, Finnegan P, Cormican M, et al. Lyme disease and glomerulonephritis. Ir Med J 1999; 92(5):372.

25. Callaghan JT, Bergstrom RF, Ptak LR, et al. Olanza-pine. Pharmacokinetic and pharmacodynamic pro-file. Clin Pharmacokinet 1999;37(3):177–93.

26. Yingling VR, Callaghan JP, McGill SM. The porcine cervical spine as a model of the human lumbar spine: an anatomical, geometric, and functional comparison. J Spinal Disord 1999;12(5):415–23.

27. Mayer EK, Sevdalis N, Rout S, et al. Surgical check-list implementation project: the impact of variable WHO checklist compliance on risk-adjusted clinical outcomes after national implementation: a longitu-dinal study. Ann Surg 2016;263(1):58–63.

28. van Klei WA, Hoff RG, van Aarnhem EE, et al. Effects of the introduction of the WHO "Surgical Safety Checklist" on in-hospital mortality: a cohort study. Ann Surg 2012;255(1):44–9.

29. James MA, Seiler JG 3rd, Harrast JJ, et al. The occurrence of wrong-site surgery self-reported by candidates for certification by the American Board of Orthopaedic Surgery. J Bone Joint Surg Am 2012;94(1):e2.1–2.12.

30. Urbach DR, Govindarajan A, Saskin R, et al. Intro-duction of surgical safety checklists in Ontario, Can-ada. N Engl J Med 2014;370(11):1029–38.

31. Institute of Medicine (US) Committee on Standards for Developing Trustworthy Clinical Practice Guide-lines, Graham R, Mancher M, Miller Wolman D, et al, editors. Clinical Practice Guidelines We Can Trust. Washington (DC): National Academies Press (US); 2011.

32. Woolf SH, Grol R, Hutchinson A, et al. Clinical guide-lines: potential benefits, limitations, and harms of clinical guidelines. BMJ 1999;318(7182):527–30.

33. Cook D, Giacomini M. The trials and tribulations of clinical practice guidelines. JAMA 1999;281(20): 1950–1.

34. Sabharwal S, Patel NK, Gauher S, et al. High meth-odologic quality but poor applicability: assessment of the AAOS guidelines using the AGREE II instru-ment. Clin Orthop Relat Res 2014;472(6):1982–8.

35. Appraisal of guidelines for research & evaluation II. 2013. Available at: http://www.agreetrust.org/wp-content/uploads/2013/10/AGREE-II-Users-Manual-and-23-item-Instrument_2009_UPDATE_2013.pdf. Accessed January 2, 2016.

Patient Centeredness in Total Joint Replacement
Beyond the Slogan

Hussein A. Zeineddine, MD[a],
Mouhanad M. El-Othmani, MD[b],
Zain Sayeed, MSc, MHA[b],
Monique C. Chambers, MD, MSL[b],
Khaled J. Saleh, MD, MSc, FRCS (C), MHCM, CPE[c],*

KEYWORDS

- Patient-centered care • Total joint replacement • Orthopedic surgery • Health policy

---

KEY POINTS

- PCC is a fundamental principle that, although fully developed theoretically, is still in its youth in terms of clinical application.
- PCC in orthopedics and TJR in particular still needs to be expanded and studied more thoroughly, namely at the implementation level.
- The benefits of PCC necessitates that the practice start sooner rather than later, and that governmental agencies, institutions, and various stakeholders invest in setting up dedicated centers to that end.

INTRODUCTION

Over the last decade, the notion of patient-centered care (PCC) has been gaining considerable focus among the medical community.[1] Although this concept dates back to the 1960s to 1970s and was discussed by scholars, such as Balint and Lipkin,[2,3] the term itself was coined in 1988 by The Picker Institute.[4,5] Since then, the implementation of care-delivery models in alignment with PCC concepts has been studied in various medical specialties including pediatrics, cardiology, and rheumatology.[6,7] The impact of PCC on the health care system was significant, so much so that the Institute of Medicine (IOM) designated PCC as one of the six fundamental aims of the US health care system.[8]

Total joint replacement (TJR) is considered the definite treatment of end-stage arthritis associated with certain indications to include pain, functional limitations, and stiffness.[9] The procedure is considered one of the most efficient procedures in medicine because it leads to substantial improvement in quality of life.[10] The estimated cost of primary TJR in 2015 exceeded $50 billion, and the rates are projected to increase in upcoming decades, especially with the increasing prevalence of the aging population.[11] With the current rise in health care expenditures, optimizing the quality and the economics associated with health care delivery has become a necessity. As such, the PCC model is perceived as a valid and

---

Funding Sources: No additional funding sources were used for this article.
Conflicts of Interest: No conflicts of interest are evident for authors of this article.
[a] Department of Surgery, University of Chicago, 5812 South Ellis Avenue, Chicago, IL 60637, USA; [b] Division of Orthopaedics and Rehabilitation, Southern Illinois University School of Medicine, 701 North First Street, Springfield, IL 62781, USA; [c] Department of Orthopaedic and Sports Medicine, Detroit Medical Center, 311 Mack Avenue, 5th Floor, Detroit, MI 48201, USA
* Corresponding author.
E-mail address: kjsaleh@gmail.com

Orthop Clin N Am 47 (2016) 697–706
http://dx.doi.org/10.1016/j.ocl.2016.05.012

sustainable approach that might lead to the crucially needed improvement in health care quality, while simultaneously decreasing associated costs.

This article highlights the practice of PCC in TJR by focusing on the major attributes of PCC models and providing a brief comment on PCC-based clinical care pathways in joint surgery.

DEFINING PATIENT-CENTERED CARE

A large number of institutions and experts have attempted to define and characterize PCC. The IOM defines PCC as "Health care that establishes a partnership among practitioners, patients, and their families (when appropriate) to ensure that decisions respect patients' wants, needs, and preferences and that patients have the education and support they need to make decisions and participate in their own care."[12]

Along the same lines, the American Academy of Orthopedic Surgeons defines PCC as "the provision of safe, effective, and timely medical care achieved through cooperation among the physician, an informed and respected patient (and family), and a coordinated healthcare team."[13]

The Picker Institute, one of the leaders in the patient-centeredness field, defines PCC based on eight fundamental dimensions: (1) respect for patient-centered values, (2) coordination and integration of care, (3) information and communication, (4) physical comfort, (5) emotional support, (6) involvement of family and friends, (7) transition and continuity of care, and (8) access to care.[14,15]

Other definitions include that of the Planetree model health care, which "cultivate the healing of mind, body, and spirit; that are patient-centered, value-based, and holistic; and that integrate the best of Western scientific medicine with time-honored healing practices."[15,16] The Planetree model is based on nine integral attributes that significantly overlap with other institutions' definitions. Other characterizations include those of the Ontario Medical Association,[17] International Alliance of Patients' Organizations,[18] Institute for Family-Centered Care Model (family-centered care),[19] and many others.[20]

Even with this multitude of definitions and organizations associated with the conceptualization of PCC, the key attributes remain solid and constant throughout with substantial convergence. As such, it is evident that the insight on, definition of, and concept of PCC are widely established and available, whereas

the challenge at hand remains to design the optimal delivery system.

THE BENEFITS OF PATIENT-CENTERED CARE

Multiple studies have highlighted the positive impact of PCC on improving health care delivery models and patient outcomes.[21–30] One of the main impacts of implementing PCC is the reduction of morbidity and mortality through targeting integral points in the treatment process, such as physician-patient relationship, communication, and active participation.[21,22] Furthermore, there is better overall compliance with the course of therapy, a reduction in the impact of symptoms on the quality of life, and improvement of health care efficiency by limiting the underuse and overuse of available resources.[23–30] Kim and colleagues,[31] in an interview of more than 500 patients, reported that patient-perceived physician empathy improved patient satisfaction and compliance. In another study, PCC was shown to improve objective outcomes in which patients with type 2 diabetes achieved better control of glucose levels.[32] Bertakis and Azari,[33] in a randomized trial of more than 500 participants, noted a 51% decrease in expenses for patients that were treated with a more extensive PCC approach. As such, PCC has been proven to improve patients' health status over a variety of value-metrics and variables, such as lessening discomfort along with better mental health, while simultaneously improving health care efficiency.[21]

PATIENT CENTERED CARE IN ORTHOPEDIC SURGERY

Orthopedic surgeons are advocating for PCC as a successful care-delivery model that focuses on the patient's needs, understanding, expectations, and preferences. The TJR literature still suffers from paucity in assessing and reporting patient satisfaction, choice of intervention, role of the patient in the decision-making process, and other integral parameters related to PCC. However, available research has shown that PCC positively impacts orthopedics and TJR patients, and additional efforts are currently underway to gain further knowledge.[34–36] Even though various protocols and guidelines exist for standardizing certain aspects of care in TJR (ie, deep vein thrombosis perioperative prophylaxis), limited guidelines are available to provide physicians and institutions with appropriate means to establish and implement PCC in TJR.[37]

PATIENT SATISFACTION

Patient satisfaction is one of PCC's dimensions and is sometimes used as a proxy to assess the success of PCC implementation.[6,38] Physicians who attain the highest rates of patient satisfaction are rewarded by their hospitals, and the government, through new reimbursement models.[6] Although it is challenging to define, satisfaction is an integration of various experiences the patient handles in relation to preset expectations.[39,40] Aside from expectations, other factors, sometimes unrelated to the disease process, also alter this parameter.[41] A study by Bourne and colleagues[42] has shown that living alone is one of the variables that correlate with patient dissatisfaction after TJR. Other factors that correlate with dissatisfaction following TJR, which ranges from 10% to 30%, are summarized in Table 1, and include preoperative expectations and pain relief.[42–48] There is substantial disparity in variables used to assess satisfaction as a TJR outcome.

Among the available measurements, many are structured to focus on what surgeons deem important in affecting postoperative satisfaction, rather than centering on the patient's values and perspective. Studies have established that patient satisfaction is a critical instrument in improving patient care and outcomes[49–51] and positively impacting physicians' job satisfaction, and reducing stress and burnout.[52] Yet, measuring patient satisfaction in TJR, orthopedics, or medicine as a whole has always been a challenge.[53–55] The American Academy of Orthopedic Surgeons was among the first within the surgical field to exhibit interest in measuring satisfaction using the Musculoskeletal Outcomes Data Evaluation and Management System questionnaire. Unfortunately, the project was later discontinued,[54] in part because of lack of interest among orthopedic surgeons.[56] However, analysis of this experience did provide valuable lessons for future large-scale data collection. Methods to minimize respondents' burden, approaches to motivate physicians, and recommendations to expand the scope of involvement to include the community and government arose from this exercise.[56] Other measurements currently in use include the Picker patient satisfaction tool, the Pay-for-Performance initiative tools, the Press Ganey Survey, and the Consumer Assessment of Healthcare Providers and Systems. Patient-reported measurement instruments routinely incorporated in perioperative outcomes assessment in orthopedics include the Oxford Hip and Knee Scores, Western Ontario and McMaster Universities Arthritis Index, Knee injury and Osteoarthritis Outcome Score, and Hip Disability and Osteoarthritis Outcome Score. Clinician-completed scores, such as the Knee Society Score, MAYO Wrist Score, and Harris Hip Score, are also available.[57] Although these measures have been validated and are being used in research, they are widely heterogeneous in terms of collected variables.[58] In addition, many of the validated measurements, such as the Oxford Hip Scores, are not designed to assess patient satisfaction primarily.[54]

The implementation of patient-reported outcome measures in nationwide registries is an integral component of assessing the quality of TJR, and will form the major cornerstone in achieving an accurate assessment of patient satisfaction.[36] However, the current variability and discrepancies in available instruments

Table 1 Factors associated with dissatisfaction after TJR		
Patient-Specific	**Patient-Physician**	**Surgeon-Specific**
Preoperative condition (pain at rest, comorbidities, avascular necrosis)	Unmet expectations (the most consistent variable and one with highest impact)	Surgical approach (conflicting evidence)
Age at surgery (conflicting evidence)	Low functional outcome and residual symptoms	Complexity of the case (conflicting evidence)
Living alone, lack of social support	Postoperative complications	Hospital and surgeon volume (conflicting evidence)
Mental health status at baseline	Revision surgery	
Female gender (conflicting evidence)		
Low income		

remains challenging, and research should continue, as described later, to develop the optimal tool for the specific measure in question.

Graham and coworkers[54] highlight an integral issue concerning patient satisfaction measurement, emphasizing the need for a "right measure of outcome" tailored to the question to be answered. Adding to the current ongoing lack of a standardized instrument that assesses patients-perceived satisfaction, a clear distinction should be made between "satisfaction with the process of care and satisfaction with the outcome of care."[54] The outcome of care consists of factors that are influenced by the surgeon, such as patient expectations and physician-patient communication. However, the process of care is a more global and multidisciplinary series of events that span different departments and involve variables that are beyond the physician's influence. Graham and coworkers[54] indicate that orthopedic surgeons should focus on the measurement of factors on which they can have an impact.[54] Although this is true, we advocate that the physician plays a much larger role and contribution to patient satisfaction with the entire process of care. Because this task might be daunting, future goals of the health care system should include designating specialized units with well-structured care pathways to achieve satisfaction with the entire spectrum of care delivery, including outcome and process of care. In relation to TJR, more extensive research is needed, and specific tools should be developed to take into account variables perceived as significant by patients. As Graham and coworkers[54] eluded, these tools should distinguish between outcome and process of care satisfaction. Within the PCC context, future research should also focus on the factors that the patient recognizes as integral to satisfaction (eg, psychosocial, cognitive). Efforts should be invested in constructing centers capable of achieving patient satisfaction. Optimal care should be based on parameters, such as patient expectations, communication, follow-up care, and others that research might reveal to be of significance (eg, patient-surgeon interaction; staff hospitality and attitude; logistics of the center, such as parking spaces; presence of support group).

COMMUNICATION

Communication is one of the dimensions of PCC set forth by the IOM.[12] Successful communication is attained when a physician and a patient achieve a partnership in care, decision-making, and understanding of the disease, treatment options, and other aspects of the care process. Communication with patients should be based on sound, well-articulated skills that account for values, such as empathy, compassion, and humanism. Based on these values, the content of the communication should include the diagnosis, prognosis, and available disease-management options. Regardless of the method of communication, any interaction should be "attentive, responsive and tailored to an individual's needs."[12] Available evidence highlights the benefits of optimizing communication and correlates it with an improved understanding of medical information, increased compliance with treatment, and increased likelihood of having more realistic expectations.[52,59–61] More importantly, good communication culminates in increased patient satisfaction with the process of care.[54] Ha summarizes many other beneficial outcomes of good physician-patient communication, such as improved recovery and psychological adjustments of the patients.[52]

Similarly, studies have shown that communicating with patients and educating them about TJR leaves a positive impact before and after the surgical procedure.[34,62] One study has shown that TJR candidates enrolled in a presurgical class focusing on patient needs, education, and potential benefit have an improved health quality.[34] Communicating with family members and other patients with similar experiences also proved to improve health-quality.[34] However, the level of communication in orthopedic surgery remains surprisingly suboptimal. In a study that assessed the implementation of informed decision by orthopedic surgeons, only 9% met the criteria of informed decision.[63] In another study by Tongue and colleagues,[64] patients reported that only around 30% of surgeons took enough time to communicate with them. Interestingly, 75% of orthopedic surgeons believed they were taking the time needed to communicate properly with patients, whereas only 20% of surgeons believed that their peers spent enough time and practice proper communication techniques with patients.[64] These alarming results emphasize the lack of proper communication between orthopedic surgeons and their patients.

A study assessing factors affecting a patient's decision to undergo a TJR showed that one of the main reasons to avoid surgery is the false perception of the low impact of the procedure on current health status.[65] Other factors correlating with unwillingness to undergo TJR include low expectations in relation to postoperative pain relief and improved functionality.[66,67] Because current evidence supports the substantial improvement in quality of life following TJR, the results of the aforementioned studies indicate a huge gap in communication between patients and their care providers, whether surgeons or primary care physicians (PCP).[45,68] Communication between patients and orthopedic surgeons is also needed to guarantee a solid understanding and more realistic expectations by the patient of what the intervention may and may not provide. In a study assessing patient satisfaction following TJR, a major reason for dissatisfaction was the failure to meet preoperative expectations, which may be easily avoided using proper preoperative communication.[42]

Communication is a multifaceted process and also involves the PCP-patient interaction as previously suggested. Schonberg and colleagues[69] reported that the surgical option as a treatment modality for patients with severe osteoarthritis was neglected and never discussed by the PCP in many cases. The authors also noted that patients were more likely to undergo the procedure when the PCP presented surgical intervention as a viable option.[69] Some studies attribute the PCP's omission of TJR as a treatment modality for severe osteoarthritis to the underestimation of the procedure's effectiveness and respective impact.[70] There is a crucial need for establishing a better communication between the PCP and the patient, and also between various providers and stakeholders in the health care delivery loop. The patient must remain centralized in these interactions.

Communication requires the combined efforts and active participation of the patient, PCP, surgeon, family, administrators, and anyone involved in the health care system (Fig. 1). Even though communication should always cover the essentials of informed consent (diagnosis, prognosis, alternatives), it should also include the patient's expectations, needs, perspectives, social values, and other aspects of care. Communication involves educating the patient and also serves as an educational process to the surgeon and the PCP to treat the patient rather than the disease. Finally, the gap in communication between PCP and orthopedic surgeons should also be filled to avoid delay in patient care. To that end, the health care system should invest in centers dedicated to PCC. These centers should tie together the different variables in this complex equation. It should also oversee and guide the communication needed, by the different technologies at hand, in a coherent integrated flow that is evidence-based and patient-centered.

PATIENTS (AND FAMILY) AS PARTNERS IN CARE

The IOM asserts the necessity that "patient values guide all clinical decisions."[12] This statement emphasizes the need for cooperation between the physician and the patient to reach the optimal personalized treatment. This inherently implies the need for abandoning the paternalistic approach adopted over the past decades. A paternalistic approach has been shown to negatively impact the patient's experience with the health care system, ranging from psychosocial effects and ending in abuse and ethical maltreatment.[71] Involving the patient (and possibly the family) in the process of care requires an active engagement by the patient that should also be facilitated by the mantra and structure of the health care system. Eddy[72] argues that an intervention should be classified as the "standard" of care only if there is "virtual unanimity among patients about the overall desirability." However, much of the treatment modalities lack this universal agreement and so the treatment plan should be centered and tailored to the preferences and values of the patient.[4] Rather than focusing on a gold-standard of treatment that is common to all, the focus should shift toward an individualized-standard. An individualized standard would stem from the patient's beliefs, values, and expectations. It will be in coherence with centralizing health care delivery around the patient along with acknowledging the unique individual needs. This goal is best achieved through the process of shared decision making (SDM), with the patient being an equal partner and contributor as the rest of the members of the health care system. This would involve an in-depth discussion between the physician and the patient including the risks and benefits of the surgery, alternative options (balanced review of conservative and invasive modalities), patient values, concerns, and preferences. These discussions constitute the basis of the selected treatment modality.[73,74] Whenever applicable, family members are included in the process of care.[75] Once this information has been shared and explained, a decision is made. The implementation of SDM in clinical scenarios has been associated with a multitude of rewarding outcomes. These outcomes included increased knowledge of the process of care, accurate perception of risks, decisions in coherence with patient's values, decreased decisional conflict for patients,

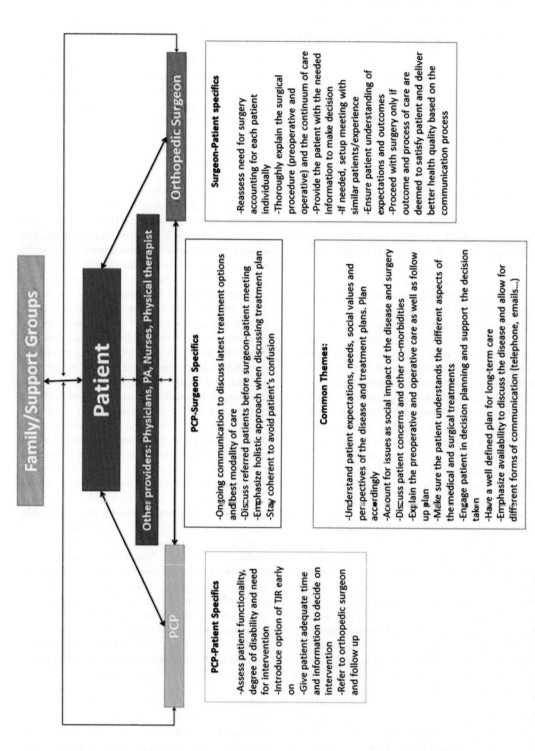

Fig. 1. Communication in a patient-centered setting.

decreased number of undecided patients,[76] greater satisfaction, and increased compliance.[77]

SHARED DECISION MAKING IN ORTHOPEDICS AND TOTAL JOINT REPLACEMENT

The nature of orthopedic surgery lends itself for SDM. Different pathologies afford conservative and surgical management, and as such, the process of SDM should be an integral part of our practice. However, orthopedic literature about SDM and decision aids is not as extensive as in other fields of medicine.[78] Patient satisfaction, which has been linked to preoperative expectations, can be exponentially improved by explaining the potential outcomes of the procedure and providing the patient with the liberty of choice.

Patients considering TJR would need to establish their decision based on their expectations, understanding, aims, preferences, coping ability, need for pain relief, and quality of life.[79] A recent systematic review by Page and Moulton[78] about SDM and decision aids found few examples in orthopedics. Interestingly, among the available models, SDM in TJR has shown that age, gender, socioeconomic status, social networks, and ethnicity impact the patient's decision to undergo surgery.[79] This study highlights the complex nature of the decision-making process and the need to improve understanding of the various factors that might influence that decision.

Recent studies assessing the effect of SDM on TJR outcomes re-emphasized the positive impact of SDM and its implications on patient decisions.[80,81] PCC is based on collaboration between the patient and the health care system with the physician being a central modulating hub for all interactions (Fig. 2). The concept of SDM overlaps with that of patient activation. Patient activation is a form of engagement where the patient plays an important role in health management and is knowledgeable and confident to take on responsibility and action.[82,83] This practice was shown to positively influence the cost, quality, and outcomes of health care.[82,84,85] Within the realm of orthopedic surgery, implementing patient activation has shown to reduce anxiety and improve functional ability in patients suffering from back pain.[86] Similarly, preoperative orthopedic patients were more confident in performing perioperative tasks when the activation model was applied.[85] The plasticity of choices in orthopedics and TJR makes it even more reasonable to adopt the SDM strategy. However, there is a lack in the ultimate tool for SDM in TJR, and studies should be conducted to improvise and validate new tools that maximize patient involvement, with minimal interruption of the clinical workflow. Finally, we re-emphasize that SDM is not a one-time event and any decision (medical, surgical, financial, and so forth) involving patient care should be subjected to the same principles. Physicians should also attempt to involve families as

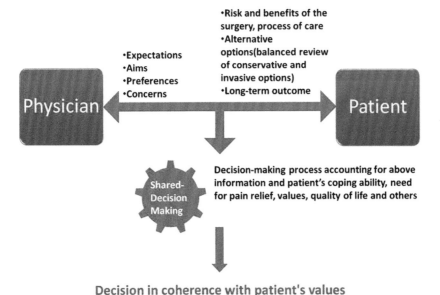

Fig. 2. Decision-making process in the patient-centered setting.

part of the patient- and family-centered care when judged as beneficial to the patient.[87] The composite nature of medical care and the increased righteous demand in involving the patient in all aspects of care necessitates designing specialized, state-of-the-art centers dedicated to PCC in orthopedics.

SUMMARY

PCC is a fundamental principle that, although fully developed theoretically, is still at its youth in terms of clinical application. So far, PCC in orthopedics still needs to be expanded and studied more thoroughly. However, investing in research on PCC in orthopedics will not have any impact if there is a lack of solid commitment in implementation. The practice of PCC should start sooner rather than later, and governmental agencies, institutions, and all stakeholders should invest in setting up dedicated centers to that end. The process of PCC in TJR spans the whole clinical spectrum from interaction with the patient, the family, and care providers. It is also an ongoing and continuous endeavor, starting in the preoperative period and extending toward undergoing surgery and long-term follow-up. If any progress in the field is expected, clinicians should start planning toward implementing it side-by-side with ongoing research at centers of excellence.

ACKNOWLEDGMENTS

The authors thank Dr Peter Wong for presenting this topic during the Central Illinois Healthcare Management Summit chaired by Dr K.J. Saleh.

REFERENCES

1. Epstein RM, Street RL Jr. The values and value of patient-centered care. Ann Fam Med 2011;9(2): 100–3.
2. Sia C, Tonniges TF, Osterhus E, et al. History of the medical home concept. Pediatrics 2004;113(5 Suppl):1473–8.
3. Saha S, Beach MC, Cooper LA. Patient centeredness, cultural competence and healthcare quality. J Natl Med Assoc 2008;100(11):1275–85.
4. Barry MJ, Edgman-Levitan S. Shared decision making–pinnacle of patient-centered care. N Engl J Med 2012;366:780–1.
5. Conway J, Johnson B, Edgman-Levitan S, et al. Partnering with patients and families to design a patient- and family-centered health care system: background paper for invitational meeting of patient-centered care leaders. Massachusetts, June 2, 2006.
6. Heidenreich PA. Time for a thorough evaluation of patient-centered care. Circ Cardiovasc Qual Outcomes 2013;6:2–4.
7. El Miedany Y. Adopting patient-centered care in standard practice: PROMs moving toward disease-specific era. Clin Exp Rheumatol 2014; 32(5 Suppl 85):S-40–6.
8. Institute of Medicine. Crossing the quality chasm: a new health system for the 21st century. Washington, DC: National Academies Press; 2001.
9. Mandl LA. Determining who should be referred for total hip and knee replacements. Nat Rev Rheumatol 2013;9(6):351–7.
10. Losina E, Walensky RP, Kessler CL, et al. Cost-effectiveness of total knee arthroplasty in the United States: patient risk and hospital volume. Arch Intern Med 2009;169(12):1113–21.
11. Kurtz S, Ong K, Lau E, et al. Projections of primary and revision hip and knee arthroplasty in the United States from 2005 to 2030. J Bone Joint Surg Am 2007;89:780–5.
12. Institute of Medicine. Envisioning the national health care quality report. Washington, DC: National Academies Press; 2001.
13. Farley FA. The case for patient-centered care in orthopaedics. J Am Acad Orthop Surg 2006;14:447–51.
14. Available at: http://www.pickerinstitute.com/. Accessed September 10, 2015.
15. Shaller D. Patient-centered care: what does it take?. Shaller Consulting. 2007. Available at: http://www. commonwealthfund.org/publications/fund-reports/ 2007/oct/patient-centered-care–what-does-it-take. Accessed September 10, 2015.
16. Available at: http://planetree.org/. Accessed September 10, 2015.
17. Ontario Medical Association. OMA policy on patient-centred care. Ont Med Rev 2010;34–49. Available at: https://www.oma.org/resources/ documents/patient-centredcare,2010.pdf.
18. Declaration on Patient-Centred Healthcare. What is patient-centred healthcare?: a review of definitions and principles. London: IAPO; 2005.
19. Available at: www.familycenteredcare.org. Accessed September 10, 2015.
20. Cronin C. "Patient-centered care: an overview of definitions and concepts," prepared for the National Health Council. 2004.
21. Stewart M, Brown JB, Donner A, et al. The impact of patient-centered care on outcomes. J Fam Pract 2000 Sep;49(9):796–804.
22. Anderson EB. Patient-centeredness: a new approach. Nephrol News Issues 2002;16(12):80–2.
23. Michie S, Miles J, Weinman J. Patient-centeredness in chronic illness: what is it and does it matter? Patient Educ Couns 2003;51(3):197–206.
24. Little P, Everitt H, Williamson I, et al. Observational study of effect of patient centredness and positive

approach on outcomes of general practice consultations. BMJ 2001;323(7318):908–11.

25. DiMatteo MR. The role of the physician in the emerging health care environment. West J Med 1998;168(5):328–33.

26. Beck RS, Daughtridge R, Sloane PD. Physician-patient communication in the primary care office: a systematic review. J Am Board Fam Pract 2002;15(1):25–38.

27. Rhoades DR, McFarland KF, Finch WH, et al. Speaking and interruptions during primary care office visits. Fam Med 2001;33(7):528–32.

28. Berry LL, Seiders K, Wilder SS. Innovations in access to care: a patient-centered approach. Ann Intern Med 2003;139(7):568–74.

29. Bechel DL, Myers WA, Smith DG. Does patient-centered care pay off? Jt Comm J Qual Improv 2000;26(7):400–9.

30. Saha S, Beach MC. The impact of patient-centered communication on patients' decision making and evaluations of physicians: a randomized study using video vignettes. Patient Educ Couns 2011;84(3):386–92.

31. Kim SS, Kaplowitz S, Johnston MV. The effects of physician empathy on patient satisfaction and compliance. Eval Health Prof 2004;27(3):237–51.

32. Prueksaritanond S, Tubtimtes S, Asavanich K, et al. Type 2 diabetic patient-centered care. J Med Assoc Thai 2004;87(4):345–52.

33. Bertakis KD, Azari R. Patient-centered care is associated with decreased health care utilization. J Am Board Fam Med 2011;24(3):229–39.

34. Lane-Carlson ML, Kumar J. Engaging patients in managing their health care: patient perceptions of the effect of a total joint replacement presurgical class. Perm J 2012;16(3):42–7.

35. Franklin PD, Allison JJ, Ayers DC. Beyond joint implant registries: a patient-centered research consortium for comparative effectiveness in total joint replacement. JAMA 2012;308(12):1217–8.

36. Franklin PD, Lewallen D, Bozic K, et al. Implementation of patient-reported outcome measures in U.S. Total joint replacement registries: rationale, status, and plans. J Bone Joint Surg Am 2014;96(Suppl 1):104–9.

37. Van Citters AD, Fahlman C, Goldmann DA, et al. Developing a pathway for high-value, patient-centered total joint arthroplasty. Clin Orthop Relat Res 2014;472(5):1619–35.

38. Rathert C, Wyrwich MD, Boren SA. Patient-centered care and outcomes: a systematic review of the literature. Med Care Res Rev 2013;70(4):351–79.

39. Morris BJ, Jahangir AA, Sethi MK. Patient satisfaction: an emerging health policy issue. What the orthopaedic surgeon needs to know. Available at: http://www.aaos.org/news/aaosnow/jun13/advocacy5.asp. Accessed October 10, 2015.

40. Pascoe GC. Patient satisfaction in primary health care: a literature review and analysis. Eval Program Plann 1983;6:185–210.

41. Chow A, Mayer EK, Darzi AW, et al. Patient-reported outcome measures: the importance of patient satisfaction in surgery. Surgery 2009;146(3):435–43.

42. Bourne RB, Chesworth BM, Davis AM, et al. Patient satisfaction after total knee arthroplasty: who is satisfied and who is not? Clin Orthop Relat Res 2010;468(1):57–63.

43. Anderson JG, Wixson RL, Tsai D, et al. Functional outcome and patient satisfaction in total knee patients over the age of 75. J Arthroplasty 1996;11:831–40.

44. Noble PC, Conditt MA, Cook KF, et al. The John Insall Award: patient expectations affect satisfaction with total knee arthroplasty. Clin Orthop Relat Res 2006;452:35–43.

45. Hawker G, Wright J, Coyte P, et al. Health-related quality of life after knee replacement. Results of the knee replacement patient outcomes research team study. J Bone Joint Surg Am 1998;80:163–73.

46. Heck DA, Robinson RL, Partridge CM, et al. Patient outcomes after knee replacement. Clin Orthop Relat Res 1998;356:93–110.

47. Robertsson O, Dunbar M, Pehrsson T, et al. Patient satisfaction after knee arthroplasty: a report on 27,372 knees operated on between 1981 and 1995 in Sweden. Acta Orthop Scand 2000;71:262–7.

48. Wylde V, Learmonth I, Potter A, et al. Patient reported outcomes after fixed- versus mobile-bearing total knee replacement: a multi-centre randomised controlled trial using the Kinemax total knee replacement. J Bone Joint Surg Br 2008;90:1172–9.

49. Guldvog B. Can patient satisfaction improve health among patients with angina pectoris? Int J Qual Health Care 1999;11:233–40.

50. Donabedian A. The quality of care. How can it be assessed? JAMA 1988;260:1743–8.

51. Marquis MS, Davies AR, Ware JE Jr. Patient satisfaction and change in medical care provider: a longitudinal study. Med Care 1983;21:821–9.

52. Ha JF, Longnecker N. Doctor-patient communication: a review. Ochsner J 2010;10(1):38–43.

53. Asadi-Lari M, Tamburini M, Gray D. Patients' needs, satisfaction, and health related quality of life: towards a comprehensive model. Health Qual Life Outcomes 2004;2:32.

54. Graham B, Green A, James M, et al. Measuring patient satisfaction in orthopaedic surgery. J Bone Joint Surg Am 2015;97(1):80–4.

55. Judge A, Arden NK, Price A, et al. Assessing patients for joint replacement: can pre-operative Oxford hip and knee scores be used to predict patient satisfaction following joint replacement surgery and to guide patient selection? J Bone Joint Surg Br 2011;93(12):1660–4.

56. Saleh KJ, Bershadsky B, Cheng E, et al. Lessons learned from the hip and knee musculoskeletal outcomes data evaluation and management system. Clin Orthop Relat Res 2004;429:272–8.

57. Available at: http://www.orthopaedicscore.com/. Accessed October 15, 2015.

58. Murray DW, Fitzpatrick R, Rogers K, et al. The use of the Oxford hip and knee scores. J Bone Joint Surg Br 2007;89(8):1010–4.

59. Middleton S, Gattellari M, Harris JP, et al. Assessing surgeons' disclosure of risk information before carotid endarterectomy. ANZ J Surg 2006;76(7):618–24.

60. Arora N. Interacting with cancer patients: the significance of physicians' communication behavior. Soc Sci Med 2003;57(5):791–806.

61. Bredart A, Bouleuc C, Dolbeault S. Doctor-patient communication and satisfaction with care in oncology. Curr Opin Oncol 2005;17(14):351–4.

62. Dorr LD, Chao L. The emotional state of the patient after total hip and knee arthroplasty. Clin Orthop Relat Res 2007;463:7–12.

63. Braddock CH 3rd, Edwards KA, Hasenberg NM, et al. Informed decision making in outpatient practice: time to get back to basics. JAMA 1999;282(24): 2313–20.

64. Tongue JR, Epps HR, Forese LL. Communication skills for patient-centered care: research-based, easily learned techniques for medical interviews that benefit orthopaedic surgeons and their patients. J Bone Joint Surg Am 2005;87:652–8.

65. Figaro MK, Williams-Russo P, Allegrante JP. Expectation and outlook: the impact of patient preference on arthritis care among African Americans. J Ambul Care Manage 2005;28:41–8.

66. Trousdale RT, McGrory BJ, Berry DJ, et al. Patients' concerns prior to undergoing total hip and total knee arthroplasty. Mayo Clin Proc 1999;74:978–82.

67. Wright JG, Rudicel S, Feinstein AR. Ask patients what they want: evaluation of individual complaints before total hip replacement. J Bone Joint Surg Br 1994;76:229–34.

68. Wiklunch I, Romanus B. A comparison of quality of life before and after arthroplasty in paitents who had arthrosis of the hip joint. J Bone Joint Surg Am 1991;73A:765–9.

69. Schonberg MA, Edward MR, Hamel MB. Perceptions of physician recommendations for joint replacement surgery by older patients with severe hip or knee osteoarthritis. J Am Geriatr Soc 2009;57(1):82–8.

70. Ang DC, Thomas K, Kroenke K. An exploratory study of primary care physician decision making regarding total joint arthroplasty. J Gen Intern Med 2007;22:74–9.

71. Moreno BAC, Arteaga GMG. Violation of ethical principles in clinical research. Influences and possible solutions for Latin America. BMC Med Ethics 2012;13:35.

72. Eddy DM. Designing a practice policy: standards, guidelines, and options. JAMA 1990;263:3077–84.

73. Charles C, Gafni A, Whelan T. Shared decision-making in the medical encounter: what does it

74. Fowler FJ Jr, Levin CA, Sepucha KR. Informing and involving patients to improve the quality of medical decisions. Health Aff (Millwood) 2011;30(4): 699–706.

75. Rodriguez-Osorio CA, Dominguez-Cherit G. Medical decision making: paternalism versus patient-centered (autonomous) care. Curr Opin Crit Care 2008;14(6):708–13.

76. Stacey D, Légaré F, Col NF, et al. Decision aids for people facing health treatment or screening decisions. Cochrane Database Syst Rev 2014;(1): CD001431.

77. Kaplan SH, Greenfield S, Gandek B, et al. Characteristics of physicians with participatory decision-making styles. Ann Intern Med 1996;124:497–504.

78. Page AE, Moulton B. Shared decision making in orthopaedics. Available at: http://www.aaos.org/news/aaosnow/dec14/clinical4.asp. Accessed October 10, 2015.

79. Slover J, Shue J, Koenig K. Shared decision-making in orthopaedic surgery. Clin Orthop Relat Res 2012; 470(4):1046–53.

80. Bozic KJ, Belkora J, Chan V, et al. Shared decision making in patients with osteoarthritis of the hip and knee: results of a randomized controlled trial. J Bone Joint Surg Am 2013;95:1633–9.

81. Arterburn D, Wellman R, Westbrook E, et al. Introducing decision aids at Group Health was linked to sharply lower hip and knee surgery rates and costs. Health Aff (Millwood) 2012;31(9):2094–104.

82. Tzeng A, Tzeng T, Vasdev S, et al. The role of patient activation in achieving better outcomes and cost-effectiveness in patient care. J Bone Joint Surg Rev 2015;3:e4. Available at: http://reviews.jbjs.org/content/3/1/e4.

83. Hibbard JH, Mahoney ER, Stockard J, et al. Development and testing of a short form of the patient activation measure. Health Serv Res 2005;40(6 Pt 1): 1918–30.

84. Skolasky RL, Mackenzie EJ, Wegener ST, et al. Patient activation and functional recovery in persons undergoing spine surgery. J Bone Joint Surg Am 2011;93(18):1665–71.

85. Pellino T, Tluczek A, Collins M, et al. Increasing self-efficacy through empowerment: preoperative education for orthopaedic patients. Orthopaedic Nurs 1998;17(4):48–59.

86. Von Korff M, Moore JE, Lorig K, et al. A randomized trial of a lay person-led self-management group intervention for back pain patients in primary care. Spine 1998;23(23):2608–15.

87. DiGioia A 3rd, Greenhouse PK, Levison TJ. Patient and family-centered collaborative care an orthopaedic model. Clin Orthop Relat Res 2007;463: 13–9.

Affordable Care Organizations and Bundled Pricing: A New Philosophy of Care

Gonzalo Barinaga, MD[a],
Monique C. Chambers, MD, MSL[a],
Mouhanad M. El-Othmani, MD[a],
Richard B. Siegrist, MBA, MS, CPA[b],
Khaled J. Saleh, MD, MSc, FRCS (C), MHCM, CPE[c],*

KEYWORDS

• ACOs • Bundle payments • Episode of care • Gainsharing • TJA

KEY POINTS

- When bundling is used in an affordable care organization (ACO) model of delivery, there is the potential to improve quality of care and reduce economic burden.
- Gainsharing agreements between providers and ACOs can be challenging, but present a tremendous opportunity for orthopedic surgeons.
- Although ACOs and bundle payment models seem to conflict, both are attempts to facilitate and encourage coordinated and integrated care while simultaneously reducing cost.
- As implementation of various measures unfold, research is necessary to determine the success of these models and the possibility of integrating them for arthroplasty patients.

INTRODUCTION

Hip and knee arthroplasties are among the most common surgical procedures performed for Medicare patients; more than 400,000 procedures were performed in 2013, with a total cost of more than $7 billion.[1] It is estimated that the prevalence of hip and knee osteoarthritis will increase by 18.2% by 2020 owing to the aging US population.[2] The number of total joint arthroplasty (TJA) procedures will follow the trend, and is projected to reach 4 million procedures by 2030.[1] Under the current fee-for-service (FFS) economic model of health care, financial reimbursements are partitioned for each service provided and billed as a separate service. This fragmented approach has led in part to an uncontrolled increase in national health care expenditures.

The average cost of arthroplasty procedures ranges from $16,500 to $33,000 across various geographic areas in the United States.[3] This clear variation in cost is mirrored by a disparity in the quality of care and postoperative course. The rate of readmission, for example, varies significantly between geographic locations, adding to the financial burden associated with a single episode of care.[3] Although Medicare reimbursements did not cover readmission within the first 24 hours after discharge, the estimated expenditure for unplanned rehospitalization exceeded

Funding Sources: No additional funding sources were used for this article.
Conflicts of Interest: No conflicts of interest are evident for authors of this article.
[a] Division of Orthopaedics and Rehabilitation, Southern Illinois University School of Medicine, 701 North First Street, Springfield, IL 62781, USA; [b] Harvard T.H. Chan School of Public Health, Harvard University, 677 Huntington Ave, Boston, MA 02115, USA; [c] Department of Orthopaedic and Sports Medicine, Detroit Medical Center, 311 Mack Avenue, 5th Floor, Detroit, MI 48201, USA
* Corresponding author.
E-mail address: kjsaleh@gmail.com

$12 billion under the FFS system.[3] In response, a greater emphasis on providing a continuum of care and establishing coordination between providers has been the focus in the design of new payment models. This vision is planned to be imposed through risk-sharing payment models that reward cost reduction and penalize overexpenditure, across the entire episode of care.

Under the Patient Protection and Affordable Care Act (ACA), the Centers for Medicare and Medicaid Services' (CMS) Innovation was chartered to develop new models of health care delivery.[4] Bundled payments can have a substantial effect on the national health care expenditures, with a projected decrease of 5.4%.[5] This payment model imposes a preset single collated sum of reimbursement for the entire episode of care. As such, the total cost of care delivery will be reconciled against a fixed reimbursement for that episode, and the organization will realize either a savings or a loss. Shifting risk onto providers creates an incentive to improve health care efficiency, which includes improved collaboration and decreased fragmentation of health care delivery.

The development of bundled reimbursement models has also created a dynamic relationship between providers by means of gainsharing. Previously suppressed by the Department of Justice, gainsharing programs are now being incorporated into bundle payment strategies with CMS oversight. This scenario will create new opportunities for providers to realize benefits from high-quality care and create new strategies to leverage during contract negotiations. This review examines new developments in bundle payments, affordable care organizations (ACOs), and gainsharing agreements as they pertain to arthroplasty.

HISTORICAL PERSPECTIVE

The concept of bundling in health care services has been introduced as a proposed costs-saving approach. Between 1983 and 1987, the Reagan administration focused on CMS expenditures with the development of the prospective payer system. Reimbursement into diagnosis related groups allow bundling of inpatient-hospital costs into a single payment. A decade later, the 1997 Balanced Budget Act curtailed postacute care (PAC) costs with prospective payments.[6] Both programs represent early attempts at bundling to decrease costs nationally, albeit the continuous fragmentation of care delivery. Providers were still reimbursed under the FFS model, which encourages providers

based on quantity rather than quality of care and limits their ability to value the total cost for patient care. Patients received multiple bills from various providers involved in their care, which created an extremely complicated billing system. As costs continued to increase, CMS reimbursements continued to decrease and thus the costs were shifted to private insurers.[6]

Throughout the late 1980s and 1990s, various programs that included some principles of bundled payment were initiated by CMS and some hospitals. Between 1990 and 1994, CMS trailed bundle payments with coronary bypass surgery. This approach increased savings for CMS from 1 side, and increased profits for physicians and hospitals from the other side.[7] At the turn of the century, CMS designated Orthopaedics and Cardiac Centers of Excellence as a foundation for bundled payments.[8] Hospitals also attempted bundling payments with orthopedic device manufacturers. The Lahey Clinic, in 1997, established a single price for arthroplasty implants, and decreased cost by 32% per total hip case and 23% per knee arthroplasty procedure.[9] The implementation of ACA incited a new wave of pilot programs, among which the Prometheus Bundled payment program, created by the Health Care Incentives Improvements Institute, was the most prominent. As a pioneer, the program faced several challenges early on, raising concerns about the potential of dissemination on a nationwide scale.[10] Most recently, in 2013, the Bundled Payment Care Initiative (BPCI) developed by CMS's Innovation Center, created 4 models to compare different structures of retrospective and prospective bundled payments (Table 1).[11] Implementation of the various models occurred over 2 phases, including the preparation period in phase 1 and the accepted 2115 participants that entered phase 2. Phase 2 increases the risk sharing associated with loss and gains related to bundling of the episode of care.[4] CMS has developed future pilot programs that will be implemented in the coming years, most notably the Comprehensive Care of Joint Replacement.[12]

CONSIDERING A BUNDLE PAYMENT SERVICE LINE

Developing a bundle payment service line for arthroplasty procedures requires investment and commitment from all providers and institutions involved in the process of care delivery. There are several considerations that must be addressed when contemplating the implementation of a bundled reimbursement model. First,

Table 1
Bundled Payment Care Initiative models

Model Type	Payment Type	Episode of Care	Care Delivery Services	Awardee Phase
1	Retrospective payment via MS-DRG	Inpatient acute care hospital stay	Part A Services	April 2013–June 2015
2	Retrospective payments via FFS model	Inpatient acute care hospital stay + postacute care 90 d postdischarge	Nonhospice part A and B services	June 2015-Present
3	Retrospective payments via FFS model	Postacute care services with SNF/ rehabilitation	Nonhospice part A and B services	TBD
4	Prospective payments from CMS to hospital	Entire inpatient stay and readmissions	All Services by hospital, physician, other providers	TBD

Abbreviations: CMS, Centers for Medicare and Medicaid Services; FFS, fee for service; MS-DRG, Medicare severity-diagnosis related group; SNF, skilled nursing facility; TBD, to be determined.

Data from Bundled payments for care improvement (BPCI) initiative: general information. Available at: https://innova-tion.cms.gov/initiatives/bundled-payments/. Accessed November 20, 2015.

participants willing to provide care and to commit to the success of the program should be identified. The involvement of administrators, nursing coordinators, anesthesia providers, physical and occupational therapists, discharge coordinators, and PAC leadership, among others, is crucial for the program. Financial and legal representation may also be required for negotiations between various providers. The next step is to determine the capability of an individual organization to undergo a transition into bundled payments. Health care systems that include physician network groups allow for the coordination of care and risk distribution among providers within the network. Increased risk by hospitals and physicians can lead to substantial losses in a poorly managed service line. As such, a thorough historical analysis of claims data within a provider group is essential to determine the success of model implementation. If a particular provider or service line has a trend of increased costs over several years, then a bundle payment plan would be detrimental to the organization. It is recommended that cost analysis of providers be historically neutral or down-trending before developing a bundle payment model. The American Association of Medical Colleges also recommends that a minimum volume of 100 cases per year is essential to reduce the effect of variability and outliers on bundles.[1] Once the decision to implement bundle payments reaches agreement between various stakeholders, the focus shifts toward determining the components of the bundle.

DEFINING THE BUNDLE

TJA procedures are well-suited for bundled payments, because they satisfy several criteria for successful bundling. Arthroplasty procedures are highly prevalent, making cost analysis and interventions reliably predictable. Among Medicare cases, TJA accounts for 4.7% and consumes the greatest proportion of Medicare expenditures with costs reaching as high as 6.3%. The coefficient of variation for arthroplasty is 0.42, which is low relative to other medical conditions such as heart failure and shock (coefficient of variation, 0.80).[13] This coefficient of variation allows for greater payment predictability while simultaneously representing enough variation to improve efficiency. Finally, major joint arthroplasty procedures have clear evidence-based guidelines, which are ideal for accurate and measurable outcomes.[13]

Determining which patients are eligible for bundling in arthroplasty procedures can minimize risk of outliers. Patient risk factors for readmission, infection, and increased resource-consumption must be evaluated thoroughly in the preoperative period. Inneh and colleagues,[14] analyzed the readmission rates, length of stay, and rates of reoperation in 5314 TJA patients. Patient risk factors associated with worse outcomes included prior genitourinary, circulatory, and respiratory conditions; an American Society of Anesthesiologists score of N2; advanced age; and prolonged operation time. Mental health conditions and the metabolic syndrome also demonstrated a strong predictive correlation with serious complications in TJA patients.[14,15] Risk factors for surgical site infection after TJA include revision surgery, higher Charlson comorbidity index, and male gender.[16] Our institution recommends considering bundling for primary unilateral arthroplasty procedures of patients with a body mass index of less than 35, an American Society of Anesthesiologists score equal to or less than 2, hemoglobin A1C of less than 7.9, and nonsmokers. Patients with higher American Society of Anesthesiologists scores, modifiable medical comorbidities, social factors, and psychiatric illness can be considered for the program once appropriate preoperative medical optimization has been conducted. In addition to protecting the organization from potential financial loss, this approach allows patients the opportunity to engage in shared responsibility in an effort to improve their health and outcomes.[17]

DETERMINING THE LENGTH OF EPISODE

Defining the episode of care is another variable that should be assessed and defined to mitigate financial risks associated with an episode of care. Shorter episodes (ie, <30 days) reduce risk of postoperative complications by decreasing the window of potential exposure. However, shorter episodes also have lower reimbursement rates and smaller profit margins compared with longer 60-or 90-day episodes.[1] With regard to TJA, the greatest proportion of cost lies within the first 30 days after the procedure and then decreases significantly.[1] Thus, longer episodes are more attractive owing to the decreased rate of complications and increased profit potential. For percutaneous cardiac procedures, a 90-day episode was noted to have a 30% higher reimbursement when compared with a 7-day episode.[1]

The BPCI model 2, which was selected as the framework for the Comprehensive Care of Joint Replacement program starting in 2016, uses a 90-day TJA episode, with the hospital admission day representing the start point. Early results from phase 2 demonstrate a decrease in length of stay from 4.6 to 4.3 days, and a decrease in PAC used from 66% to 47%.[4] Although there was no change in mortality and 30-day readmission rates, emergency department visits within 30 days increased from 6.9% to 8.7%.[4] Early results from the New York University Hospital for Joint Surgery, a model 2 BPCI participant, also revealed decreased readmission rates and cost throughout the 90-day episode.[18] Although

these are early and preliminary results, a 90-day episode for TJA procedures seems to present a reasonable option for risk management and predicting postoperative outcomes.

PRICING THE BUNDLE

The transition from FFS to a bundled payment system will entail a learning curve for both CMS and private payers. In the FFS model, services are marketed individually to payers and beneficiaries, which complicates the decision making process for consumers. Bundled payments, on the other hand, coalesce fragmented services into a single marketable entity introducing more competition into the market. Orthopedic TJA providers will be in a position to influence price setting owing to the high demand and predictive nature of the procedures.

The BPCI pilot programs use retrospective payments (models 1–3) and prospective payments (model 4) to establish reimbursement strategies. Retrospective payment models allow risk adjustment using the current FFS infrastructure, while also providing a method to reconcile outlier episodes of care. Prospective payments would require revamping internal accounting systems and is perceived as a high-risk approach by BPCI model 2 participants.[4] Beneficiary characteristics should be risk-adjusted for more accurate price fixation. The Medicare severity diagnosis related group system in conjunction with the hierarchal condition category allows for more accurate prediction of cost for specific conditions and appropriate inpatient risk adjustment. Hospital characteristics, such as the percent of indirect medical education and disproportionate share hospital payments should also be received to further adjust payments.[13] First, postacute setting accounts for the largest proportion of total cost, and thus demands that stratification considers place of discharge as well.[13] The average CMS payment for 470 Medicare severity diagnosis related groups patients discharged to home health agency averaged $14,901, whereas it was $21,742 for those to SNF, and long-term care hospital episodes averaged $43,772.[13] Therefore, bundles should also be adjusted retrospectively based on destination after hospital disposition. Model 2 of the BPCI uses risk adjusted payments, which are later reconciled against the CMS's predicted price. Appropriate risk stratification with private payers will likely follow a similar approach. However, price settlements will have greater variation depending on the payer type. CMS reimbursements are inflexible and leave no room for negotiation or price manipulation. Private insurers will allow for greater manipulation based on market share, leverage, and economic outcomes. Surgeons can increase their leverage and market share through contracting in ACOs or physician networks. Independent surgical groups may remain independent, but are encouraged to partner with physician groups for greater leverage in contract negotiations.

DEVELOPING PATIENT CARE PATHWAYS

Several studies have demonstrated decreases in cost and waste, and improved patient outcomes as a result of integrated care pathways.[19–21] Establishing standardized management guidelines can be challenging among surgeons owing to variation in level of comfort with recommendations based on individual experience or training. A cost analysis based on provider-specific and patient-related variables should be performed to identify sources of variation and financial waste. All stakeholders involved in the management of the patient's care episode should be involved in the process to determine which treatment should be standardized among providers.[22] Important areas to discuss include surgical timing, therapy protocols, required medications, expected implants, and discharge plans. In the inpatient setting, standardizing implants can have a substantial effect on cost reduction, although this would be expected to face a strong surgeon and patient preference-based opposition.[9] The American Academy of Orthopedic Surgery has also published several clinical practice guidelines for TJA, which may be of assistance when creating integrated care pathways.[23] Once in-hospital integrated care pathways are established, attention to PAC should also be highlighted.

POSTACUTE CARE

Before the 1997 PAC, cost increased exponentially, with reimbursements based on individual services rendered rather than prospective payments. The Balanced Budget Act of 1997 was aimed at addressing the growing disparity with prospective payments for PAC providers.[24] However, despite early evidence of decreased wasteful resource consumption, PAC reimbursements continued to vary by provider type. As a result, patients were often discharged to high level of care facilities motivated by the higher reimbursement rate.[7] The BPCI model 2 aims to join inpatient costs with PAC under a single bundled payment to improve care coordination and patient outcomes throughout the entire cycle of care. The majority of TJA patients will require some level of PAC rehabilitation (inpatient or outpatient), or home health services. Lavernia and colleagues[25] in 2006 estimated that $3.2 billion are spent annually in PAC after TJA. Home health services cost about $8300 less compared with acute care facilities. Ong and colleagues[26] found in a database study from 1997 to 2010 that more than 50% of TJA patients were discharged from the hospital to an inpatient facility. There was also an increase in the number of discharges to skilled nursing units and a reduced rate to rehabilitation facilities. In contrast with physician reimbursement and implant cost for hospitals, the average annual physical therapy cost per patient increased by more than $648 million a year.[26] The BPCI significantly altered PAC eligibility by waiving the Medicare 3-day inpatient stay requirement. Among BPCI participants in phase 2, institutional PAC discharges decreased by 14.8% points compared with the control group. However, the number of PAC days remained similar between BPCI and the control group throughout the intervention period.[4] Failure in managing PAC appropriately will ultimately lead to failure in a bundled payment system. Coordination with PAC providers within ACOs will be critical in improving patient care and decreasing cost, and must be at the forefront during the planning phase.

AFFORDABLE CARE ORGANIZATIONS IN THE BUNDLED CARE MARKET

The changes brought about through the ACA meant a drastic need to restructure the health care system. In an effort to minimize cost, while optimizing quality of care at lower costs, new laws encourage continuity in health care delivery within an integrated system. The development of an ACO provided a model of high-quality care, while simultaneously reducing costs associated with the multiple aspects of the care cycle.[27] However, early quality and cost results are mixed. An ACO is a network of physicians, hospitals, and other health care stakeholders collaborating to provide coordinated high quality care to Medicare patients. The primary care physician is an essential component of this model and serves as the central point of contact through which all other providers can coordinate care. Physicians and hospitals share the responsibility of providing care for a group of patients with incentives to maximize shared savings and maintain a healthy patient population.[28] Similarly, the participants in the ACO network also share the risk of any loss associated with providing care that is costly and unnecessary.

Several types of prior delivery systems would be conducive for the ACO model based on eligibility criteria for each organization (Table 2). These include integrated delivery systems, multispecialty group practices, physician hospital organizations, independent practice associations, and virtual physician organizations. Forming an ACO allows small provider groups to join forces and compete with larger institutions that could otherwise dominate the market. A large emphasis is placed on care coordination, continuity of care, and managing disease as part of an integrated system. For the provider, this means that there is centralized contracting for each patient that combines horizontal consolidation of care among all providers involved in the patient's management and vertical integration between care providers among different levels of the health care team. The ACO adopts the concepts behind bundled payments and provides a foundation for efficient care that expands beyond a single episode of care.

Major differences in the ACO model rely on capitation of risks in contract and redefining the relationship between providers and the hospital. Rather than being contracted individually with a hospital or outpatient surgical center, physicians would be employed by the ACO. Reimbursements and quality of care recommendations are based on broader governance by population health management. This is reflected in risk management that is based on performance rather than insurance risk.

For successful integration of the ACO model into care delivery, organizations should focus on improving quality measurements and not profitability. Often, efforts to improve quality also result in improved profit margins. Administrators should accurately assess the health status for the majority of patients that would receive care within the ACO. Outliers should also be identified and accounted for to manage appropriately the risk associated with care for such patients. Additionally, key decision makers should understand the total cost of care provided across various settings, including the inpatient, outpatient clinical care or rehabilitation, and urgent care settings. Clinicians should also be empowered with information that allows them to understand the cost associated with an episode of care and equipped with the necessary tools to incorporate costs in management decisions. Finally, an ACO will not be effective without investing in the patient and adopting a patient-centered approach. This effectiveness requires the patient to provide feedback on factors and variables in the health care experience that contribute to patient satisfaction. Early ACOs should focus on communication with all members of the health care delivery team, including the patients and family members involve in the postdischarge care process.

Affordable Care Organization Limitations

Care coordination is often challenging, and although theoretically appealing, there remains lack of evidence on positive impact of this approach on realization of cost reduction. Even with all the right tools in place, the implementation of ACOs carries considerable challenges. Pay-for-performance and shared savings programs may not lead to improved quality of care. Additionally, the ability of orthopedic surgeons to provide quality care coordination is highly dependent on the primary care physician, who acts as the central physician for all of the patient's care. With a shortage of primary care physicians able to cover the large increase in patients eligible for Medicare, the surgeon's role may be compromised. As such, there is a great need to establish patient care pathways that will improve efficiency and outcomes for beneficiaries.

GAINSHARING

The definition of gainsharing has evolved from a nebulous concept of profit sharing between hospitals and physicians to a highly attractive incentive in new bundle payment models. The concept of gainsharing is based on hospitals and physicians working together to reduce cost, and any realized savings are shared among the parties.[29] Historically, the Office of the Inspector General discouraged gainsharing in 1999 by stating that it violated the Federal Civil Monetary Penalty Statute.[29] However, gainsharing has again gained favor throughout the last decade as a tool for incentivizing higher quality at a decreased cost. In the 1990s, gainsharing gained traction as a response to orthopedic manufactures inflating costs. In 1997, orthopedics service lines were 25% hospital profit. However, only a 2% profit was being realized by 2001. From 1991 to 2006, CMS payments for TJA increased by 19%, the list price for implants increased by 171%, and the average implant selling price increased by 117%. This dramatic increase in cost fostered hospital–physician partnerships to reduce implant costs.[9] The Office of

Table 2	
Criteria for ACO eligibility	
Domain	**Standard**
ACO structure and operations	• Defines its organizational structure. • Demonstrates capability to manage resources. • Aligns provider incentives through payment arrangements and other mechanisms to promote the delivery of efficient and effective care.
Access to needed providers	• Has sufficient numbers and types of practitioners. • Provides timely access to culturally competent health care.
Patient-centered primary care	Primary care practices within the organization act as medical homes for patients.
Care management	• Collects, integrates, and uses data from various sources for care management, performance reporting, and identifying patients for population health programs. • Provides resources to patients and practitioners to support care management activities.
Care coordination and transitions	Facilitates timely exchange of information between providers, patients, and their caregivers to promote safe transitions.
Patient rights and responsibilities	• Informs patients about the role of the ACO and its services. • Provides transparency of clinical performance and performance-based financial incentives offered to practitioners.
Performance reporting and quality improvement	• Measures and publically reports performance on clinical quality of care, patient experience and cost measures. • Identifies opportunities for improvement. • Brings together providers and stakeholders to collaborate on improvement initiatives.

Abbreviation: ACO, affordable care organization.
From National Committee for Quality Assurance (NCQA). ACO eligibility criteria. Available at: www.ncqa.org/tabid/1456/Default.aspx.

the Inspector General has revisited gainsharing programs, and in 2005 it examined the effects of 13 gainsharing programs on coronary stent patients. Gainsharing hospitals reduced cost 7.4%, of which 91% attributed to lower prices, and 9% to lesser use.[30] Gainsharing continued to gain support from hospitals systems and Medicare Payment Advisory Commission as a future tool to curtail costs.[29,31] The growing evidence in support of gainsharing from pilot programs and providers has led to its inclusion in the BPCI.

Gainsharing within the BPCI and Comprehensive Care of Joint Replacement has been permitted by CMS to promote "care redesign." To preserve quality standards and decrease patient risk, gainsharing arrangements under CMS must be disclosed and transparent. Providers must apply for a waiver that would protect applicants from fraud and abuse penalties. A physician payment limit of 50% of the savings is also enforced by CMS. Owing to the strict guidelines of federal and state laws, including the federal Anti-Kickback Law, the Stark Physician Self-Referral Law, the Federal Civil Monetary Penalties Law, and the False Claims Act, the authors recommend seeking experienced legal counsel when establishing gainsharing agreements.

Gainsharing agreements between providers and ACOs can be challenging, but present a tremendous opportunity for orthopedic surgeons. There is currently no standard for these agreements as long as they follow legal regulations and ethical standards. Considerations for gainsharing agreement should begin by establishing a time period. For example, every month total claims paid are compared against the contracted bundled price. Any savings are entered into a pool and become available upon meeting quality criteria. Within an ACO, physician groups can have collective benchmarks, making them eligible for a portion of the total savings. Within orthopedic groups, criteria for the division of savings may be equivalent among participants based on physician criteria. Examples of physician criteria may include: passed Surgical Care Improvement Project, mortality, Western Ontario and McMaster Osteoarthritis Index scores, readmissions, length of stay, and patient education classes. It is important for physicians to enter gainsharing agreements with hospitals and ACOs to further engage participants in a high quality program.

UNDERSTANDING THE PAYMENT MODELS

In April 2015, Congress passed the Medicare Access and Children's Health Insurance Program Reauthorization Act of 2015 (MACRA). MACRA combines 3 arms of health care reform: merit-based incentive payment system, alternative payment models (APMs), and a physician-focused payment model. Bundle payment models are considered APMs under MACRA. In January 2015, the CMS set goals with the hopes that 30% of traditional Medicare payments would contribute to APMs, such as bundled payments, ACOs, or medical homes by the end of 2016.[32] Further expansion is expected by 2018, with 50% of such payments allocated to these models.[32] The Department of Health and Human Services has already made significant progress in reaching these goals. In 2011, no Medicare payments were made through APMs; however, approximately 20% of CMS payments are currently being put toward APMs. The BPCI pilot program is the prototype APM program for bundled payment systems under CMS and will

continue to serve as an efficiency and quality measure of the programs' success in the future.[32]

SUMMARY

Although ACOs and bundle payment models may seem to conflict, both are attempts to facilitate and encourage coordinated and integrated care while simultaneously reducing cost. ACOs carry a broader scope of services for arthroplasty patients, with part A and part B services included in the shared savings program. Organizations that participate in bundling can choose the bundled services and have an active role in determining several aspects related to the episode of care. ACOs also cross a more expansive time period of care, whereas bundling focuses more on specific services to a specific patient. Additionally, ACOs are specific to Medicare providers/patients and only certain types of sponsors can participate. For bundling, all eligible awardees can participate, which may include physicians, hospitals, and different health systems. Finally, the savings for ACOs are shared between the ACO and Medicare, while the savings and losses in bundling systems are dependent upon the type of bundling and the target price. When bundling is used in an ACO model of care delivery, there is the potential to improve quality of care and reduce economic burden on health care institutions. As implementation of various ACA measures

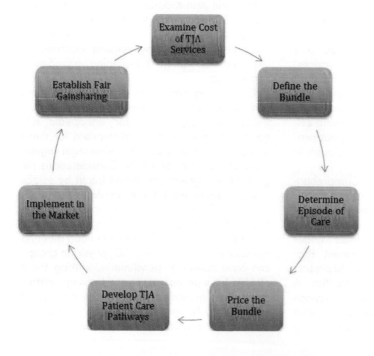

Fig. 1. Progression of implementing bundle payment models in affordable care organizations and hospital services. TJA, total joint arthroplasty.

unfold, further research is necessary to determine the success of these models and the possibility of integrating the models for arthroplasty patients (Fig. 1).

ACKNOWLEDGMENTS

The authors thank Mr R.B. Siegrist for presenting this topic during the *Central Illinois Healthcare Management Summit* chaired by Dr K.J. Saleh.

REFERENCES

1. Comprehensive care for joint replacement payment model proposed rule, File code CMS-5516-P. Available at: www.aamc.org/download/442290/data/aamccommentsontheccjrproposedrule.pdf. Accessed November 20, 2015.

2. Helmick CG, Lawrence RC, Pollard RA, et al. Arthritis and other rheumatic conditions: who is affected now, who will be affected later? National Arthritis Data Workgroup. Arthritis Care Res 1995; 8(4):203–11.

3. Jencks SF, Williams MV, Coleman EA. Rehospitalizations among patients in the Medicare Fee-for-Service Program. N Engl J Med 2009;360(14): 1418–28.

4. Lewin's Group. CMS Bundled Payments for Care Improvement (BPCI) Initiative Models 2-4: Year 1 Evaluation & Monitoring Annual Report. Available at: https://innovation.cms.gov/Files/reports/BPCI-EvalRpt1.pdf. Accessed October 17, 2015.

5. Hussey PS, Eibner C, Ridgely MS, et al. Controlling U.S. health care spending–separating promising from unpromising approaches. N Engl J Med 2009;361(22):2109–11.

6. Frakt AB. How much do hospitals cost shift? A review of the evidence. Milbank Q 2011;89(1):90–130.

7. Sood N, Huckfeldt PJ, Escarce JJ, et al. Medicare's bundled payment pilot for acute and postacute care: analysis and recommendations on where to begin. Health Aff (Millwood) 2011;30(9):1708–17.

8. Ronning PL, Meyer JW. Centers of excellence: an assessment tool for cardiovascular and orthopedic programs. Hosp Technol Ser 1996;15(13):1–29.

9. Healy WL, Iorio R, Lemos MJ, et al. Single price/Case price purchasing in orthopaedic surgery: experience at the Lahey Clinic. J Bone Joint Surg Am 2000;82A(5):607–12.

10. Hussey PS, Ridgely MS, Rosenthal MB. The PROMETHEUS bundled payment experiment: slow start shows problems in implementing new payment models. Health Aff (Millwood) 2011;30(11):2116–24.

11. Bundled Payments for Care Improvement (BPCI) initiative: general information. Available at: https://innovation.cms.gov/initiatives/bundled-payments/. Accessed November 20, 2015.

12. Comprehensive care for joint replacement. Available at: www.cms.gov/Newsroom/MediaReleaseDatabase/Fact-sheets/2015-Fact-sheets-items/2015-07-09.html. Accessed November 20, 2015.

13. Medicare payment bundling: from claims data and policy implications: analyses of episode-based payment. Available at: www.aamc.org/download/312462/data/ahaaamcfullreport.pdf. Accessed November 20, 2015.

14. Inneh IA, Lewis CG, Schutzer SF. Focused risk analysis: regression model based on 5,314 total hip and knee arthroplasty patients from a single institution. J Arthroplasty 2014;29(10):2031–5.

15. Gage MJ, Schwarzkopf R, Abrouk M, et al. Impact of metabolic syndrome on perioperative complication rates after total joint arthroplasty surgery. J Arthroplasty 2014;29(9):1842–5.

16. Rasouli MR, Restrepo C, Maltenfort MG, et al. Risk factors for surgical site infection following total joint arthroplasty. J Bone Joint Surg Am 2014; 96A(18):e158.

17. Froimson MI, Rana A, White RE Jr, et al. Bundled payments for care improvement initiative: the next evolution of payment formulations: AAHKS Bundled Payment Task Force. J Arthroplasty 2013; 28(8 Suppl):157–65.

18. Iorio R, Clair AJ, Inneh IA, et al. Early results of Medicare's bundled payment initiative for a 90-day total joint arthroplasty episode of care. J Arthroplasty 2016;31(2):343–50.

19. Van Citters AD, Fahlman C, Goldmann DA, et al. Developing a pathway for high-value, patient-centered total joint arthroplasty. Clin Orthop Relat Res 2014;472(5):1619–35.

20. Goldstein W. CORR Insights(R): developing a pathway for high-value, patient-centered total joint arthroplasty. Clin Orthop Relat Res 2014;472(5):1636–7.

21. Mertes SC, Raut S, Khanduja V. Integrated care pathways in lower-limb arthroplasty: are they effective in reducing length of hospital stay? Int Orthop 2013;37(6):1157–63.

22. Froemke CC, Wang L, DeHart ML, et al. Standardizing care and improving quality under a bundled payment initiative for total joint arthroplasty. J Arthroplasty 2015;30(10):1676–82.

23. Evidence-based clinical practice guidelines. Available at: www.aaos.org/research/guidelines/guide.asp. Accessed November 20, 2015.

24. Chandra A, Dalton MA, Holmes J. Large increases in spending on postacute care in Medicare point to the potential for cost savings in these settings. Health Aff (Millwood) 2013;32(5):864–72.

25. Lavernia CJ, D'Apuzzo MR, Hernandez VH, et al. Postdischarge costs in arthroplasty surgery. J Arthroplasty 2006;21(6):144–50.

26. Ong KL, Lotke PA, Lau E, et al. Prevalence and costs of rehabilitation and physical therapy

after primary TJA. J Arthroplasty 2015;30(7): 1121–6.

27. Kocot SL, Dang-Vu C, White R, et al. Early experiences with accountable care in Medicaid: special challenges, big opportunities. Popul Health Manag 2013;16(Suppl 1):S4–11.

28. Issar NM, Jahangir AA. The Affordable Care Act and orthopaedic trauma. J Orthop Trauma 2014; 28(Suppl 10):S5–7.

29. Healy WL. Gainsharing: a primer for orthopaedic surgeons. J Bone Joint Surg Am 2006;88(8): 1880–7.

30. Ketcham JD, Furukawa MF. Hospital-physician gainsharing in cardiology. Health Aff (Millwood) 2008;27(3):803–12.

31. Hackbarth G, Reischauer R, Mutti A. Collective accountability for medical care - toward bundled Medicare payments. N Engl J Med 2008;359(1):3–5.

32. MACRA: new opportunities for Medicare providers through innovative payment systems (updated). Available at: http://healthaffairs.org/blog/2015/09/28/macra-new-opportunities-for-medicare-providers-through-innovative-payment-systems-3/. Accessed November 28, 2015.

Big Data, Big Research

Implementing Population Health-Based Research Models and Integrating Care to Reduce Cost and Improve Outcomes

Afshin A. Anoushiravani, MD[a], Jason Patton, MD[a],
Zain Sayeed, MSc, MHA[a], Mouhanad M. El-Othmani, MD[a],
Khaled J. Saleh, MD, MSc, FRCS (C), MHCM, CPE[b,*]

KEYWORDS

• Big data • NIS • NSQIP • Medicare data • Research advances

KEY POINTS

- Big data, in the health care setting, may be defined as a collection of information extracted from traditional and digital sources used to drive future discoveries and analyses.
- Awareness of advantages and limitations of large data registries, such as Medicare claims data, National Surgical Quality Improvement Program, National Inpatient Sample, Kid's Inpatient Database, and private alternatives, are necessary for orthopedic surgeons to conduct meaningful outcomes research.
- Use of the International Society of Arthroplasty Registries' recommendations on creation of registries will enable orthopedic surgeons to target quality improvement initiatives and better track patient outcomes.

INTRODUCTION

In the early twentieth century, Dr Codman became the first advocator for the collection and analysis of patient outcomes.[1] With the aid of medical and technological advancements throughout the century, the collection, analysis, and interpretation of collected data gave rise to an era of Big Data.[2] Simply put, big data is a collection of information extracted from traditional and digital sources used to drive medical advancements.[3] Over the past decade, several factors have converged allowing for the rise of big data and its implementation in clinical research.[4] Advanced electronic devices with data mining capabilities as well as the reduced cost of data storage and analysis has provided clinicians with the capabilities to answer questions beyond the scope of randomized controlled trials and meta-analyses.[4,5]

Big Data: Big Business

In the last 5 years, big data research applications are quickly turning into big business. International Business Machine, a prominent leader in information technology (IT), recently reported that 90% of the world's data was collected within the last 2 years, further demonstrating the rapid

---

Funding Sources: No additional funding sources were used for this article.

Conflicts of Interest: No conflicts of interest are evident for authors of this article.

[a] Division of Orthopaedics and Rehabilitation, Southern Illinois University School of Medicine, 701 North First Street, Springfield, IL 62781, USA; [b] Department of Orthopaedic and Sports Medicine, Detroit Medical Center, 311 Mack Avenue, 5th Floor, Detroit, MI 48201, USA

* Corresponding author.

E-mail address: kjsaleh@gmail.com

http://dx.doi.org/10.1016/j.ocl.2016.05.008

rate at which information is being collected.[6] Within the next 5 years this IT sector is projected to grow by 400% to $50 billion annually.[7] As a result, many corporations and entrepreneurs are focusing on IT applications in health care. Early leaders in this emerging sector have been large hospital organizations who have used patient data to implement population-based health care initiatives. Through this approach, clinical and economic advantages in the form of improved quality of care, increased efficiency, and reduced resource consumption have been realized.[8–10] Although big data can be beneficial to patients, health care providers must use this information in an appropriate manner, as improper use may lead to harmful outcomes and clinical practices.

Large national databases have emerged as a viable means of reporting surgical outcomes and resource consumption patterns within orthopedic surgery. In the United States, several large publically governed patient registries exist. The strengths and limitations of each database depend on the purpose and design of the database. Before incorporating data from a specific database, an investigator must have a good understanding of the research question being asked as well as strengths and limitations associated with available databases.[11] The purpose of this article is to review various advantages and disadvantages of large data sets available for orthopedic use, examine their ideal use, and report how they are being implemented nationwide. Improvements that can be made to more efficiently collect relevant data and introducing model orthopedic practices that have embraced the big data big research model are also presented. Throughout this article, the reader should also be mindful that clinicians cannot ignore big data. Furthermore, clinicians must ensure that it is used in an ethical manner to improve patient outcomes.[12]

CURRENT BIG DATA REGISTRIES
International Databases

The first national orthopedic registry was created in Sweden in 1975 to collect information on total knee arthroplasty (TKA).[13] Since then, all Scandinavian and several English-speaking countries have developed independent total joint registries.[14] The Swedish joint registry assigns each patient a single national health identifier ensuring that a given primary prosthesis implanted at one institution can be connected to subsequent revisions at a different institution.[14] In 2007, the Nordic Arthroplasty Register Association (NARA) was created to enable collaboration among the TKA and total hip arthroplasty (THA) registries of Sweden, Denmark, and Norway.[15] Although the collaboration has allowed for a robust analysis of total joint arthroplasty (TJA) outcomes, NARA demonstrates how intraoperative techniques, such as cement fixation during THA, depend on regional norms rather than evidence-based practices.[14] Additionally, infrequently used implants have been removed from the Swedish market because of insufficient outcomes data.[14] Ultimately, the relatively small sample size and national tendencies in regard to surgical technique and prosthesis selection may limit the comparative capabilities of Scandinavian TJA registries.[14] Although not without limitation, these evidence- and population-based international registries have served as prototypes for several American data sets.

Medicare Claims Data

The United States has assigned specific governmental agencies with the task of collecting orthopedic care administrative data, whereas European registries were developed under the impetus of professional societies.[14] In 1965, the US Congress established Medicare as Title XVII of the Social Security Act; on July 1, 1966 the program was initiated.[10,16] The Centers for Medicare and Medicaid Services (CMS) is the national insurance program offering health care to 4 groups of US citizens: those 65 years or older, the disabled, those with end-stage renal disease, and those with amyotrophic lateral sclerosis.[16] The Medicare claims data set has recorded administrative claims data, reimbursement, and payment information on more than 45 million beneficiaries; therefore, it is the most robust nationwide database available to clinicians.[10,16] However, it is primarily limited to elderly and disabled patients and is not representative of the US population.

Additionally, the database has the ability to track beneficiaries through both ambulatory and inpatient settings. This feature enables researchers to assess short- and long-term outcomes and trends in resource utilization. Although the Medicare data set is considered the most comprehensive and robust database available in the United States, it is heavily regulated and is associated with significant up-front costs ranging from $3000 to $20,000 per data file.[10] Furthermore, the data set relies heavily on *International Classification of Disease* (ICD) codes and is ineffective at assessing nonbillable events. It should also be noted that the Medicare database does not include information on implant type, surgical approach, or laterality. This lack of data is particularly relevant as CMS shifts away from a fee-for-service model to value-based reimbursement models.

National Surgical Quality Improvement Program

The National Veterans Affair Surgical Risk Study (NVASRS) was developed as an outcomes-based database and was a congressional response to the high surgical mortality rate among the Veteran Health Administration.[17] Following the NVASRS success, the program expanded to all 132 Veterans Affairs hospitals and was renamed the National Surgical Quality Improvement Program (NSQIP).[17] Since its inception, NSQIP has been credited with reducing the 30-day postoperative mortality and morbidity by 47% and 43%, respectively.[17,18] In 1999, NSQIP was piloted at several academic medical centers and has since been implemented at more than 650 medical institutions worldwide.[19,20] NSQIP is unique in that trained Surgical Clinical Reviewers collect a continuum of data from admission up to 30 days postoperatively.[20] The collected data are based on the review of patient charts, not insurance or administrative data.[20] Additionally, all surgical patients, including those undergoing elective orthopedic procedures, are included in NSQIP.[20] Thus, NSQIP is particularly well designed at assessing postoperative outcomes and resource utilization among various medical centers while having the added capability of evaluating patients' postoperative course and complications. Notably, large national and statewide databases are an accessible low-cost alternative to the Medicare database.

Discharge Databases

In 1988, the federal government charged the Agency for Healthcare and Research Quality (AHRQ) with collecting in-hospital outcomes and resource utilization through the Healthcare Cost and Utilization Project (HCUP).[21] Deidentified patient information was gathered from participating medical centers and organized into state and national databases. These data sets were further separated into emergency department (National Emergency Department Sample), ambulatory care center (State Ambulatory Surgery and Services Database), or inpatient hospital stays. The most commonly used HCUP databases include the Kid's Inpatient Database (KID), National Inpatient Sample (NIS), and State Inpatient Database (SID). Although these discharge databases are relatively low cost and accessible, they rely heavily

on ICD coding practices to identify patients of interest.

The NIS is the largest all-payer inpatient database and is updated annually. The entries in the NIS include up to 15 ICD diagnostic and procedural codes.[21] The patient samples are reported in a uniform and deidentified manner, making them ideal for retrospective observational cohort studies.[22,23] Before 2012, the NIS was referred to as the Nationwide Inpatient Sample; however, the sampling methodology was modified in 2012 to reflect a more nationally representative model; hence, the nomenclature changed to highlight this modification. Historically, the NIS has incorporated up to 8 million discharges from approximately 4000 hospitals across the United States. Hospitals are stratified by size, geographic location, and academic affiliation.[23] The NIS incorporates 20% of all US discharges, and a multiplier is used to provide national estimates. Major limitations of the NIS include its inability to report on short- and long-term outpatient outcomes as well as its heavy reliance on proper coding practices.[23] Furthermore, discrepancies between the NIS and the NSQIP revealed that the NIS is not well suited in reporting short-term outcomes related to infection (sepsis, pneumonia, urinary tract infection, surgical site infections) and 30-day patient mortality.[11] Bozic and colleagues[24] noted that patients' postoperative complications recorded in administrative databases were comparable and in high concordance with patient charts. Although the NSQIP is similar in cost and usability to the NIS, NSQIP incorporates fewer patient samples and is by no means a nationally representative data set.

The KID is very similar to the NIS except in that it focuses on the pediatric population. It was developed in 1997 as a means of providing a national pool that can be used to assess and analyze rare pediatric disorders.[25] The database is updated every 3 years and has not been well adopted within the orthopedic community. Another HCUP database, the SID, is representative of statewide hospital discharges that have been consolidated in a uniform manner, facilitating its comparison and incorporation into the NIS.[26] Although the SID is overseen by the HCUP, differences in data set variables, length of follow-up, and complication data exist and vary by state.[26] California and New York are considered to have larger and more comprehensive databases.

Although well powered, these large national and statewide databases have historically been used to evaluate epidemiologic patterns. More recently, a trend toward assessing postoperative in-hospital outcomes and resource consumption among patient cohorts has emerged. Investigators have used the Charlson Score and Elixhauser Comorbidity Index as a means of reporting cohort comorbidity profiles. Some studies have matched comorbidity profiles among cohorts reducing confounding bias, allowing for a more accurate comparison of postoperative outcomes and resource utilization patterns.[27,28]

Other Databases

Alternatives to large government-funded and administered databases are those curated by private insurance providers and large medical entities.[10] Within the last few years, insurance claims data from major insurers have been available for purchase.[10] As medical providers and insurers continue to merge, there is considerable potential for medical research.[10] However, these administrative and insurance claims databases gather patient information from many sources increasing the data sets heterogeneity, ultimately making generalizations difficult to substantiate.

Currently, many private databases, including PearlDiver, MarketScan, and Premier, are available for purchase.[10] Although these databases provide access to massive amounts of information through a simplified platform, their higher costs ($5000 to $50,000) serve as a significant barrier.[10] Additionally, the data incorporated into these databases are extracted and compounded from numerous sources (ie, NIS, CMS, insurance providers) reducing the uniformity of variables comprising the database.[10]

EXAMINING THE IDEAL USE OF BIG DATA

Big data is currently used in orthopedics to assess trends that may not be apparent in lower-powered population samples. Grauer and Leopold[5] proposed that studies using big data play a role in relating less common events with previously unidentified risk factors. Although registry data are less satisfactory, meaningful long-term prospective studies are difficult to perform in orthopedic surgery and require significant resources.[29,30] Notably, Robertsson[13] demonstrated that 4000 patients had to be randomized and followed for 10 years to obtain 80% power for detecting a significant difference in an implant whose revision rate is 30% more than the mean (5.0% vs 6.5% revision rate).[13] Thus, registry-based studies are particularly well suited for postmarket surveillance of

orthopedic devices, postoperative clinical outcomes, as well as short- and long-term resource utilization trends.

Studies using big data enable researchers to uncover and detect rare events, evaluate resource utilization without ethical compromise, and assess safety of care.[5,31] Large databases including the NIS, NSQIP, National Hospital Discharge, National Trauma Databank, and Medicare databases have aided orthopaedic surgeons in assessing population-based trends and guide advancements in orthopaedic care. Large database studies are able to identify provider- or hospital-specific variables associated with postoperative complications, and compare resource consumption among various geographic regions or practice types.[32]

Clinical cost and performance data may support employers in deciding which orthopedic surgeons are available to supply care to their organization. Although such performance expectations may place strain on surgeons, there is greater potential professional adoption of standard practices and quality improvement (QI) techniques.[33] Within the past decade, several regional or enterprise joint replacement registries are in place, including those at Kaiser Permanente and Massachusetts General Hospital. Their data entry includes standard patient-specific information, procedures, and device characteristics as well as a uniform battery of outcome measures, including preoperative and postoperative functional and symptom scores.[9,34,35]

In 1994 the American Academy of Orthopaedic Surgeons (AAOS) established a Musculoskeletal Outcomes Data Evaluation and Management System in order to create gold standard patient-based functional health questionnaires and to collect data from orthopedic surgeons using such instruments.[36] Although this early initiative demonstrated success in initial data collection, 30% complete follow-up was reported for a given TJA procedure.[37] The current emergence of patient-reported outcome measures (PROMs) is also adding several additional capabilities to registries.[36] In the PROMs framework, detailed data describing the relief of symptoms, restoring or improving functional ability, restoring quality of life, and reassuming social roles are collected.[36] Such measures offer a more subjective approach to the quality of care delivered by orthopedic surgeons but may result in a closer inspection of what enhances patient satisfaction. Currently, the CMS is identifying methods to use PROMs in TJA to assess the value of each procedure, with the goal of ultimately linking their findings with reimbursement models. Large registries, including Function and Outcomes Research for Comparative Effectiveness in Total Joint Replacement (FORCE-TJR), the American Joint Replacement Registry, Michigan Arthroplasty Registry Collaborative for Quality Improvement, and the California Joint Registry, have incorporated outcome measures, such as the Short Form Health Survey, the Western Ontario and McMaster University Osteoarthritis Index, or the hip-specific Oxford index into their data tracking systems.[38]

A MACRO-PERSPECTIVE ON BIG DATA MEASUREMENTS IN ORTHOPEDICS

Big data is also used on national circuits and affects varying health care policies. The AHRQ reports that quality problems are reflected in practice variation within several health care settings. As big data collection and analysis continues, performance measures are being applied to orthopedic practices as markers of effective health care delivery. Bozic and Chiu[39] examined broad categories of performance that are monitored by public and private reporting programs, such as the AHRQ and the CMS.[16] The investigators demonstrated that 5 broad categories of appraisal exist for identifying quality of health care delivery and include *structural*, *process*, *outcome*, *patient experience*, and *efficiency*.[16] Furthermore, outcome measures, including health-related quality of life, infection rate, dislocation rate, readmission rate, and reoperation rate, have shown to be the most direct measure of quality.[39,40] As such, these categories are currently identified as markers of hospital and physician performance and are being targeted by various QI methodologies in an attempt to improve the quality of care delivery.

Assessing National and Local Performance Measurement Initiatives

Over the past decade, numerous organizations have attempted to create tools that allow various quality-reporting agencies to measure the aforementioned performance metrics. Press Ganey Inc is an organization providing access to publicly reported quality standards and survey results.[10] One such example includes the hospital-acquired conditions (HAC) score, which has been recognized as a national performance benchmark.[10] Such benchmarks cannot be overlooked, as they may result in the withholding of health care funds because of poor performance scores.[10] Over a 2-year period, fiscally rooted

penalties have been credited with halving the in-hospital mortality rate, decreased length of stay by 9%, and reduced the variable costs per case by 4%.[10]

The National Quality Forum (NQF) is presented as a tool that provides consumers with data that can assist in the decision-making process.[41] As a federally recognized endorser of performance measures, the NQF oversees and promotes QI initiatives of various institutions. As demonstrated by the Medicare Improvements and Extension Act of 2006, the NQF became an authority in selecting measures for use in programs, such as the CMS Physician Quality Reporting System and the CMS Electronic Health Records Incentive Program. Once a performance measure is submitted to the NQF, an expert panel evaluates its value, scientific accuracy, usability, and feasibility.[41] These metrics are then reported on the national health arena and presented for public comment and input.

State and local agencies also aimed toward assessing big data by measuring state-specific performance. One example includes the Minnesota Health Scores initiative, which assesses hospital quality and patient experience ratings focusing on patient satisfaction and whether or not they received recommended care.[42] The Minnesota Community measurement collects and reports data on population health, health conditions, procedures, and location of care delivery to offer a statewide quality reporting system.[42] In Illinois, the Department of Public Health issues a hospital report per institution depending on several quality characteristics resulting from various collected performance metrics.[43] Such use of big data has resulted in publicly available information that may alter patient choices for provider as well as institution.

The availability of online information regarding quality reporting has increased interest in the development of grading systems that compare outcomes and resource consumption of hospitals and physicians. HealthGrades.com Inc has developed hospital report cards to offer information about the quality of health care providers via the Internet.[44] One study assessed online ratings of orthopedic surgeons to identify variables that affect a surgeon's score. Investigators concluded that 5 variables resulted in higher ratings, including ease of scheduling, time spent with patient, wait time, surgeon proficiency, and bedside manner.[45] Although these variables have been shown to affect patient satisfaction, no database in the United States incorporates all 5 variables, hence, demonstrating a limitation to the utilization of large databases. In a general sense, the primary sponsor of the data set, whether it is CMS or another medical entity, may elucidate the goal behind the establishment of the data set. The use of such databases is of national importance because of public reporting of surgical outcomes and the financial repercussions bestowed on underperforming organizations.

A MODEL FOR BIG DATA RESEARCH

As more orthopedists incorporate electronic medical records (EMRs) into their practice, widespread clinical data collection will ensue and may result in surgical outcomes improvement. To date, clinical data have been primarily limited to large national or institutional registries. Data collection has been hindered by personnel requirements and workflow disruptions and ultimately resulting in increased costs.[2] In addition, there are increasing concerns over electronic security and data collection techniques, especially in light of costly security breaches at the University of California, Los Angeles.[2,46] Although, a consensus among orthopedic surgeons is needed before the implementation of standardized orthopedic data collection guidelines, the AAOS and the American Orthopaedic Association should play a leadership role in the development of such data registries. Here the authors make recommendations implemented by early pioneers in orthopedic clinical data registries.

The Basic Model
Large orthopedic registries collect data from multiple sources throughout a vast EMR network. Thus, it is essential that efforts be made to standardize registries. Because of limited resources, all patient variables cannot realistically be collected in an organized fashion. Hence, the International Society of Arthroplasty Registries (ISAR) has recommended 14 basic variables that should be included in all orthopedic registries.[3] The ISAR's minimum requirements enable orthopedic surgeons to follow through in their dedication to continuous QI, enhancing patient outcomes.[14]

The Goal
Collection of the ISAR's minimum requirements is feasible; however, establishment of comprehensive data registries requires a partnership with programmers. The objective of such a relationship should be to develop an efficient means of extracting clinically relevant data while minimizing resources utilization. To achieve such a solution, an institution's EMR needs to readily populate the registry.[2] Well-designed electronic data collection protocols not only reduce human input error and permit patient participation but they also provide a viable and standardized means of collecting clinical data.[47,48] The active patient involvement (ie, PROMs) in orthopedic care has the added benefit of improved postoperative outcomes and patient satisfaction.[49] These comprehensive and detailed data sets can then be used in more elaborate studies evaluating surgical outcomes as they relate to patient-specific factors. Such studies will better elucidate the different modalities of failure, enhancing postoperative outcomes while minimizing resources utilization.

The Electronic Medical Record
In the era of big data, new technologies are allowing orthopedic surgeons to collect and compute all patient data. The EMR will serve as the conduit between patient registries and clinicians, and as a result EMR functionality will be of utmost importance. The content and design of health care IT systems should be guided by the clinicians and not by administrators and their financially motivated concerns. The rigidity of medical records should give way to readily programmable and adaptable EMRs tailored to orthopedic surgeons. Lastly, EMRs should have a continuum capability in an effort to avoid the repopulation of previously collected data. As orthopedic surgeons attempt to create physician-owned medical facilities and ambulatory surgery centers, choice of EMR with such capabilities becomes a necessity.

SUMMARY

As big data continues to gain momentum in the clinical research arena, orthopedic surgeons must have a thorough understanding of the advantages and limitations associated with large databases, particularly in the era of value-based health care. The implementation of standardized national orthopedic registries in conjunction with readily programmable and adaptable EMRs tailored to orthopedic surgeons will ultimately improve patient outcomes while minimizing the economic burden.

ACKNOWLEDGMENTS

The authors would like to thank Dr Marc Swiontkowski for presenting this topic during the Central Illinois Healthcare Management Summit chaired by Dr K.J. Saleh.

REFERENCES

1. Codman EA. The classic: the registry of bone sarcomas as an example of the end-result idea in hospital organization. 1924. Clin Orthop Relat Res 2009;467(11):2766–70.

2. Goldstein J. Private practice outcomes: validated outcomes data collection in private practice. Clin Orthop Relat Res 2010;468(10):2640–5.

3. Arthur L. What is big data? 2013. Available at: http://www.forbes.com/sites/lisaarthur/2013/08/15/what-is-big-data/. Accessed November 12, 2015.

4. Nash DB. Harnessing the power of big data in healthcare. Am Health Drug Benefits 2014;7(2):69–70.

5. Grauer JN, Leopold SS. Editorial: large database studies–what they can do, what they cannot do, and which ones we will publish. Clin Orthop Relat Res 2015;473(5):1537–9.

6. Stevens JA, Ballesteros MF, Mack KA, et al. Gender differences in seeking care for falls in the aged Medicare population. Am J Prev Med 2012;43(1):59–62.

7. B U. Visualizing the big data industrial complex [Infographic]. 2013. Available at: http://www.forbes.com/sites/bruceupbin/2013/08/30/visualizing-the-big-data-industrial-complex-infographic/. Accessed November 12, 2015.

8. Groves P, Kayyali B, Knott D, et al. The big data revolution in healthcare. 2013. Available at: http://www.pharmatalents.es/assets/files/Big_Data_Revolution.pdf. Accessed November 12, 2015.

9. Paxton EW, Inacio MC, Khatod M, et al. Kaiser Permanente National Total Joint Replacement Registry: aligning operations with information technology. Clin Orthop Relat Res 2010;468(10):2646–63.

10. Pugely AJ, Martin CT, Harwood J, et al. Research in orthopaedic surgery: part I: claims-based data. J Bone Joint Surg Am 2015;97(15):1278–87.

11. Bohl DD, Basques BA, Golinvaux NS, et al. Nationwide Inpatient Sample and National Surgical Quality Improvement Program give different results in hip fracture studies. Clin Orthop Relat Res 2014;472(6):1672–80.

12. Helfet DL, Hanson BP, De Faoite D. Big data: the paradigm shift needed to revolutionize musculoskeletal clinical research. Am J Orthop 2014;43(9):399–400.

13. Robertsson O. Knee arthroplasty registers. J Bone Joint Surg Br 2007;89(1):1–4.

14. Delaunay C. Registries in orthopaedics. Orthop Traumatol Surg Res 2015;101(1 Suppl):S69–75.

15. Havelin LI, Robertsson O, Fenstad AM, et al. Scandinavian experience of register collaboration: the Nordic Arthroplasty Register Association (NARA). J Bone Joint Surg Am 2011;93(Suppl 3):13–9.

16. Marjoua Y, Butler CA, Bozic KJ. Public reporting of cost and quality information in orthopaedics. Clin Orthop Relat Res 2012;470(4):1017–26.

17. Khuri SF, Daley J, Henderson W, et al. The Department of Veterans Affairs' NSQIP: the first national, validated, outcome-based, risk-adjusted, and peer-controlled program for the measurement and enhancement of the quality of surgical care. National VA Surgical Quality Improvement Program. Ann Surg 1998;228(4):491–507.

18. Khuri SF. The NSQIP: a new frontier in surgery. Surgery 2005;138(5):837–43.

19. Fink AS, Campbell DA Jr, Mentzer RM Jr, et al. The National Surgical Quality Improvement Program in non-Veterans Administration hospitals: initial demonstration of feasibility. Ann Surg 2002;236(3):344–53 [discussion: 353–4].

20. Jiranek WA, Hanssen AD, Greenwald AS. Antibiotic-loaded bone cement for infection prophylaxis in total joint replacement. J Bone Joint Surg Am 2006;88(11):2487–500.

21. Chiu FY, Chen CM, Lin CF, et al. Cefuroxime-impregnated cement in primary total knee arthroplasty: a prospective, randomized study of three hundred and forty knees. J Bone Joint Surg Am 2002;84-A(5):759–62.

22. Neuhaus V, King J, Hageman MG, et al. Charlson comorbidity indices and in-hospital deaths in patients with hip fractures. Clin Orthop Relat Res 2013;471(5):1712–9.

23. Karpanen TJ, Worthington T, Conway BR, et al. Permeation of chlorhexidine from alcoholic and aqueous solutions within excised human skin. Antimicrob Agents Chemother 2009;53(4):1717–9.

24. Bozic KJ, Bashyal RK, Anthony SG, et al. Is administratively coded comorbidity and complication data in total joint arthroplasty valid? Clin Orthop Relat Res 2013;471(1):201–5.

25. Malinzak RA, Small SR, Rogge RD, et al. The effect of rotating platform TKA on strain distribution and torque transmission on the proximal tibia. J Arthroplasty 2014;29(3):541–7.

26. Malinzak RA, Ritter MA, Berend ME, et al. Morbidly obese, diabetic, younger, and unilateral joint arthroplasty patients have elevated total joint arthroplasty infection rates. J Arthroplasty 2009;24(6 Suppl):84–8.

27. D'Apuzzo MR, Novicoff WM, Browne JA. The John Insall Award: morbid obesity independently impacts complications, mortality, and resource use after TKA. Clin Orthop Relat Res 2015;473(1):57–63.

28. Ladha KS, Zhao K, Quraishi SA, et al. The Deyo-Charlson and Elixhauser-van Walraven comorbidity indices as predictors of mortality in critically ill patients. BMJ Open 2015;5(9):e008990.

29. Stanton T. OREF Award goes to SPORT project. AAOS Now 2014. Available at: http://www6.aaos.org/news/PDFopen/PDFopen.cfm?page_url=http://www.aaos.org/news/aaosnow/apr14/research5.asp. Accessed October 8, 2015.

30. Maloney WJ. National joint replacement registries: has the time come? J Bone Joint Surg Am 2001; 83-A(10):1582–5.

31. Belmont PJ Jr, Goodman GP, Kusnezov NA, et al. Postoperative myocardial infarction and cardiac arrest following primary total knee and hip arthroplasty: rates, risk factors, and time of occurrence. J Bone Joint Surg Am 2014;96(24):2025–31.

32. Bozic KJ, Kurtz SM, Lau E, et al. The epidemiology of revision total knee arthroplasty in the United States. Clin Orthop Relat Res 2010; 468(1):45–51.

33. Lansky D, Milstein A. Quality measurement in orthopaedics: the purchasers' view. Clin Orthop Relat Res 2009;467(10):2548–55.

34. Hauser DL, Wessinger SJ, Condon RT, et al. An electronic database for outcome studies that includes digital radiographs. J Arthroplasty 2001; 16(8 Suppl 1):71–5.

35. Malchau H, Garellick G, Eisler T, et al. Presidential guest address: the Swedish Hip Registry: increasing the sensitivity by patient outcome data. Clin Orthop Relat Res 2005;441:19–29.

36. Brinker MR, O'Connor DP. Stakeholders in outcome measures: review from a clinical perspective. Clin Orthop Relat Res 2013;471(11):3426–36.

37. Saleh KJ, Bershadsky B, Cheng E, et al. Lessons learned from the hip and knee musculoskeletal outcomes data evaluation and management system. Clin Orthop Relat Res 2004;(429):272–8.

38. Franklin PD, Lewallen D, Bozic K, et al. Implementation of patient-reported outcome measures in U.S. total joint replacement registries: rationale, status, and plans. J Bone Joint Surg Am 2014;96(Suppl 1): 104–9.

39. Bozic KJ, Chiu V. Quality measurement and public reporting in total joint arthroplasty. J Arthroplasty 2008;23(6 Suppl 1):146–9.

40. Bozic KJ, Smith AR, Mauerhan DR. Pay-for-performance in orthopedics: implications for clinical practice. J Arthroplasty 2007;22(6 Suppl 2):8–12.

41. O'Brien JM, Corrigan J, Reitzner JB, et al. Will performance measurement lead to better patient outcomes? What are the roles of the National Quality Forum and Medical Specialty Societies? Chest 2012;141(2):300–7.

42. Quality measures for public reporting: final recommendations to the Minnesota Department of Health. 2009. Available at: http://www.health.state.mn.us/healthreform/measurement/QualityMeasures_FinalRecs.pdf. Accessed September 21, 2015.

43. Illinois hospital report card: where the data comes from. 2015. Available at: http://www.healthcarereportcard.illinois.gov/contents/view/data_sources. Accessed September 21, 2015.

44. Morrissey J. Internet company rates hospitals. Mod Healthc 1999;29(33):24–5.

45. Bakhsh W, Mesfin A. Online ratings of orthopedic surgeons: analysis of 2185 reviews. Am J Orthop 2014;43(8):359–63.

46. Shively N. UCLA sued over recent hospital records hacking. 2015. Available at: http://www.latimes.com/business/la-fi-ucla-hack-lawsuit-20150811-story.html. Accessed September 3, 2015.

47. Wang YC, Hart DL, Stratford PW, et al. Clinical interpretation of computerized adaptive test-generated outcome measures in patients with knee impairments. Arch Phys Med Rehabil 2009;90(8):1340–8.

48. Lee SJ, Kavanaugh A, Lenert L. Electronic and computer-generated patient questionnaires in standard care. Best practice & research. Clin Rheumatol 2007;21(4):637–47.

49. Larsson US, Svardsudd K, Wedel H, et al. Patient involvement in decision-making in surgical and orthopaedic practice: the Project Perioperative Risk. Soc Sci Med 1989;28(8):829–35.

Big Data, Big Problems

Incorporating Mission, Values, and Culture in Provider Affiliations

Steven H. Shaha, PhD, DBA[a], Zain Sayeed, MSc, MHA[b],
Afshin A. Anoushiravani, MD[b],
Mouhanad M. El-Othmani, MD[b],
Khaled J. Saleh, MD, MSc, FRCS (C), MHCM, CPE[c],*

KEYWORDS

- Big data • Comparative effectiveness • Orthopedics • Total joint arthroplasty
- Administrative database • Clinical database

KEY POINTS

- Big data refers to electronic health data sets so large and diverse that they cannot be easily managed with traditional software.
- Orthopedic data are often reported in five broad measures: structural, process, outcome, patient experience, and efficiency.
- On selection of electronic health record (EHR) systems, orthopedic surgeons must consider the capability of an EHR to ensure data quality, interoperability, and assistance at point of musculoskeletal care.

INTRODUCTION

Among the more compelling trends in health care is the rising use of big data. Driven by health care reform and efforts to improve delivery of care by cost-effective means, immense quantities of data ("big data") are being collected over extensive periods of time.[1] These initiatives support wide ranges of health care function, such as population health management and clinical decision support (CDS).[2,3] By definition, big data refers to electronic health data sets so large and diverse that they cannot be easily managed with traditional software.[4] Inputs from clinical support systems, patient health records, sensor data, and patient-specific variables all contribute to big data in the health care industry.[4] As such, big data enables regulatory agencies to assess the performance of organizations, while allowing communities to understand specific population patterns and needs.

For health care providers amidst such complexity lies the opportunity to use big data to aid in assessment of practice patterns and predict future needs.[4] At a macro level, governmental and organizational leadership have acquired the ability to assess performance maximization with use of big data analytics.[5,6] Such evaluation will continue to grow, because it is reported that big data for US health care will soon reach to yottabytes (10^{24} gigabytes) in size.[7] Furthermore, efforts have been made to integrate computer technology, mobile applications, and electronic health record (EHR) software to store and track data.[5,6] These inputs, collectively termed health information technology, have

---

Funding Sources: No additional funding sources were used for this article.

Conflicts of Interest: No conflicts of interest are evident for authors of this article.

[a] Center for Public Policy and Administration, 260 South Central Campus Drive, Room 214, University of Utah, Salt Lake City, UT 84112, USA; [b] Division of Orthopaedics and Rehabilitation, Southern Illinois University School of Medicine, 701 North First Street, Springfield, IL 62781, USA; [c] Department of Orthopaedic and Sports Medicine, Detroit Medical Center, 311 Mack Avenue, 5th Floor, Detroit, MI 48201, USA

* Corresponding author.

E-mail address: kjsaleh@gmail.com

added to more than 120 patient registries either being developed or in operation.[8] This exponential rise in big data initiatives draws the question of whether big data is truly an asset, at the grandeur often promoted for a new capability, for meeting needs within a host of more real-time and granular realities.

Despite the intentions of big data initiatives, some argue that for the past several decades improved health care delivery to patients has been limited, that health care reform has added little value to patient care.[9] In part, the challenge results from the fact that the types of the data being collected are without proper context and compare outcomes over extended time periods. This purpose contrasts with the information needs of surgeons and patients in real-time. Within the orthopedic community use of big data analytics may allow surgeons to reach a deeper understanding of outcomes that can be applied at the point of musculoskeletal care. Specific population data may determine appropriate treatment options for particular patients, enhancing the decision-making process.

This article explores how integration of data from clinical registries and EHRs produces a quality impact within orthopedic practices. We differentiate data from information, and define several types of data that are collected and used in orthopedic outcome measurement. Furthermore, we assess the concept of comparative effectiveness and its impact on orthopedic clinical research. This article also places emphasis on how the concept of big data produces health care challenges balanced with benefits that may be faced by patients and orthopedic surgeons. Finally, we review essential characteristics of an EHR that interlinks musculoskeletal care and big data initiatives.

DIFFERENTIATING DATA AND INFORMATION

A large driver behind big data initiatives is the nationwide shift from a volume-based to value-based health care system.[9] Adding value to musculoskeletal care cannot avoid collection and reporting of cost and quality information of orthopedic procedures.[10] This perspective has lent toward objectifying value assessment by health outcomes per dollar spent.[10,11] Thus, within the past decade an increasing tendency is noted toward public reporting of outcomes-based performance measures.[12] Consequently, it has become imperative for hospitals, providers, and patients to differentiate data from information. Data are simply the building blocks

by which information is built, whereas information gives data meaning and context.[13] In some discussions data are raw, and have not been molded into information.[13] Information gathered from such data may be used clinically, to aid in treatment of patients; administratively, to charge a patient or insurance party; and macroscopically, to analyze trends between hospitals or the competency of clinicians. Until data are rendered to generate information, they do not provide answers, or aid in clinical decision-making.[13]

TYPES OF DATA COLLECTED AND A BRIEF OVERVIEW OF LARGE DATASETS

Several types of data continue to be collected nationwide. Marjoua and colleagues[10] demonstrate that orthopedic data are often reported in five broad measures: (1) structural, (2) process, (3) outcome, (4) patient experience, and (5) efficiency. Table 1 provides definitions and examples of these types of measures.[10] Such data are recorded in clinical databases that come in two forms: administrative databases and clinical registries. Administrative databases store insurance claims and reimbursement data, whereas clinical databases collect data specific to a disease process or procedure.[14,15] The federal government afforded early efforts at reducing health care costs and driving outcomes research primarily focused on large administrative claims data.

These administrative datasets have been updated and maintained by the Centers for Medicare and Medicaid services and the Agency for Healthcare and Research Quality.[14,15] The Agency for Healthcare and Research Quality is a federal agency charged with collecting and analyzing in-hospital outcomes and resource utilization trends nationally. Interestingly, federally curated datasets have been primarily used to report epidemiologic resource utilization analyses. Furthermore, claims data are limited in that they do not capture information on patient comorbidities, disease severity, conditions present during admission, patient satisfaction, and socioeconomic factors.[14,15] Currently there are several databases available for the evaluation of administrative variables, with the ones most frequently used in orthopedics being the Medicare claims dataset, National Inpatient Sample, and Kid's Inpatient Database.[14,15] The Medicare claims dataset is the most comprehensive database for inpatient and outpatient claims, with greater than 45 million identifiable patient samples.[14,15] Although highly powered, the dataset

Table 1		
Types of data collected in musculoskeletal care		
Type of Data	**Definition**	**Example**
Structural	Refer to provider infrastructure, such as type of medical facility, availability of level one trauma resources, and use of electronic medical record.	Patient chart information, electronic medical record usage
Process	Measurements that assess adherence to evidence-based practice guidelines.	Surgical site marking, thromboprophylaxis
Outcome	Measurement of postoperative events in administrative claims data; require risk adjustment.	Readmission rate, reoperation rate, rates of postoperative infection
Patient experience	Patient-centered measurement of subjective experience.	Patient satisfaction surveys, patient-reported outcome measures
Efficiency	Cost analysis as it pertains to episode of care. Measured with ease, but often poorly relates with quality and requires risk adjustment for comparison.	Costs of imaging and physical therapy service per episode of care

Adapted from Marjoua Y, Butler CA, Bozic KJ. Public reporting of cost and quality information in orthopaedics. Clin Orthop Relat Res 2012;470(4):1019.

is limited by its inherent design.[14,15] The dataset is heavily reliant on International Classification Diagnosis-9-Clinical Modification codes, thus it is ineffective at assessing nonbillable outcomes. Furthermore, Medicare claims data lack basic information on implant type, surgical approach, laterality, and patient-reported outcome measures.

Within the past two decades further expansion of clinical registries has gained significant notoriety. An example is the Function and Outcome Research for Comparative Effectiveness in Total Joint Replacement Program.[16,17] This program encompasses data from orthopedic practices in the United States including academic centers, community hospitals, and private practice.[8] The program focuses on collecting patient-centered outcome measures, such as range of motion scores, complications and adverse events, patient-specific characteristics, and clinical examination data.[8] Another clinical registry produced by a single institution is the Hospital for Special Surgery Total Joint Replacement registry.[18] Since 2007, this registry has been able to enroll more than 10,000 patients with total joint replacement.[18] Patient data regarding preoperative characteristics (demographics, activity scores, expectations, and other questionnaires), intraoperative findings (implant type, surgical approach, and so forth), and postoperative outcomes (complications, length of stay, and so forth) are also recorded, with extensive follow-up (at least 2 years).[18] Furthermore, research assistants enter patient information into a secure World Wide Web–based database system that is designed to gather registry inputs.[18] Thus, clinical registries have the capability to gather several variables that will likely have substantial impact on comparative value of varying orthopedic practice trends.

UNDERSTANDING COMPARATIVE EFFECTIVENESS RESEARCH IN ORTHOPEDICS

As the ascendancy of big data ensues, the characteristics of orthopedic clinical research have expanded to incorporate the concept of comparative effectiveness.[19] Comparative effectiveness research aims to assist patients, clinicians, and policy makers to make informed decisions on how to improve individual and population-based musculoskeletal care.[19] Hence, recent literature has shifted focus on evaluating current treatments in varying populations to identify specific characteristics of providers and organizations that affect health care delivery and outcome. Effectiveness research requires accurate measurement, powered sample sizes, and data that describes specific characteristics of patient and provider in each episode of musculoskeletal care.[20,21]

At present, no standardized method exists that enables capturing data on the scale and scope required by various stakeholders in orthopedics. Another component of effectiveness research is its ability to assess and quantify the quality of care delivered to varying patient populations, resulting in adjusted reimbursement, accordingly.[12] Such a change in direction for the health care industry has resulted in publically reported data regarding the comparative value of involved stakeholders.

Patients, surgeons, researchers, payers, policy makers, and other related parties (pharmacologic, device manufacturers, academic institutions, and so forth) approach outcomes reporting with varying perspectives. Specifically, orthopedic outcome reporting requires data collected consistently from surgeons that practice in a variety of settings including community hospitals, private practice, and academic institutions.[22] Several barriers exist that affect the ability to obtain meaningful data across populations including, but not limited to, resource constraints and issues related to data management.[20,21] In particular, community surgeons often do not use outcome measures routinely to aid in clinical decision-making for musculoskeletal care.[20,21] Thus, it becomes difficult to impart routine data collection methods without adopting new costs and practice burdens in such settings.[20,21]

Furthermore, clinical practice often focuses on delivery of optimal musculoskeletal care without research embedded in the process. Collection of varying outcome measures and meaningful information involves abstraction of data from clinical and administrative databases that are subject to lack of structure and format across providers.[23,24] Such variability introduces retrieval errors that may be costly in terms of patient care. An example of such issues is reflected in the extensive reprogramming required by statisticians in the analysis of diverse data sets.

Although the ability of comparative effectiveness studies to propel orthopedic research has yet to be fully elucidated, certain contextual parameters must be understood by patients, providers, and health care institutions. Contextual factors including specialty of providers, types of EHR system, institutional characteristics, and patient-specific factors as they relate to an episode of musculoskeletal care hold tremendous impact in outcome measurement and data-reporting.[25] Because comparative effectiveness research intends to determine the effect of characteristics of providers, facilities, and systems on treatment outcomes, ignoring contextual factors in observational studies lends to confounded interpretation.[18,20] Accordingly, data on specified characteristics must be thoroughly collected to avoid introduction of bias that may limit the generalizability of reported results.

UNDERSTANDING BIG DATA STRENGTHS AND CHALLENGES FOR THE PATIENT AND THE PROVIDER

The strengths and limitations of big data are best considered through a variety of perspectives. First, one can visualize the real-time delivery of musculoskeletal care as it pertains to the patient. In an episode of care in which patients and orthopedists interact, the information they need is personal and immediate. Big data knowledge of community needs, population characteristics, and proven best practices can add enormous insight and assist in making best decisions. Thus, each patient and episode of care must be addressed by context and not a "one size fits all" approach. A list of contextual considerations for patients, providers, and institutions is provided in Table 2.

In the past decade patients are more inclined to select surgeons and institutions with

Table 2		
Contextual parameters to consider for patients, surgeons, and health care organizations		
Patient	**Orthopedic Surgeon**	**Health Care Organization**
Demographics: age, race, sex, employment, household income, relationship status	Geographic location: rural, urban, suburban	Geographic location: rural, urban, suburban
Geographic location: rural, urban, suburban	Experience: years in practice, fellowship training, board certifications	Hospital system: trauma center, community, private surgical group
Diagnosis: stage and prognosis of disease	Practice setting: community hospital, academic medical center, private practice	Technology: medical supplies, implants, disposables, type of information system used
Comorbidities: injury, acute condition, chronic condition	Case volume: number of cases, case mix	Payers and payment type: private, public, Medicare, workers compensation
Risk factors and behaviors: obesity, illicit drug use, activity level, diet, tobacco use, alcohol use		

information provided by big data reporting. Although such research is available for patients to aid in decision-making, patients must be cognizant of missing data and patient dropout that is not entirely clear in reported clinical research.[26–29] In either consumer or regulatory scenarios involving comparative reporting, big data can provide information far beyond what any individual (practitioner or patient) could readily discern. For example, HealthGrades, an online health care rating World Wide Web site, uses publicly available data sets to analyze rates of readmission and infection.[11] As such, patients select providers or institutions based on administrative data that represent an oversimplified view of patient care. Because big data registries continue to report clinical statistics, such as rates of postoperative infection, readmission, and length of hospital stay, little focus is placed on patient-centered outcomes.[22] Essentially, amid more wholesome contextual reporting, combining cost and utilization data with functional recovery scores may provide more robust information for patients to decide elective care.

For orthopedic surgeons, big data evidence at times may represent simplified, aggregate variables. This intentionally summarizes data from masses of detail to enable appropriate comprehension at varying levels of musculoskeletal care.[30] Often orthopedic literature incorporates the use of comorbidity indices, such as the Charlson Score, to allow for outcome analysis.[31] The Charlson Score predicts 10-year mortality for 22 common comorbid conditions, while effectively deidentifying the comorbidity. Simply put, a past diagnosis of diabetes is not necessarily the same as a past history of congestive heart failure. Nonetheless, each diagnosis is weighted similarly in calculation of Charlson Score. Although such a tool enables stratification of cohort samples for statistical validity and comparison, it does not take into consideration contextual data that are necessary for generalization across varying clinical settings, inherently confounding reported results. To validate orthopedic evidence abstracted from big data registries, guidelines for design and reporting of quality observational trials have been made.[32] This includes strengthening the reporting of observational studies in epidemiology criteria.[32] Use of such design criteria and appropriate methodology can mitigate the limitations of observational research and depict realistic clinical practice, resulting in higher external validity.[33]

Another challenge faced by orthopedic surgeons is that big data is statistically lagged and may represent findings from time periods that are outdated. Several observational studies assess outcome analysis from select time frames that are restricted by the type of data set used. For example, a study Westermann and colleagues[34] assessed the epidemiology of reverse shoulder arthroplasty in the United States using National Inpatient Sample. The study was inherently limited by coding practices in that before 2011 total shoulder arthroplasty and reverse shoulder arthroplasty were coded identically; however, after 2011 separate codes were formed for each procedure. Therefore, any study assessing shoulder arthroplasty dating before 2011 must be closely assessed by practicing surgeons. Seldom does big data information represent anything in real-time and therefore must be thoroughly investigated before application in clinical settings.

ELECTRONIC MEDICAL RECORD: CAPTURING CONTEXT AND BIG DATA

Big data encompasses many benefits and challenges for patients and providers. The study of big data cannot be fully investigated without discussing the role EHR plays for applied big data initiatives. EHR surpasses many existing registries and large data sets in volume and provider usability.[23] The data from EHR also offer perspective of real-time musculoskeletal care and outcomes of diverse patient populations that represent actual practice.[23] As orthopedic surgeons continue to play administrative roles in health care organizations and private groups, the process of EHR selection often becomes a conversation of ensuring data quality, interoperability, and assistance at point of musculoskeletal care.

The ability of electronic medical records (EMRs) to capture quality data depends on several factors including completeness, correctness, concordance, plausibility, and currency (Table 3). Although each characteristic aids in determining data quality, orthopedists must focus extensively on completeness and correctness when evaluating an EMR for big data and research initiatives, because these variables aid in contextual comparison. Data completeness is defined by how well an EHR is able to capture data that represents routine clinical care and serve a purpose for secondary analyses.[35] Data correctness measures the proportion of true data elements present in a given EMR.[36] Hogan and Wagner[36] assessed the quality of data recorded by EMR systems to range between 44% and 100% in correctness, and 1.1% and

Table 3 Characteristics of EHR data input	
Correctness	Is what is recorded in the EHR accurate?
Completeness	Is the entire clinical episode properly recorded in the EHR?
Concordance	Is there agreement between elements in the EHR and other clinical records?
Plausibility	Does what is recorded in the EHR make sense in light of other contextual data regarding the episode of care?
Currency	Is what is present in EHR a relevant representation of the episode of care at a given time point?

100% in completeness. More recently, Chan and colleagues[37] demonstrate that EHR data are variable across clinical settings and multiple institutions because of differences in measurement, recording, and clinical focus. Therefore, it is imperative that the orthopedist develop a full understanding of the interrelationship of patient care, research tasks, and data quality when selecting an EMR for their respective health care institution.

Another major concept of EMR is the ability of recorded data to have an interoperability function. In 2009, the US Congress allocated $19 billion to promote use of EHR as a component of the Affordable Care Act.[38] Additionally, meaningful use clauses have arisen as major components of newer reimbursement models as a result of such resource allocation.[38] Despite such investment, the problem remains in the inability of EHRs to communicate with one another.[39] Interoperability, defined as a continuity function of EHR, allows data to be mobilized from one institution or provider to another, without loss of data.[40] Furthermore, in a position statement by the American Academy of Orthopaedic Surgeons, it was strongly recommended that all EHR develop interoperability functions to improve patient safety, increase clinical efficiency, reduce costs, and allow transfer of patient information.[41] In alignment with big data initiatives, interoperability allows for integration of varying EHR data across institutions. Further research is necessary in assessing the quality impact of interoperability of EMR in orthopedic practice.

Finally, the highest function of EHR is to aid in CDS.[42] CDS is the ability of EMR to use passive or active decision support to modify provider behavior.[42] Studies have shown that CDS is able to aid in varying clinical settings. Zaouter and colleagues[43] assessed the use of a decision support system in the management of hemodynamic and respiratory events in orthopedic patients under propofol sedation and spinal anesthesia.

Investigators reported that of the 150 patients enrolled in their study, 100% of respiratory and hemodynamic critical events were detected in the group using the CDS function, whereas the non-CDS group missed 26% of such critical events. Zaouter and colleagues[43] concluded that CDS may help clinicians detect and treat critical events more efficiently. The ability of big data and EHR to effectively aid orthopedic surgeons in real time has yet to be fully elucidated; however, such EHR capability holds substantial benefit in orthopedic practice across settings.

SUMMARY

As the rise of big data continues to affect orthopedic practice, it is imperative that surgeons be aware of benefits and challenges associated with such initiatives. Attention to methods of how to integrate EHR and big data capability may provide substantial benefit to orthopedic surgeons and their patients. As health reform continues to assess value in musculoskeletal care, further research is necessary in assessing the effects of big data initiatives on orthopedic practices nationwide.

REFERENCES

1. Mathias B, Lipori G, Moldawer LL, et al. Integrating "big data" into surgical practice. Surgery 2015; 159(2):371–4.
2. Fernandes L, O'Connor M, Weaver V. Big data, bigger outcomes: healthcare is embracing the big data movement, hoping to revolutionize HIM by distilling vast collection of data for specific analysis. J AHIMA 2012;83(10):38–43 [quiz: 4].
3. Feldman B, Martin EM, Skotnes T. Big data in healthcare hype and hope 2012. Available at: http://www.west-info.eu/files/big-data-in-healthcare.pdf. Accessed November 6, 2015.
4. Perry DC, Parsons N, Costa ML. 'Big data' reporting guidelines: how to answer big questions, yet avoid big problems. Bone Joint J 2014;96-b(12):1575–7.

5. Wasser T, Haynes K, Barron J, et al. Using 'big data' to validate claims made in the pharmaceutical approval process. J Med Econ 2015;18(12):1013–9.
6. Berger ML, Doban V. Big data, advanced analytics and the future of comparative effectiveness research. J Comp Eff Res 2014;3(2):167–76.
7. Drowning in big data? Reducing information technology complexities and costs for healthcare organizations. Frost and Sullivan - website. Available at: http://www.emc.com/campaign/global/healthcare/reduce-health-it-costs-complexity.htm. Accessed November 6, 2015.
8. Association AM. An inventory of national clinical registries 2014. Available at: http://www.abms.org/media/1356/nqrn-registry-inventory.pdf. Accessed November 6, 2015.
9. Porter ME, Teisberg EO. Redefining competition in health care. Harv Bus Rev 2004;82(6):64–76, 136.
10. Marjoua Y, Butler CA, Bozic KJ. Public reporting of cost and quality information in orthopaedics. Clin Orthop Relat Res 2012;470(4):1017–26.
11. Saleh KJ, Bozic KJ, Graham DB, et al. Quality in orthopaedic surgery: an international perspective. AOA critical issues. J Bone Joint Surg Am 2013;95(1):e3.
12. Dranove D, Kessler D, McClellan M, et al. Is more information better? The effects of 'report cards' on health care providers. J Polit Econ 2003;111:555–88.
13. Zins C. Conceptual approaches for defining data, information, and knowledge. J Am Soc Inf Sci Technol 2007;58(4):479–93.
14. Pugely AJ, Martin CT, Harwood J, et al. Database and registry research in orthopaedic surgery. Part I: claims-based data. J Bone Joint Surg Am 2015;97(15):1278–87.
15. Pugely AJ, Martin CT, Harwood J, et al. Database and registry research in orthopaedic surgery. Part 2: clinical registry data. J Bone Joint Surg Am 2015;97(21):1799–808.
16. Ayers DC, Zheng H, Franklin PD. Integrating patient-reported outcomes into orthopaedic clinical practice: proof of concept from FORCE-TJR. Clin Orthop Relat Res 2013;471(11):3419–25.
17. Franklin PD, Harrold L, Ayers DC. Incorporating patient-reported outcomes in total joint arthroplasty registries: challenges and opportunities. Clin Orthop Relat Res 2013;471(11):3482–8.
18. Mushlin AI, Ghomrawi HM. Comparative effectiveness research: a cornerstone of healthcare reform? Trans Am Clin Climatol Assoc 2010;121:141–54 [discussion: 54–5].
19. Institute of Medicine. Initial national priorities for comparative effectiveness research. Washington, DC: The National Academic Press; 2009.
20. O'Connor DP, Brinker MR. Challenges in outcome measurement: clinical research perspective. Clin Orthop Relat Res 2013;471(11):3496–503.
21. Noble PC, Fuller-Lafreniere S, Meftah M, et al. Challenges in outcome measurement: discrepancies between patient and provider definitions of success. Clin Orthop Relat Res 2013;471(11):3437–45.
22. Franklin PD, Allison JJ, Ayers DC. Beyond joint implant registries: a patient-centered research consortium for comparative effectiveness in total joint replacement. JAMA 2012;308(12):1217–8.
23. Weiskopf NG, Weng C. Methods and dimensions of electronic health record data quality assessment: enabling reuse for clinical research. J Am Med Inform Assoc 2013;20(1):144–51.
24. Weng C, Appelbaum P, Hripcsak G, et al. Using EHRs to integrate research with patient care: promises and challenges. J Am Med Inform Assoc 2012;19(5):684–7.
25. Barrack RL. The results of TKA: what the registries don't tell us. Orthopedics 2011;34(9):e485–7.
26. Little RJ, Cohen ML, Dickersin K, et al. The design and conduct of clinical trials to limit missing data. Stat Med 2012;31(28):3433–43.
27. Wood AM, White IR, Thompson SG. Are missing outcome data adequately handled? A review of published randomized controlled trials in major medical journals. Clin Trials 2004;1(4):368–76.
28. Singhal R, Rana R. Intricacy of missing data in clinical trials: deterrence and management. Int J Appl Basic Med Res 2014;4(Suppl 1):S2–5.
29. Louie DL, Earp BE, Blazar PE. Finding orthopedic patients lost to follow-up for long-term outcomes research using the Internet: an update for 2012. Orthopedics 2012;35(7):595–9.
30. Hersh WR. Adding value to the electronic health record through secondary use of data for quality assurance, research, and surveillance. Am J Manag Care 2007;13(6 Part 1):277–8.
31. Charlson ME, Pompei P, Ales KL, et al. A new method of classifying prognostic comorbidity in longitudinal studies: development and validation. J Chronic Dis 1987;40(5):373–83.
32. Vandenbroucke JP, von Elm E, Altman DG, et al. Strengthening the Reporting of Observational Studies in Epidemiology (STROBE): explanation and elaboration. Int J Surg 2014;12(12):1500–24.
33. Hoppe DJ, Schemitsch EH, Morshed S, et al. Hierarchy of evidence: where observational studies fit in and why we need them. J Bone Joint Surg Am 2009;91(Suppl 3):2–9.
34. Westermann RW, Pugely AJ, Martin CT, et al. Reverse shoulder arthroplasty in the United States: a comparison of national volume, patient demographics, complications, and surgical indications. Iowa Orthop J 2015;35:1–7.
35. Soto M, Capurro D, Catalan S. Evaluating the data completeness in the electronic health record after the implementation of an outpatient electronic

health record. Stud Health Technol Inform 2015; 216:885.

36. Hogan WR, Wagner MM. Accuracy of data in computer-based patient records. J Am Med Inform Assoc 1997;4(5):342–55.

37. Chan KS, Fowles JB, Weiner JP. Review: electronic health records and the reliability and validity of quality measures: a review of the literature. Med Care Res Rev 2010;67(5):503–27.

38. Jha AK, Burke MF, DesRoches C, et al. Progress toward meaningful use: hospitals' adoption of electronic health records. Am J Manag Care 2011; 17(12 Spec No.):Sp117–24.

39. Wilkonson J. Electronic medical records. 2015. Available at: http://www.aaos.org/AAOSNow/2015/May/managing/managing1/?ssopc=1. Accessed November 6, 2015.

40. Balas A, Al Sanousi A. Interoperable electronic patient records for health care improvement. Stud Health Technol Inform 2009;150:19–23.

41. Surgeons AAoO. Position statement on electronic health record. 2015. Available at: http://www.aaos.org/CustomTemplates/Content.aspx?id=5619&ssopc=1. Accessed November 6, 2015.

42. Rothman B, Leonard JC, Vigoda MM. Future of electronic health records: implications for decision support. Mount Sinai J Med 2012;79(6): 757–68.

43. Zaouter C, Wehbe M, Cyr S, et al. Use of a decision support system improves the management of hemodynamic and respiratory events in orthopedic patients under propofol sedation and spinal analgesia: a randomized trial. J Clin Monit Comput 2014;28(1):41–7.

Trauma

Tibial Stress Fractures in Athletes

John J. Feldman, MD[a],*, Eric N. Bowman, MD[b], Barry B. Phillips, MD[c],
John C. Weinlein, MD[d]

KEYWORDS

- Tibia • Stress fracture • Athlete • Intramedullary fixation • Tension band plate

---

KEY POINTS

- Tibial stress fractures are common in the athlete. There are various causes of these fractures, the most common being a sudden increase in training intensity.
- Most of these injuries are treated conservatively; however, some may require operative intervention. This is mostly dictated by location of the fracture, as well as failure of conservative treatment.
- There are several surgical options available to the treating surgeon, each with advantages and disadvantages.
- The physician must understand the nature of the fracture and the likelihood for it to heal in a timely manner in order to best treat these fractures in this patient subset.

Tibial stress fractures are relatively common in athletes, with a reported incidence as high as 10% to 20% in runners.[1] Treatment varies based on a number of factors, including cause, location, and duration of symptoms. Most tibial stress fractures heal uneventfully with conservative treatment; however, some can be more challenging, ultimately requiring surgery. In athletes, time to recovery is a strong consideration in the decision algorithm. Missing competition for an extended period of time can have a psychosocial impact, and, in the case of professional athletes, an economic impact. Physicians must know which fractures will likely heal in a reasonable time period and which fractures are prone to delayed union or nonunion.

Tibial stress fractures are caused by repetitive microtrauma that results in increased osteoclastic activity and an imbalance between resorption and regeneration of bone.[2] They commonly occur in individuals participating in strenuous activity such as military training and athletics. Certain sports such as running have a high occurrence of stress fractures, with the tibia being the most common site.

Underlying intrinsic and extrinsic factors can predispose individuals to developing these fractures.[3] Intrinsic factors include hormonal imbalances, nutritional deficiencies, metabolic bone diseases, relative avascularity of an area of bone, and muscle imbalances. Extrinsic factors include sudden increases in the intensity of an exercise regime. Often the intrinsic and extrinsic causes are related and may occur simultaneously. The female athletic triad of amenorrhea, disordered eating, and low bone mineral density results from an excessive training regimen coupled with decreased caloric intake.

Disclosures: B.B. Phillips is a paid presenter or speaker for Arthrex, Incorporated, and receives publishing royalties from Saunders/Mosby-Elsevier. J. Weinlein receives publishing royalties from Saunders/Mosby-Elsevier.
[a] Department of Orthopaedics, University of Tennessee-Campbell Clinic, 49 South 4th Street, Apartment 208, Memphis, TN 38103, USA; [b] Department of Orthopaedics, University of Tennessee-Campbell Clinic, 170 Alexander Street, Memphis, TN 38111, USA; [c] Department of Orthopaedics, Campbell Clinic Orthopaedics, University of Tennesee-Campbell Clinic, 1400 South Germantown Road, Germantown, TN 38138, USA; [d] Department of Orthopaedics, University of Tennessee–Campbell Clinic, 145 Greenbriar Drive, Memphis, TN 38117, USA
* Corresponding author.
E-mail address: feldman.john@gmail.com

Low body fat percentage leads to a decrease in estrogen levels with resultant osteoporosis and a propensity toward stress fracture.

Stress fractures commonly occur in 3 areas of the tibia: posteromedial cortex, anterior cortex, and tibial plateau. The posteromedial cortex is the most common site. Stress fractures in the anterior cortex are less common, with an incidence of around 4% of all tibial stress fractures.[1] The anterior tibial cortex is the tension side of the bone, and stress fractures in this area can be more problematic, as the healing potential is lower. The dreaded black line has been described as a V or wedge-shaped defect in the anterior cortex[1] (Fig. 1). They tend to be more common in athletes who participate in jumping and leaping activities, such as gymnasts and basketball players,[4] but they also occur in runners.

HISTORY

Appropriate treatment depends on prompt and accurate diagnosis. Patients report insidious onset of pain without a history of trauma. Pain is worsened by activity, particularly repetitive loading. Initially, pain increases at the end of activity and may be relieved with rest. Gradually, symptoms worsen and may persist beyond activity, frequently at night. Patients often describe an acute change in training regimen with an increase in activity.[3]

The physician should elicit a complete history related to diet, menstrual function, athletic background, and training regimen. Dietary factors to consider extend beyond disordered eating. Low calcium intake and insufficient vitamin D have been associated with lower extremity stress fractures.[5] Low-fat diets also have been shown to increase risk.[6] Low energy availability and excessive exercise, in addition to disordered eating, alter menstrual function and lead to low bone mineral density (BMD).[7]

Females with low body-mass index, amenorrhea, and low mean muscle mass are at increased risk of stress fracture.[6] One or more components of the female athletic triad—amenorrhea, disordered eating, and low BMD—often are present. Of the three, menstrual dysfunction has been implicated as the most important.[5]

Gymnasts, cross country runners, and dancers are at increased risk as well.[8] Attention should be paid to both volume and intensity of workouts. Abrupt changes or increases in training often precipitate a stress fracture.[9] Physicians should recognize conditions associated with osteoporosis or osteopenia including vitamin deficiencies, endocrinopathies, alcoholism, and renal dysfunction.[3]

PHYSICAL EXAMINATION

Tenderness typically is localized with palpation over a diaphyseal stress fracture. Percussion away from the fracture often causes pain. Specific examination tests have been described and can be useful. The hop test, single leg hopping, and the fulcrum test, performed by placing a bending moment on the tibia against either the end of the examination table or the physician's knee or arm, produce severe localized pain in patients with tibial stress fractures. Swelling and overlying skin changes such as bruising should be noted. Possible causative factors should be examined. Structural malalignment, leg length discrepancy, foot deformities,

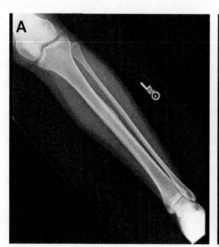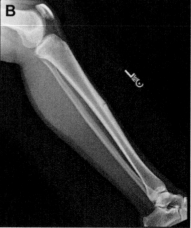

Fig. 1. (A) AP and (B) lateral radiographs of a left tibia demonstrating an anterior cortical stress fracture (dreaded black line) in 16-year-old gymnast.

low lean muscle mass, and smaller calf girth can predispose to increased tibial stress.[6]

DIFFERENTIAL DIAGNOSIS

Stress fractures are the result of normal bone being subjected to abnormal stress. By contrast, insufficiency fractures refer to normal stress applied to abnormal, pathologic, or osteoporotic bone. Pathologic fractures should always be considered, paying particular attention to any history of cancer and other constitutional systemic symptoms. Significant pain without fracture may be present with an osteoid osteoma or other bone tumors.

Medial tibial stress syndrome (MTSS) or traction periostitis (shin splints) causes medial leg pain that usually resolves promptly with conservative treatment. Exertional compartment syndrome and nerve entrapment also should be excluded. A high index of suspicion for infection, both superficial and osteomyelitis, should be maintained, particularly in children and adolescents. Common conditions such as sprains, strains, tendonitis, contusions, and muscle soreness must be excluded. Finally, stress reactions, which are prefractures, present with progressive symptoms.

Among the differential diagnosis for tibial stress fractures, distinguishing posteromedial stress fractures from medial tibial stress syndrome can be challenging. The 2 entities are sometimes grouped together in the literature as part of a continuum of stress reactions.[10] Distinctions have been made with regard to etiology and pathology. MTSS is theorized to be a traction-induced periositis of the medial tibia combined with repetitive bending loads across the tibia.[11] The soleus, which originates from the medial aspect of the tibia along with the flexor digitorum longus, acts as an inverter of the foot and contracts eccentrically during midstance as the foot pronates.[12] Studies have demonstrated that athletes who have increased pronation during midstance are more at risk for MTSS.[2]

MTSS is diagnosed based on history and physical examination. Clinically, the distal two-thirds of the posteromedial border of the tibia are diffusely tender to touch, and soft tissue swelling may be present. Advanced imaging should be used only when the diagnosis is in question or when conservative treatment fails to relieve symptoms. On MRI, MTSS appears as diffuse periosteal edema. Bone scanning has proven to be sensitive in diagnosing MTSS, with a longitudinal area of uptake present on the delayed phase of a triple-phase scintigraphy[13] corresponding to the diffuse area of periostitis. In contrast, all 3 phases of the scan are positive in acute stress fractures.[14]

IMAGING

Plain radiographs often are the first imaging modality used; however, radiographs have a low sensitivity (10% to 50%) for detecting stress fractures, particularly early in the clinical course.[15,16] Predictable progression in findings includes pretibial swelling, thickening of the cortex, and finally a visible fracture on plain films.[15] If initial films are negative, repeat imaging in 2 weeks is indicated. Anteroposterior, lateral, and oblique films should be taken.

MRI has proven to be the best imaging modality for diagnosing fractures that are not visible on plain films, as it is both highly sensitive and specific (Figs. 2 and 3). One study

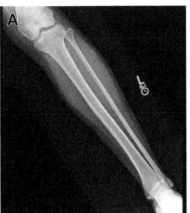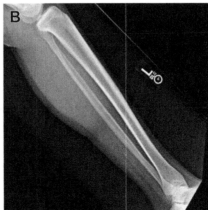

Fig. 2. (A) AP and (B) lateral radiographs of a 47-year-old runner with left tibial pain that do not demonstrate obvious pathology.

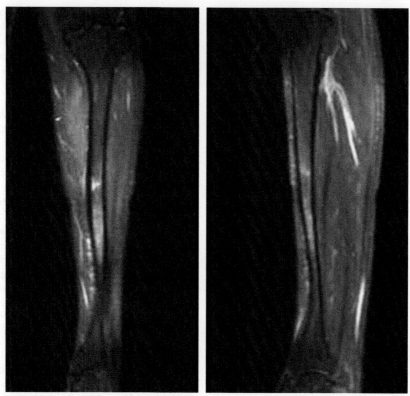

Fig. 3. MRI of the same 47-year-old runner demonstrating increased signal indicative of an occult stress fracture.

comparing MRI with bone scan and computed tomography (CT) showed the sensitivity and specificity of MRI to be 82% and 100%, respectively.[16] Increased signal in the endosteum[16] on fat-suppressed T2-weighted images occurs shortly after the onset of symptoms, prior to evidence on plain radiographs. MRI also provides bony and soft tissue detail that can help differentiate stress fractures from other pathology. This ability can prove especially important in distinguishing tibial stress fractures from MTSS. More severe fractures will have a distinct fracture line apparent on both T1-and T2-weighted sequences.[16]

Before the widespread usage of MRI, radionucleotide bone scanning was the gold standard in diagnosing stress fractures. Like MRI, bone scans are positive within the first several days following the onset of symptoms, often weeks prior to any evidence on plain radiographs. As mentioned previously, all 3 phases of the scan are positive in the presence of a stress fracture. Although sensitive, bone scans lack the specificity of MRI, as any pathology associated with bone remodeling may cause the bone scan to be positive. The exposure of the patient to radiation with bone scanning is another disadvantage compared with MRI.

CT scanning shows great bony detail and is good at demonstrating fractures once the microfractures have consolidated. This process of consolidation, however, may take weeks to occur after the onset of symptoms. For this reason, MRI is better as a diagnostic tool.

OTHER STUDIES

Vitamin D deficiency has been identified in patients with lower extremity stress fractures and should be evaluated.[17,18] Further endocrine or infection work-up may be indicated if history warrants further investigation.

TREATMENT

The consideration of time to return to play is unique to athletes and is a major factor when considering treatment options. For professional athletes, missed time often means missed financial opportunity. For amateur athletes, whose competitive clock is counting down, missed time means missed opportunities. Therefore, the treating physician must recognize fractures that are likely to heal promptly and those that may require longer healing times or may result in a nonunion.

Fortunately, the most common site of tibial stress fractures, the posteromedial cortex, also is the most likely to heal with conservative treatment, most within 4 to 8 weeks. After a thorough history and physical examination, the physician should identify causative factors, and treatment should focus on those factors. Many of these fractures are caused by a sudden change or increase in training regimen. In this scenario, treatment should consist of a period of rest followed by a return to low-impact training and finally high-impact training. The mantra of "let pain be the guide" is the correct approach for this subset of tibial stress fractures, and the athlete may return to full sport once he or she is able to participate in high-impact training without pain.

For female athletes, a history of amenorrhea or oligomenorrhea should prompt a referral to an endocrinologist or gynecologist. A dual-energy x-ray absorbtiometry (DEXA) scan in this patient population also is prudent to screen for osteopenia or osteoporosis. Delayed healing or repeat stress fractures should raise the suspicion of metabolic bone disease and should prompt an endocrinology referral.

In the authors' experience, conservative treatment tends to me more successful with females and patients with low body mass, and so they tend to be more conservative in treating these patients, regardless of where the stress fracture has occurred.

In an effort to expedite return to play, other strategies can be employed such as the use of a pneumatic brace. The brace theoretically neutralizes forces that cause extra strain at the fracture site, helping to reverse the imbalance of osteoclastic and osteoblastic activity and leading to quicker healing. Reported results of the use of pneumatic braces are mixed. One randomized prospective study comparing athletes with tibial stress fractures treated with a pneumatic brace to athletes treated with no brace found a mean return to full activity of 21 days in the brace group and 77 days in the nonbrace group.[19] Another randomized prospective study in military recruits was not as promising, finding no difference in outcomes when comparing time to pain-free hop and time to pain-free 1-mile run.[20] A pneumatic brace has also been reported to be successful in treating delayed union in anterior cortical stress fractures.[21]

Another strategy is the use of extracorporeal tools such as low-intensity pulsed ultrasound (LIPUS) and extracorpeal shockwave therapy (ECST). LIPUS has been shown to increase bone healing in animal models,[22] and has shown some promise in treating fractures in vivo.[23] The results of its use in treating patients with stress fractures are mixed, with the most comprehensive studies showing no difference between ultrasound treatment and controls.[24] Ultrasound has been used with some success in the treatment of delayed union and nonunion of stress fractures of the anterior tibial cortex in athletes.[25] ECST is another treatment modality that, like LIPUS, has shown some promise in the laboratory as well as in treating other forms of nonunion.[26] However, there is sparse literature with regard to its efficacy in treating stress fractures.

Pharmacologic interventions also have utility in the treatment of tibial stress fractures. There has been some evidence to suggest that low levels of vitamin D or calcium may play a role in predisposing athletes to stress fractures.

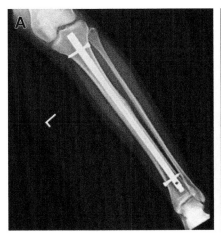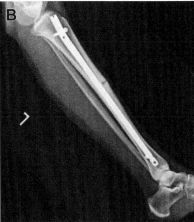

Fig. 4. (A) AP and (B) lateral of left tibia in 16-year-old gymnast with anterior cortical stress fracture treated with intramedullary nail.

Pharmacologic interventions should first be used to correct these deficiencies. Bisphosphonates also have been tried as both treatment[27] and prophylaxis in high-risk populations.[28] In theory, by targeting osteoclasts, bisphosphonates could help tip the balance in favor of healing of stress fractures. Although there is some evidence that bisphosphonate therapy may have some benefit in treating early diagnosed stress fractures,[29] the best evidence to date has not shown a difference in either prevention or treatment when compared with controls.[28,30] Better powered studies are needed to answer this question.

SURGICAL TREATMENT

Surgical treatment typically is reserved for fractures that are deemed at high risk for delayed union or nonunion or for which a prolonged period of conservative treatment has failed to obtain union. In the tibia, the high-risk fractures occur in the anterior cortex, an area notorious for the dreaded black line. For this reason, many physicians have used this radiographic

marker as an indication for surgery. Although the black line is ominous, it does not necessarily mean a nonunion is imminent. Several small series have shown successful conservative treatment of these fractures, employing strategies such as LIPUS, pneumatic braces, and shockwave therapy. The largest series of anterior tibial stress fractures with an attempt at conservative treatment was 50 patients, 40% of whom successfully returned to full activity.[31] Although these studies show that some percentage of these anterior stress fractures can heal with conservative treatment, those that did took an average of about a year.[21,32] In athletes, missing a full year of sports participation can mean missing large parts of 2 athletic seasons depending on the timing of the injury. That much time off could have major ramifications from a financial standpoint for professional athletes and could be career ending for amateur athletes. For this reason, there must be clear communication between the physician and the athlete about goals of treatment and timing of return to play.

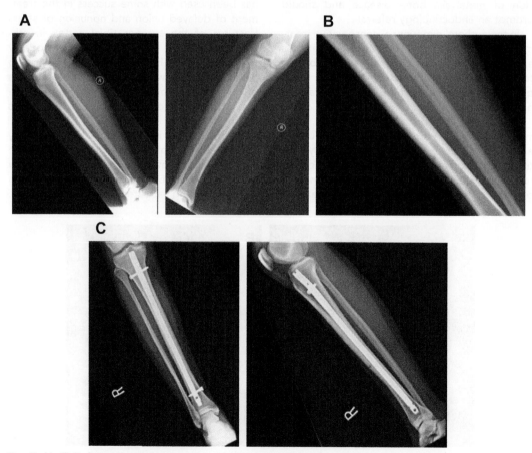

Fig. 5. (A–C) Radiographs of the contralateral tibia in the previously referenced 16-year-old gymnast demonstrating multiple anterior cortical stress fractures treated with an intramedullary nail.

If it is decided that surgery is be the best option, several techniques are available. Intramedullary fixation is one that is frequently used (Fig. 4). Published data reflect positively on this option, with high overall union rates as well as decreased time to union relative to conservative treatment. One study with 11 athletes treated with intramedullary nailing for chronic anterior midtibial stress fractures showed a 100% healing rate, with a mean clinical healing time of 2.7 months and a mean return to sports at 4 months.[33] This technique has not been universally successful, and there have been case reports of acute fractures in tibias treated with intramedullary nails for stress fractures.[34] The major downside to treating athletes with tibial nails is the high incidence of anterior knee pain following surgery. The frequency of moderate pain has been reported to be as high as 80% with conventional infrapatellar nailing at early to near-term follow-up, with 1 study showing improvement to 29% of patients at 8-year follow-up.[35] The effect that this pain has on athletic performance is not clear, but must be a consideration. Commonly, patients with tibial stress fractures have thickened cortices, and, therefore, narrow canals. This reality places a premium on preoperative planning, with special attention to canal size measurement. When treating these fractures with intramedullary nailing, the authors ream up in an effort to debulk some of the thickened cortex. They also use this technique in some cases in which there are multiple stress fractures along the anterior cortex that are not suitable for plate fixation (Fig. 5).

In an effort to treat these fractures without the sequela of anterior knee pain, tension band plating has gained recent popularity. The goal behind this technique is to counteract the tension forces along the anterior cortex and heal the fracture through absolute stability. A recent study of 13 tibial stress fractures treated with tension band plating showed a 100% union rate with union occurring at an average of 9.6 weeks and return to training at an average of 11.1 weeks.[36] The authors used a 2.7 mm or 3.5 mm plate that was contoured and placed in compression mode. The fracture site was debrided, and demineralized bone matrix was used to promote healing (Fig. 6). The downside to this technique is hardware prominence. In this study, 5 of the 13 plates were subsequently removed because of prominence. More long-

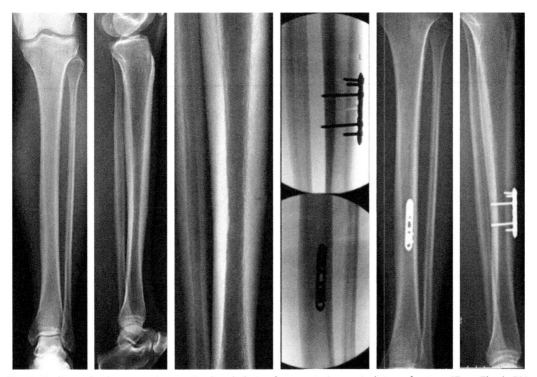

Fig. 6. Radiographs demonstrating tension band plating for an anterior cortical stress fracture. (*From* Zbeda RM, Sculco PK, Urch EY, et al. Tension band plating for chronic anterior tibial stress fractures in high-performance athletes. Am J Sports Med 2015;43(7):1715; with permission.)

term results are needed to determine if there is a risk of refracture around the plate as well following plate removal. There has been 1 case report of a new fracture occurring around the proximal screw within the zone of the plate necessitating revision to an intramedullary nail.[37] Additionally, tension band plating may not be ideal when multiple stress fractures are present.

Other techniques that have been described include drilling and debridement of the fracture site with bone grafting. The authors prefer a technique that uses some form of fixation as it helps both heal the fracture and prevent fracture progression.

SUMMARY

Tibial stress fractures are common in athletes, and most can be treated conservatively. A small subset can be problematic, and physicians must be able to recognize these fractures. Treatment should focus on addressing the cause of the injury. The physician must have a clear understanding of the patients' goals in terms of timing to return to play, as these goals may dictate how aggressive the treatment approach will be. Several surgical options are available, including intramedullary nailing and tension band plating, and it is important for the surgeon to understand the advantages and disadvantages of each to help guide appropriate treatment.

REFERENCES

1. Boden BP, Osbahr DC. High-risk stress fractures: evaluation and treatment. J Am Acad Orthop Surg 2000;8(6):344–53.
2. Bennett JE, Reinking MF, Pluemer B, et al. Factors contributing to the development of medial tibial stress syndrome in high school runners. J Orthop Sports Phys Ther 2001;31:504–10.
3. Shindle MK, Endo Y, Warren RF, et al. Stress fractures about the tibia, foot, and ankle. J Am Acad Orthop Surg 2012;20(3):167–76.
4. Orava S, Hulkko A. Stress fracture of the mid-tibial shaft. Acta Orthop Scand 1984;55:35Y37.
5. Kelsey JL, Bachrach LK, Proctor-Gray E, et al. Risk factors for stress fracture among young female cross-country runners. Med Sci Sports Exerc 2007; 39(9):1457–63.
6. Bennell KL, Malcolm SA, Thomas SA, et al. Risk factors for stress fractures in track and field athletes: a twelve-month prospective study. Am J Sports Med 1996;24(6):810–8.
7. Nattiv A, Loucks AB, Manore MM, et al. American College of Sports Medicine position stand: the female athlete triad. Med Sci Sports Exerc 2007; 39(10):1867–82.
8. Changstrom BG, Brou L, Khodaee M, et al. Epidemiology of stress fracture injuries among US high school athletes, 2005-2006 through 2012-2013. Am J Sports Med 2015;43(1):26–33.
9. Shaffer RA, Rauh MJ, Brodine SK, et al. Predictors of stress fracture susceptibility in young female recruits. Am J Sports Med 2006;34(1):108–15.
10. Fredericson M, Bergman AG, Hoffman KL, et al. Tibial stress reaction in runners. Correlation of clinical symptoms and scintigraphy with a new magnetic resonance imaging grading system. Am J Sports Med 1995;23(4):472–81.
11. Reshef N, Guelich DR. Medial tibial stress syndrome. Clin Sports Med 2012;31(2):273–90.
12. Pell RF 4th, Khanuja HS, Cooley GR. Leg pain in the running athlete. J Am Acad Orthop Surg 2004; 12(6):396–404.
13. Holder LE, Michael RH. The specific scintigraphic pattern of "shin splints in the lower leg": concise communication. J Nucl Med 1984;25:865–9.
14. Fredericson M, Jennings F, Beaulieu C, et al. Stress fractures in athletes. Top Magn Reson Imaging 2006;17(5):309–25.
15. Swischuk LE, Jadhav SP. Tibial stress phenomena and fractures: imaging evaluation. Emerg Radiol 2014;21(2):173–7.
16. Gaeta M, Minutoli F, Scribano E, et al. CT and MR imaging findings in athletes with early tibial stress injuries: comparison with bone scintigraphy findings and emphasis on cortical abnormalities. Radiology 2005;235(2):553–61.
17. Smith JT, Halim K, Palms DA, et al. Prevalence of vitamin D deficiency in patients with foot and ankle injuries. Foot Ankle Int 2014;35(1):8–13.
18. McCabe MP, Smyth MP, Richardson DR. Current concept review: vitamin D and stress fractures. Foot Ankle Int 2012;33(6):526–33.
19. Swenson EJ Jr, DeHaven KE, Sebastianelli WJ, et al. The effect of a pneumatic leg brace on return to play in athletes with tibial stress fractures. Am J Sports Med 1997;25(3):322–8.
20. Allen CS, Flynn TW, Kardouni JR, et al. The use of a pneumatic leg brace in soldiers with tibial stress fractures–a randomized clinical trial. Mil Med 2004;169(11):880–4.
21. Batt ME, Kemp S, Kerslake R. Delayed union stress fractures of the anterior tibia: conservative management. Br J Sports Med 2001;35(1):74–7.
22. Wang SJ, Lewallen DG, Bolander ME, et al. Low intensity ultrasound treatment increases strength in a rat femoral fracture model. J Orthop Res 1994;12:40–7.
23. Kinami Y, Noda T, Ozaki T. Efficacy of low-intensity pulsed ultrasound treatment for surgically managed fresh diaphyseal fractures of the lower

extremity: multi-center retrospective cohort study. J Orthop Sci 2013;18(3):410–8.

24. Rue JP, Armstrong DW 3rd, Frassica FJ, et al. The effect of pulsed ultrasound in the treatment of tibial stress fractures. Orthopedics 2004;27(11):1192–5.

25. Uchiyama Y, Nakamura Y, Mochida J, et al. Effect of low-intensity pulsed ultrasound treatment for delayed and non-union stress fractures of the anterior mid-tibia in five athletes. Tokai J Exp Clin Med 2007;32(4):121–5.

26. Cacchio A, Giordano L, Colafarina O, et al. Extracorporeal shock-wave therapy compared with surgery for hypertrophic long-bone nonunions. J Bone Joint Surg Am 2009;91(11):2589–97.

27. Stewart GW, Brunet ME, Manning MR, et al. Treatment of stress fractures in athletes with intravenous pamidronate. Clin J Sport Med 2005;15(2):92–4.

28. Milgrom C, Finestone A, Novack V, et al. The effect of prophylactic treatment with risedronate on stress fracture incidence among infantry recruits. Bone 2004;35(2):418–24.

29. Simon MJ, Barvencik F, Luttke M, et al. Intravenous bisphosphonates and vitamin D in the treatment of bone marrow oedema in professional athletes. Injury 2014;45(6):981–7.

30. Shima Y, Engebretsen L, Iwasa J, et al. Use of bisphosphonates for the treatment of stress fractures in athletes. Knee Surg Sports Traumatol Arthrosc 2009;17(5):542–50.

31. Beals RK, Cook RD. Stress fractures of the anterior tibial diaphysis. Orthopedics 1991;14(8):869–75.

32. Rettig AC, Shelbourne KD. McCarroll history and treatment of delayed union stress fractures of the anterior cortex of the tibia. Am J Sports Med 1988;16(3):250–5.

33. Varner KE, Younas SA, Lintner DM, et al. Chronic anterior midtibial stress fractures in athletes treated with reamed intramedullary nailing. Am J Sports Med 2005;33(7):1071–6.

34. Baublitz SD, Shaffer BS. Acute fracture through an intramedullary stabilized chronic tibial stress fracture in a basketball player: a case report and literature review. Am J Sports Med 2004;32(8): 1968–72.

35. Väistö O, Toivanen J, Kannus P, et al. Anterior knee pain after intramedullary nailing of fractures of the tibial shaft: an eight-year follow-up of a prospective, randomized study comparing two different nail-insertion techniques. J Trauma 2008;64(6): 1511–6.

36. Zbeda RM, Sculco PK, Urch EY, et al. Tension band plating for chronic anterior tibial stress fractures in high-performance athletes. Am J Sports Med 2015;43(7):1712–8.

37. Hattori H, Ito T. Recurrent fracture after anterior tension band plating with bilateral tibial stress fracture in a basketball player: a case report. Orthop J Sports Med 2015;3(10):1712–8.

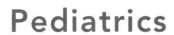

Pediatrics

Pediatric Elbow and Wrist Pathology Related to Sports Participation

Matthew D. Ellington, MD, Eric W. Edmonds, MD*

KEYWORDS

• Little league elbow • Gymnast wrist • Overuse injuries

KEY POINTS

- Upper extremity overuse injuries in the pediatric athlete have become increasingly more common.
- The identification and treatment of childhood elbow and wrist injuries are crucial to prevent long-term damage to growth and limb alignment.
- Gymnast wrist may be related to a traction injury caused by hyperextension of the wrist.
- Most of the overuse injuries at the skeletally immature elbow are associated with valgus overload syndrome.
- Osteochondrosis and osteochondritis dissecans may represent a spectrum of disease based on comparative anatomy studies.

LITTLE LEAGUE ELBOW

The term Little League elbow was originally used in 1960 by Brogdon and Crow to describe a medial epicondyle fracture seen in adolescent pitchers.[1] Although the term has been used to refer to a constellation of injuries to the pediatric elbow, many authors have tried to associate the terminology with only medial epicondyle apophysitis. For the sake of this review, the constellation of injuries will be discussed, as many of them likely represent a spectrum of elbow overuse in children.

Little League elbow has been described as a valgus overload syndrome. This is defined as repetitive throwing that imparts a tensile fore on the medial epicondyle and a compressive force at the lateral epicondyle.[2] Twenty-eight percent of youth pitchers report a history of elbow pain.[3] There is a spectrum of injuries that can occur from medial to lateral on the elbow and even posterior. Medial injuries are the most common, especially with valgus overload during the early and late cocking phases of throwing.[4] This force is transferred to the medial epicondyle, leading to apophysitis in younger children (Fig. 1) and epicondyle avulsion fractures in those nearing skeletal maturity. Lateral side injuries also occur, such as Panner disease and octeochondritis dissecans (OCD) of the capitellum and radial head. These occur slightly later in the throwing cycle from compressive forces during late cocking and early acceleration phases. Posterior injury patterns also occur, including olecranon apophysitis and posteromedial impingement, along with flexion and capsular contractures, often seen in conjunction with either medial and/or lateral pathology.

Medial Injures

Medial injuries of the elbow can range from irritation of the flexor–pronator mass to avulsion of the medial epicondyle. Patients typically present with medial elbow pain usually associated with increases in pitch count or training intensity. Although it has been hinted that pitch type may

---

Disclosure Statement: The authors have nothing to disclose.
Division of Orthopedic Surgery, Rady Children's Hospital, 3030 Children's Way Suite 410, San Diego, CA 92123, USA
* Corresponding author.
E-mail address: ewedmonds@rchsd.org

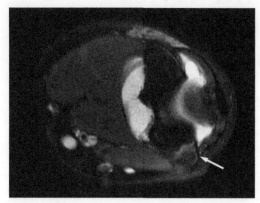

Fig. 1. MRI axial T2 FAT SATURATED image of a 12-year-old girl who plays year-round softball demonstrating elbow medial epicondyle apophysitis. Note the edema within the epicondyle and bright signal at the apophysis (*arrow*). (*Courtesy of* San Diego Pediatric Orthopedics, San Diego, CA; with permission.)

be related to an increase in injuries, this has not been born out in the literature. They typically have decreased throwing velocity and medial elbow pain that is tender to palpation.[5] Avulsion of the medial epicondyle has been reported to occur in athletes who have not adhered to the USA Baseball youth baseball pitching guidelines. Treatment of these injuries is controversial also, but most authors agree that nondisplaced or minimally displaced fractures (0-5 mm) can be treated nonoperatively with immobilization. Operative

intervention is indicated for those with displaced fractures (> 5 mm), incarcerated fragment, or those associated with an elbow dislocation.[6]

Lateral Injuries

Lateral injuries of the elbow typically are caused by either Panner disease or OCD. Panner disease, named after the Danish radiologist Hans Jessen Panner, is an osteochondrosis of the capitellum of the elbow typically seen in younger athletes (< 10 years) with no history of trauma. It causes pain and stiffness that may limit extension. They typically have a good prognosis with full return of function (Fig. 2A). OCD (Fig. 2B), however, presents in an older patient population (typically > 13 years). This has been theorized to occur secondary to a disruption in the subchondral blood flow to the capitellum.[7] The radial head can then become secondarily involved. Pain usually occurs at late cocking through acceleration when the compressive forces are the greatest at the elbow.[7]

Posterior Injuries

Posterior injuries typically occur because of shear forces during both the acceleration and deceleration phases of throwing. The main area of injury is to the olecranon apophysis (Fig. 3). These injuries typically present as localized tenderness and pain with elbow extension. Imaging may demonstrate widening of the

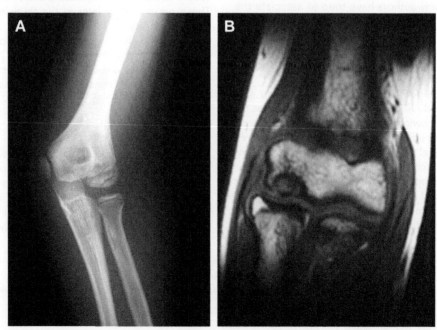

Fig. 2. Radiograph of elbow capitellum Panner disease (*A*) in a younger patient and an MRI image of OCD (*B*) in an older patient. (*Courtesy of* San Diego Pediatric Orthopedics, San Diego, CA; with permission.)

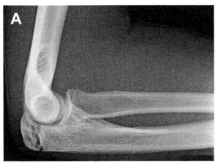 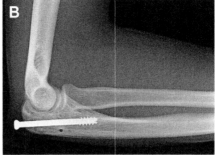

Fig. 3. Olecranon apophysitis on lateral radiograph of a 15-year-old baseball player (A); the contralateral elbow demonstrated a closed apophysis. (B) 3 months after screw fixation with tension band construct demonstrating apophyseal closure. (*Courtesy of* San Diego Pediatric Orthopedics, San Diego, CA; with permission.)

apophysis. Displacement more than 2 mm necessitates open reduction internal fixation.

Imaging
Hang, Chao, and Hang looked at 343 Little League players and found hypertrophy of the medial humeral epicondyle in all pitchers and catchers and 90% of fielders. They also found separation of the medial epicondyle in 63% of pitchers, 70% of catchers, and 50% of pitchers, while fragmentation was seen in 19% of pitchers, 40% of catchers, and 15% of fielders.[8] MRI of patients with Little League elbow demonstrates frequent abnormal findings; however, these do not seem to change clinical management.

Specific evaluation of the ulnar collateral ligament (UCL) in these athletes showed no damage to the structure and distance from the physis of 0 to 4 mm.[9]

Treatment
The most important key to treatment of these overuse injuries is prevention; this can be achieved by adhering to proper pitch count guidelines and teaching proper mechanics. After the injury has occurred, treatment needs to be hardline rest and activity modification. This should include parental education regarding cross-training and expectation management. There are no defined guidelines for how long to set the expectation for return to play.

ELBOW OSTEOCHONDRITIS DISSECANS

As discussed previously, OCD of the humeral capitellum and radial head is typically a result of lateral compression injuries. This differs from Panner disease, which is an osteochondrosis, as OCD refers to inflammation of the osteochondral articular surface, while osteochondroses are primarily unilateral, affect boys in the first decade, and occur shortly after the appearance

of the ossific nucleus at a time when the cells are vulnerable to various hormonal, nutritional, and mechanical insults.[10,11] Veterinary studies suggest that osteochondrosis and OCD may actually be a continuum of disease; wherein, at younger ages and/or smaller effect size of vascular injury, there may be an auto-resolving osteochondrosis compared with a larger effect size vascular insult that develops into OCD.[12–14]

OCD lesions have also been found in the trochlea. These usually also present in throwing athletes who present with medial elbow pain and flexion contracture/extension block. Medial lesions are usually a result of posteromedial olecranon abutment, while lateral lesions occur in a vascular watershed zone resulting from the blood supply of the trochlea.[15]

Imaging
There is commonly a focal area of lucency seen in the subchondral bone in the anterior aspect of the capitellum on radiographs. Chronic lesions will have a sclerotic border.[5] The classic crescent sign identifies a focal lesion in the capitellum surrounded by subchondral sclerosis demarcated by a semilunar rarefied zone.[16]

MRI is the study of choice to fully delineate the extent of the lesion. Early on in the process there are changes of marrow edema identified by decreased signal intensity with chondroepiphysis of the capitellum on T1-weighted images and increased signal on T2-weighted images and fast spin-echo sequences.[17,18] Unstable lesions show fluid under the lesion on T2-weighted images. False positives have been reported with MRI because of the normal anatomic sulcus between the capitellum and lateral condyle. This pseudo-defect mimics an OCD. One key difference is that the pseudo-defect is posterior, while OCD lesions are typically more anterior.[18]

Treatment

Classifying these lesions is an important adjunct for treatment. Baumgarten and colleagues[19] proposed an arthroscopic classification of the lesions that parallels that for talar lesions. Difelice and colleagues[16] also devised a classification basically showing the stability of the fracture is the most important factor for treatment.

Intact/stable lesions are best treated nonoperatively. Peterson proposed a nonsurgical treatment algorithm for these lesions consisting of a hinged elbow brace combined with rest for 3 to 6 weeks followed by return to activity in 3 to 6 months.[20] The crucial aspect of nonsurgical management is activity modification to reduce axial load to the radiocapitellar joint.[5] Casting is not recommended because of concerns for stiffness.

Surgery is reserved for those cases with persistent pain despite nonsurgical management, symptomatic loose bodies, articular cartilage fractures, and displacement of the lesion (Fig. 4). Management typically consists of excision of the loose body or partially attached lesion followed by abrasion chondroplasty or subchondral drilling.[5] There have been variable results for internal fixation of the loose fragment.[19–22]

GYMNAST WRIST

Unique to the sport of gymnastics is the reliance of the upper extremities to support body weight. This recurrent force across the wrist joint provides an injury pattern unique to the sport. Forces of up to 16 times body weight have been reported to occur across the wrist in gymnasts with various exercises such as the back hand spring and on the pommel horse.[23,24] Wrist pain has been reportedly between 46% and 79% of athletes in high-level club and collegiate gymnasts.[25,26]

Most frequently described as a compression injury, Heuter-Volkmann's Law suggests that the radiographic findings support more of a traction injury at the physis related to weight bearing on the palms and using the wrist as an ankle joint.[27] This creates hyperextension at the wrist and increases distraction at the volar aspect of the radial physis (Fig. 5).

Difiori and colleagues[28] looked at 52 nonelite gymnasts and found that gymnasts with wrist pain, which was prevalent in 73% of their cohort, were older, trained more hours per week, trained at a higher skill level, and began training at an older age. Positive ulnar variance is a known sequela of gymnast wrist. In 1987 at the World Championship Artistic Gymnastics Rotterdam, ulnar variance in female gymnasts was measured. There was found to be a significant increase in ulnar length among adults and immature gymnasts compared with nonathletes, and this change correlated to weight, height, and skeletal age of the athletes.[29] Relatively few long-term studies on the effect of ulnar variance on gymnasts exist. Claessens in 1997 reported a negative ulnar variance that worsened with increasing age during 4- to 5-year follow-up on 36 girls 6 to 14 years of age,[30] which contrasts most literature supporting ulnar variance becoming more positive with age in skeletally immature patients.[31] Difiori in 2001 found in 28 gymnasts during a 3-year follow-up period, a

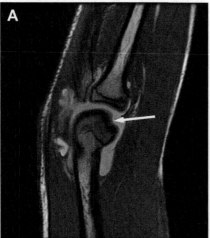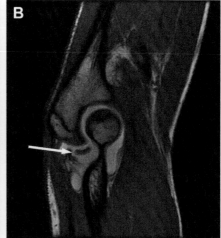

Fig. 4. MRI sagittal T1 of elbow in 14-year-old male basketball player with capitellum OCD (A, arrow) and with loose articular cartilage body (B, arrow). (Courtesy of San Diego Pediatric Orthopedics, San Diego, CA; with permission.)

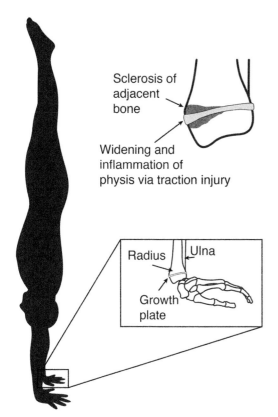

Fig. 5. Line drawing representing a novel understanding to gymnast wrist being a traction injury, rather than a compression injury. (*Courtesy of* San Diego Pediatric Orthopedics, San Diego, CA; with permission.)

mean negative ulnar variance at baseline became significantly more positive than age-appropriate controls.[32]

Imaging

Radiographs of gymnasts have shown irregular widening of the physes as well as irregularities and thickening of the zone of provisional calcification along with ulnar positive variance.[33]

Classically on MRI, the findings are edema on the metaphyseal and epiphyseal sides of the physis. Cartilaginous ingrowth can also be seen as a result of failure of ossification of the physeal cartilage in the metaphysis, which has been attributed to metaphyseal injury and bony bridging from epiphyseal trauma.[34,35] These findings are similar to those found in other traction apophysites: Osgood-Schlatter, Sindig-Larson-Johanssen, and others.[36] Triangular fibrocartilage complex (TFCC) tears may also be visualized on MRI in these same athletes.[26]

Treatment

As with most all overuse injuries traction injuries, the best treatment is prevention of the inciting event. This can be achieved with temporary relief through wrist braces that limit motion, but ultimately requires time off from the sport. Arthroscopy is warranted in those patients with TFCC tears that have failed conservative measures.[26]

REFERENCES

1. Brogdon BG, Crow NE. Little leaguer's elbow. Am J Roentgenol Radium Ther Nucl Med 1960; 83:671–5.
2. Frush TJ, Lindenfeld TN. Peri-epiphyseal and overuse injuries in adolescent athletes. Sports Health 2009;1(3):201–11.
3. Lyman S, Fleisig GS, Andrews JR, et al. Effect of pitch type, pitch count, and pitching mechanics on risk of elbow and shoulder pain in youth baseball pitchers. Am J Sports Med 2002;30(4):463–8.
4. Klingele KE, Kocher MS. Little league elbow: valgus overload injury in the paediatric athlete. Sports Med 2002;32(15):1005–15.
5. Kobayashi K, Burton KJ, Rodner C, et al. Lateral compression injuries in the pediatric elbow: Panner's disease and osteochondritis dissecans of the capitellum. J Am Acad Orthop Surg 2004;12(4):246–54.
6. Osbahr DC, Chalmers PN, Frank JS, et al. Acute, avulsion fractures of the medial epicondyle while throwing in youth baseball players: a variant of Little League elbow. J Shoulder Elbow Surg 2010;19(7):951–7.
7. Baker CL, Romeo AA. Osteochondritis dissecans of the capitellum. Am J Sports Med 2010;38(9):1917–28.
8. Hang DW, Chao CM, Hang Y-S. A clinical and roentgenographic study of Little League elbow. Am J Sports Med 2004;32(1):79–84.
9. Wei AS, Khana S, Limpisvasti O, et al. Clinical and magnetic resonance imaging findings associated with Little League elbow. J Pediatr Orthop 2010;30(7):715–9.
10. Duthie RB, Houghton GR. Constitutional aspects of the osteochondroses. Clin Orthop Relat Res 1981;158:19–27.
11. Douglas G, Rang M. The role of trauma in the pathogenesis of the osteochondroses. Clin Orthop Relat Res 1981;158:28–32.
12. Tóth F, Nissi MJ, Wang L, et al. Surgical induction, histological evaluation, and MRI identification of cartilage necrosis in the distal femur in goats to model early lesions of osteochondrosis. Osteoarthritis Cartilage 2015;23(2):300–7.
13. Tóth F, Nissi MJ, Ellermann JM, et al. Novel application of magnetic resonance imaging demonstrates characteristic differences in vasculature at predilection sites of osteochondritis dissecans. Am J Sports Med 2015;43(10):2522–7.

14. McCoy AM, Toth F, Dolvik NI, et al. Articular osteochondrosis: a comparison of naturally-occurring human and animal disease. Osteoarthritis Cartilage 2013;21(11):1638–47.

15. Marshall KW, Marshall DL, Busch MT, et al. Osteochondral lesions of the humeral trochlea in the young athlete. Skeletal Radiol 2009;38(5):479–91.

16. Difelice GS, Meunier MJ, Paletta GA Jr. Elbow injury in the adolescent athlete. In: Altcheck DW, Andrews JR, editors. The athlete's elbow: surgery and rehabilitation. 1st edition. Philadelphia: Lippincott Williams & Wilkins; 2001. p. 231–48.

17. Bowen RE, Otsuka NY, Yoon ST, et al. Osteochondral lesions of the capitellum in pediatric patients: role of magnetic resonance imaging. J Pediatr Orthop 2001;21(3):298–301.

18. Schenk M, Dalinka MK. Imaging of the elbow. An update. Orthop Clin North Am 1997;28(4):517–35.

19. Baumgarten TE, Andrews JR, Satterwhite YE. The arthroscopic classification and treatment of osteochondritis dissecans of the capitellum. Am J Sports Med 1998;26(4):520–3.

20. Peterson RK, Savoie FH, Field LD. Osteochondritis dissecans of the elbow. Instr Course Lect 1999;48: 393–8.

21. Harada M, Ogino T, Takahara M, et al. Fragment fixation with a bone graft and dynamic staples for osteochondritis dissecans of the humeral capitellum. J Shoulder Elbow Surg 2002;11(4):368–72.

22. Takeda H, Watarai K, Matsushita T, et al. A surgical treatment for unstable osteochondritis dissecans lesions of the humeral capitellum in adolescent baseball players. Am J Sports Med 2002;30(5): 713–7.

23. Koh TJ, Grabiner MD, Weiker GG. Technique and ground reaction forces in the back handspring. Am J Sports Med 1992;20(1):61–6.

24. Markolf KL, Shapiro MS, Mandelbaum BR, et al. Wrist loading patterns during pommel horse exercises. J Biomech 1990;23(10):1001–11.

25. Caine D, Cochrane B, Caine C, et al. An epidemiologic investigation of injuries affecting young competitive female gymnasts. Am J Sports Med 1989;17(6):811–20.

26. Mandelbaum BR, Bartolozzi AR, Davis CA, et al. Wrist pain syndrome in the gymnast: Pathogenetic, diagnostic, and therapeutic considerations. Am J Sports Med 1989;17(3):305–17.

27. Rang M. Syndromology. In: Wenger DR, Rang M, editors. The art and practice of children's orthopaedics. New York: Raven Press; 1993. p. 627–55.

28. DiFiori JP, Puffer JC, Mandelbaum BR, et al. Factors associated with wrist pain in the young gymnast. Am J Sports Med 1996;24(1):9–14.

29. De Smet L, Claessens A, Lefevre J, et al. Gymnast wrist: an epidemiologic survey of ulnar variance and stress changes of the radial physis in elite female gymnasts. Am J Sports Med 1994;22(6): 846–50.

30. Claessens A, Lefevre J, Philippaerts R, et al. The ulnar variance phenomenon: a study in young female gymnasts. In: Armstrong N, Kirby B, Welsman J, editors. Children and exercise XIX. London: E & FN Spon; 1997. p. 537–41.

31. DiFiori JP, Caine DJ, Malina RM. Wrist pain, distal radial physeal injury, and ulnar variance in the young gymnast. Am J Sports Med 2006;34(5):840–9.

32. DiFiori JP, Puffer JC, Aish B, et al. Ulnar variance in young gymnasts: a three-year cohort study. Med Sci Sports Exerc 2001;33(5):S223.

33. Dwek JR, Cardoso F, Chung CB. MR imaging of overuse injuries in the skeletally immature gymnast: spectrum of soft-tissue and osseous lesions in the hand and wrist. Pediatr Radiol 2009;39(12):1310–6.

34. Ecklund K, Jaramillo D. Patterns of premature physeal arrest: MR imaging of 111 children. AJR Am J Roentgenol 2002;178(4):967–72.

35. Jaramillo D, Laor T, Zaleske DJ. Indirect trauma to the growth plate: results of MR imaging after epiphyseal and metaphyseal injury in rabbits. Radiology 1993;187(1):171–8.

36. Davis KW. Imaging pediatric sports injuries: lower extremity. Radiol Clin North Am 2010; 48(6):1213–35.

Shoulder Injuries in Pediatric Athletes

James E. Moyer, MD[a,1], Jennifer M. Brey, MD[b,*]

KEYWORDS

- Pediatric shoulder injury • Shoulder overuse injuries • Adolescent shoulder instability
- Shoulder fractures

KEY POINTS

- Shoulder injuries in pediatric athletes may be acute injuries or caused by repetitive overuse.
- Acute injuries in skeletally immature shoulders tend to be fractures or sprains, as opposed to tendon or muscle injuries.
- Chronic overuse injuries tend to occur in overhead athletes. Baseball pitchers who have high pitch counts are at highest risk.

INTRODUCTION

As the number of children and adolescents participating in competitive sports has increased, especially in overhead activities, there has been a corresponding increase in the number of injuries to the shoulder.[1] Skeletally immature athletes present with many of the same complaints as more mature athletes, but differences in anatomy and technique often lead to age-specific injuries. Although traumatic injuries, such as sprains or fractures, are common across the spectrum of competitive activities, overuse injuries predominate.

Overuse injuries in young athletes are typically caused by repeated stress and cumulative trauma to the developing physis of the proximal humerus as well as adaptive changes in the soft tissue stabilizers of the glenohumeral joint. Physeal injuries are usually diagnosed by history and physical examination and may be confirmed on radiographs. Soft tissue injuries such as SLAP (superior labrum anterior and posterior) lesions, glenohumeral instability, and rotator cuff disorders may be more difficult to diagnose definitively.

Traumatic injuries to the skeletally immature shoulder may occur with any activity, but are more common with high-energy collision sports such as football.[1] Traumatic injuries include ligament sprains, muscle strains, fractures of the humerus, and fractures of the clavicle. Knowing the anatomic differences of the developing osseous structures of the shoulder girdle is key in diagnosis and management.

Anatomy

During growth, the anatomy of the proximal humerus osseous and ligamentous structures undergoes multiple changes. The proximal humeral physis typically closes at between 14 and 17 years in girls and 16 to 18 years in boys. This physis also contributes about 80% of the overall humeral length, making an injury to this area at a young age possibly more consequential but also allowing extensive remodeling of acute fractures.[2]

Any activity that involves stress of the physis, such as overhead throwing or repetitive upper extremity activities, puts the physis at risk of injury. Injuries vary from chronic stress reaction caused by overuse to acute fracture of the physis. The

Disclosure: The authors have nothing to disclose.
[a] Non-operative Pediatric Orthopedics, Kosair Children's Hospital, Children's Orthopaedics of Louisville, Louisville, KY, USA; [b] Department of Orthopaedic Surgery, Kosair Children's Hospital, Children's Orthopaedics of Louisville, University of Louisville, Louisville, KY, USA
[1] Present address: 3999 Dutchmans Lane, 6F, Louisville, KY 40207.
* Corresponding author. 3999 Dutchmans Lane, 6F, Louisville, KY 40207.
E-mail address: Jennifer.brey@gmail.com

Orthop Clin N Am 47 (2016) 749–762
http://dx.doi.org/10.1016/j.ocl.2016.05.003
0030-5898/16/$ – see front matter © 2016 Elsevier Inc. All rights reserved.

physis is thought to be a weak point of the upper arm compared with the ligamentous structures. The ligaments of the glenohumeral joint provide static stability depending on the position of the arm.[3] The rotator cuff muscles, scapular stabilizers, and long head of the biceps also contribute to dynamic stability of the shoulder.

The clavicle is the first bone in the body to start the ossification process via intramembranous ossification.[4] It shows both intramembranous and endochondral types of ossification. The lateral clavicular epiphysis typically does not ossify until 18 years of age. The medial clavicular epiphysis is the last to appear, at approximately 18 to 20 years of age, and does not fuse until 23 to 25 years of age, making the clavicle the last bone in the body to completely fuse.[5] Strong ligaments provide significant stability at the medial and lateral ends of the clavicle, thereby making fractures in the middle of the clavicle more likely.[5]

OVERUSE INJURIES
Introduction
Pediatric or adolescent athletes involved in repetitive overhead activities, such as baseball, swimming, or volleyball, are at risk for overuse injuries to the shoulder. Overuse injuries are very common, comprising approximately 60% of all sports injuries in children and adolescents. Female athletes typically present more often with overuse injuries, but male athletes participating in certain demanding team sports, such as baseball, are at highest risk.[6] It is estimated that 50% of overuse injuries in physically active children and adolescents may be preventable.[7] Volume of activity, whether measured in number of repetitions or quantity of time, may be the greatest predictor of overuse injury.[8] Shoulder pain, fatigue, and/or decreased velocity should be an indication to coaches and parents that an overuse injury may exist. Educating players, coaches, and trainers about these symptoms may help identify overuse injuries early.[9,10]

Baseball in particular has been the focus of extensive research with regard to pediatric shoulder injuries. Seasonal incidence of shoulder pain ranges from 32% to 35%, with nearly 9% of all pitching performances resulting in shoulder symptoms.[9,11] The incidence of injury for pitchers was found to be 37.4%, whereas it was only 15.3% for position players. Overall, pitchers experienced 47.1% of all shoulder injuries in baseball.[12] In a study of youth baseball players by Olsen and colleagues,[10] athletes who underwent surgery for shoulder or elbow injuries caused by pitching were more likely to have increased number of pitches thrown per inning and per game, more likely to pitch with pain, and pitched with higher velocity. There was no significant difference between injured and uninjured athletes with regard to injury prevention programs, types of pitches thrown, or private pitching instruction.

The role of specific types of pitches on shoulder pain incidence is inconclusive. Although some data exist that show higher levels of injury in curveball throwing, other studies have found higher mechanical demands with fastball throwing.[13] In general, many of the issues of the throwing shoulder are rooted in poor biomechanics, scapular dyskinesis, muscular imbalance, glenohumeral internal rotation deficit, and excessive throwing or overhead activity.[14]

Biomechanics of Throwing
The mechanism of baseball throwing is a complicated process involving the coordination of the upper and lower extremities as well as core musculature. Throwing is typically divided into 6 phases: wind-up, early cocking, late cocking, acceleration, deceleration, and follow-through (Fig. 1).[13,14]

During the late cocking phase, the arm is in an abducted and externally rotated position, creating an anteriorly directed force of the humeral head. This force is then counterbalanced by the static and dynamic stabilizers of the glenohumeral joint. During the acceleration portion of throwing, the arm moves at speeds of several thousand degrees per second, creating a large rotational force at the proximal humerus, often several times greater than the rotational strength of the proximal humeral physis.

Youth pitchers show several changes compared with mature pitchers. Younger pitchers tend to begin trunk rotation earlier in the throwing process. There is also a trend toward more open pelvic position during throwing. Both of these mechanisms have been proposed to increase the likelihood of injury to the developing physis because of higher rotational stress at the proximal humerus.[14]

LITTLE LEAGUE SHOULDER AND OVERUSE SYNDROMES

Shoulder overuse injuries are most common in boys aged 11 to 16 years. The most common age of presentation is 14 years in boys.[15] In adolescents, the most common causes of shoulder pain from overhead activities are Little Leaguer's shoulder, glenohumeral instability, and rotator cuff disorders.

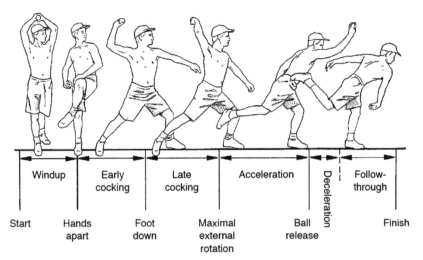

Fig. 1. Phases of throwing. (*Adapted from* DiGiovine NM, Jobe FW, Pink M, et al. An electromyographic analysis of the upper extremity in pitching. J Shoulder Elbow Surg 1992;1:16; with permission.)

Skeletally immature pitchers tend to develop problems with developing structures of the shoulder, including the proximal humeral physis, which may manifest in young pitchers with Little Leaguer's shoulder, which has been described as osteochondrosis, epiphysiolysis, and stress reaction of the proximal humerus.[15] Vertically oriented collagen fibers within the zone of hypertrophy are most susceptible to injury. Radiographs may show physeal widening and fragmentation, often appearing similar to the presentation of Salter-Harris I fractures. Repetitive stress may lead to microfractures in this area and hypertrophy seen on radiographs (Fig. 2).[16]

Once the proximal humeral physis has closed, the static and dynamic stabilizers of the shoulder are more likely to be injured. Skeletally mature pitchers more often develop disorders in the anterior and superior glenoid labrum (SLAP lesions).[17]

Glenohumeral internal rotation deficit is also seen in older throwers as a loss of internal rotation compared with the nonthrowing shoulder.[18] Alterations in shoulder and scapular motion can lead to changes in the labrum, including SLAP tears. Baseball and softball pitchers who sustained injury during the season had significantly decreased internal rotation compared with age-matched peers as well as the nondominant arm.[19] Rotator cuff disorders and impingement syndromes are also occasionally seen in overhead athletes, often related to instability.[20]

History and Physical Examination
Patients typically present with increasing shoulder pain during throwing motions, which may progress to activity at rest. Important information

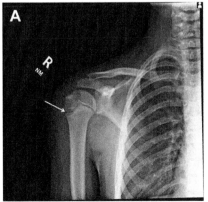
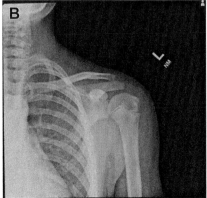

Fig. 2. (A) A 12-year-old boy with shoulder pain at the beginning of the baseball season. Radiograph of shoulder of throwing arm at presentation. White arrow shows widening of the proximal humeral physis. (B) Left shoulder radiograph taken for comparison at initial presentation.

to obtain includes the patient's sport, level of competition, previous injuries, amount of time spent playing, recent increases in activity, and pitch counts.

In skeletally immature athletes with Little Leaguer's shoulder, tenderness on palpation of the lateral proximal humerus is often seen.[14,16] Scapular dysfunction may also be noted with forward flexion and abduction of both arms. Shoulder motion, flexibility, strength, and other components of the kinetic chain should also be assessed.

Skeletally mature throwers often show increased external rotation along with decreased internal rotation of the throwing arm with the shoulder in abduction. The overall arc of motion may be maintained without corresponding pain or dysfunction.[21] Alterations in range of motion are often noted in young throwers as well, but the overall range of motion may be decreased.[22]

Radiographs of the proximal humerus in skeletally immature throwers should be obtained. Radiographs of the contralateral shoulder often aid in confirmation. Although physeal widening on radiographs is often confirmatory in patients with shoulder pain, many asymptomatic throwers also show widening.[23] It is hypothesized that physeal widening may also be caused by adaptive changes within the proximal humerus. Advanced imaging is typically reserved for patients with anterior instability or for refractory cases.

Treatment

Prevention of overuse injuries should be the goal of all athletes, coaches, and parents. Off-season condition focusing on pitching mechanics and strengthening of the kinetic chain is recommended. Monitoring players for pain during or after activities may alert coaches and parents that an overuse injury may be developing. Pitching limits should be established for players 9 to 14 years old: full-effort throwing should be limited to 75 pitches per game, 600 pitches per season, and 2000 to 3000 pitches per year.[11] Little League Baseball, with recommendations from the American Sports Medicine Institute, has instituted specific guidelines for pitch counts (Table 1) and for required days of rest (Table 2). Of note, pitchers who have pitched more than 41 pitches in a game are not permitted to switch positions to catcher.

The mainstay of treatment is rest from all throwing activities. Treatment algorithms vary, but most include a period of absolute rest from throwing, then gradual return to activities. Nonsteroidal antiinflammatory medication may also help with pain and inflammation during recovery. Strengthening exercises focusing on the

Table 1
Pitch counts for Little League Baseball

Player Age (y)	Pitches Permitted Per Day
17–18	105
13–16	95
11–12	85
9–10	75
7–8	50

Data from Little League Baseball, Incorporated. The Little League pitch count regulation guide. 2008. Available at: http://www.littleleague.org/assets/old_assets/media/pitch_count_publication_2008.pdf. Accessed November 28, 2015.

rotator cuff musculature, core strengthening, and pitching mechanics are emphasized. Stretching exercises focusing on abduction and internal rotation are also recommended.[14] Most athletes are able to return to baseball in 3 months.[15]

For patients with SLAP lesions, a short period of physical therapy and rest may help to resolve symptoms. However, when there is continued pain and MRI consistent with labral injury, surgical repair may be indicated (Fig. 3).

ANTERIOR INSTABILITY

Anterior shoulder instability is a common problem in adolescent athletes, comprising 85% to 95% of all shoulder instability. Incidence is reported to be 11.2 occurrences per 100,000 person-years.[24] Younger male athletes are at particularly high risk, because nearly 40% of

Table 2
Days of rest required after pitching

Player Age (y)	Pitches Thrown Per Day	Days of Rest Required
≤14	≥66	4
	51–65	3
	36–50	2
	21–35	1
	≤20	0
15–18	≥76	4
	61–75	3
	46–60	2
	31–45	1
	≤30	0

Data from Little League Baseball, Incorporated. The Little League pitch count regulation guide. 2008. Available at: http://www.littleleague.org/assets/old_assets/media/pitch_count_publication_2008.pdf. Accessed November 28, 2015.

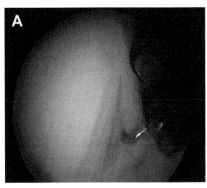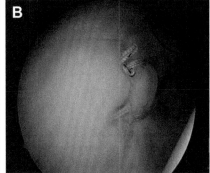

Fig. 3. (A) SLAP tear in 12-year-old baseball pitcher. (B) Labrum repaired with 2 suture anchors.

shoulder instability events occur in males athletes younger than 22 years.[25] The presence of an open physis seems to be slightly protective for anterior dislocation, with a lower percentage occurring in children younger than 13 years,[26] likely secondary to Salter-Harris fractures occurring through the proximal humeral physis rather than glenohumeral dislocation. Athletes participating in contact or collision sports are also at highest risk.[27]

Although the rates of initial anterior shoulder instability episodes are high in adolescents, perhaps more significant is the rate of recurrence. The rate of recurrence has been found to be 51% to 100%.[3,26,28,29] In a study by Lawton and colleagues,[30] of 70 shoulder dislocations in 66 patients aged 16 years or younger, 40% eventually underwent surgery. Those who underwent surgery were less likely to report continued instability at more than 2 years' follow-up compared with those treated with physical therapy alone.

A classic study by Rowe[31] of 500 shoulder dislocations found a high rate of initial dislocation in patients between 10 and 20 years old. The recurrence rate of instability in this group was 83%, with a 100% rate in patients less than 10 years old.[31] A report of 9 children with open physes and shoulder dislocation found a recurrence rate of 80%.[28]

History and Physical Examination

A history of traumatic dislocation from a single event is common in patients involved in contact or collision sports. Any reduction maneuvers performed, whether on field or in an acute care setting, should be documented. A history of pain or paresthesias with overhead activities, especially with the arm in external rotation and abduction, may be present without a frank dislocation episode. Pain with the arm in adduction and internal rotation may indicate posterior

instability. This condition may be seen in football linemen during blocking or pushing against a heavy object.[3]

Initial physical examination should include a complete neurovascular examination of both extremities. Nerve dysfunction has been seen in 5% to 25% of shoulder fractures and dislocations, most commonly axillary nerve injuries.[32] Patients should be examined for loss of motion, both active and passive. Examination should include both shoulders to evaluate for differences of range of motion, scapular motion, muscle atrophy, swelling, or bruising.

Specific shoulder tests to be performed include the anterior apprehension test, Jobe relocation test, anterior and posterior drawer test, and sulcus test. The anterior apprehension test is performed by having the patient lay supine on the examination table and slowly abducting and externally rotating the arm. Feelings of pain or instability are suggestive of anterior instability. The Jobe relocation test is then performed with the arm kept in the abducted and externally rotated position and applying a posterior-directed force on the humeral head. This test is positive if pain or feelings of instability resolve. Drawer testing is performed by placing the arm in line with the scapula and evaluating the amount of humeral head translation with force applied to the proximal humerus. Laxity is defined as grade 1 to 3 translation based on the amount of motion of the humeral head on the glenoid.

Imaging should begin with standard shoulder radiographs, including internal rotation, external rotation, and either axillary or scapular Y views. More specific imaging may include West Point view for anterior glenoid deficits or Stryker notch views for Hill-Sachs lesions. MRI with arthrography is recommended for imaging of the glenoid labrum, glenoid surface, and rotator cuff. Bankart and Hill-Sachs lesions have been noted in most first-time dislocations, with a smaller number of SLAP lesions (Fig. 4A, B).[33] Glenoid bone loss is common in adolescents and is a risk factor for recurrence.[34] Computed tomography (CT) may be performed to further delineate bone loss of the humeral head or glenoid.

Treatment

Caution should be used in initial closed reduction of presumed shoulder dislocation in young children. Many physeal fractures of the proximal humerus may appear similar to a shoulder dislocation, with swelling and internal rotation of the proximal arm.[35] Radiographs should be taken before any reduction maneuver in order to protect against iatrogenic injury to the proximal humeral physis. After initial closed reduction, a short period of immobilization is generally recommended, although there is no consensus regarding arm position.[36–38]

Because of the high risk of recurrence of instability, there is great debate regarding appropriate initial treatment of a first-time instability episode.[39] Factors that need to be taken into consideration include the patient's chosen sport, future plans in that sport, future career plans (ie, military or manual labor), history and/or success

of previous treatment, medical and psychiatric history, and expectations regarding possible outcomes.

After a short period of immobilization, nonoperative treatment usually begins with cessation of sports and an initial course of physical therapy. Therapy usually consists of shoulder range-of-motion exercises, scapular and rotator cuff strengthening, and sport-specific therapy. If the patient has a pain-free shoulder with symmetric bilateral upper extremity strength and range of motion after 4 to 6 weeks of nonoperative treatment, an attempt may be made to return to sports. Abduction shoulder bracing may be attempted, but this is usually poorly tolerated in adolescents and has limited effectiveness.[40] Pain or continued instability symptoms even after conservative treatment is prognostic for recurrence.[41]

Operative treatment of shoulder instability is recommended in patients who have failed conservative treatment and in some first-time dislocations. Adolescent patients involved in collision sports, such as ice hockey and football, may be candidates for initial surgical treatment if the patients and their families are unwilling to modify their activities. Patients may also choose to be

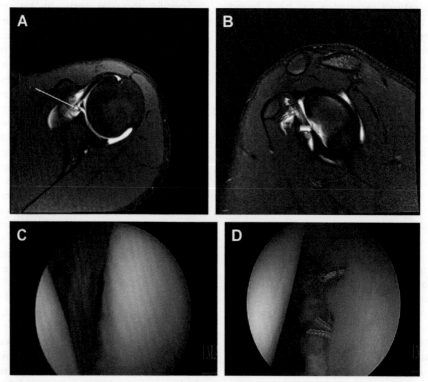

Fig. 4. (A) MRI of the left shoulder in a 13-year-old boy after dislocation from a bicycle crash. Arrow shows labrum separation from glenoid on axial view. (B) Full arrow shows labral detachment from glenoid on coronal view. (C) Arthroscopic appearance of torn labrum. (D) Suture anchors placed in anterior labrum.

treated with nonoperative therapies and delay surgery until after their sports season has finished.

Older studies in which open stabilization procedures were performed showed low recurrence rates and high rates of return to sports.[26,30,42] Arthroscopic methods of stabilization have also shown good results in the adolescent population (Fig. 4C, D). A large study of 32 shoulders treated with arthroscopic Bankart repair at an average age of 15 years showed a low recurrence rate of 15.6%.[43] A study of 65 patients with an average age of 16 years treated with arthroscopic repair found a recurrence rate of 21%. Overall, 81% of patients were able to return to their previous levels of activity.[44] Other studies in young patients have found similar results, with recurrence rates of 11% to 21%.[3]

MULTIDIRECTIONAL INSTABILITY

Approximately 5% of shoulder instability may be considered as multidirectional instability (MDI).[45,46] However, shoulder instability is difficult to classify. One large study of asymptomatic adolescents found a high rate of physical examination findings of shoulder instability without other signs of ligamentous laxity, with positive physical examination findings in 57% of boys and 48% of girls.[47] Symptomatic MDI is seen most often in patients participating in repeated overhead activities, most commonly gymnastics and swimming.[48]

As opposed to anterior shoulder instability, MDI is not typically caused by a single dislocation event. MDI may also be associated with generalized ligamentous laxity. Patients with Ehlers-Danlos syndrome and other connective tissue disorders may also present with instability symptoms. Practitioners should be aware of any medical history and make appropriate referrals to genetics if there is suspicion for underlying disorder.

History

In patients involved in overhead sports such as swimming or baseball, symptoms are usually gradual in onset. Symptoms may also correlate with a recent increase in training. A history of a traumatic dislocation may be seen in the presence of previous instability episodes. Many patients report a history of spontaneous reduction after these events. Patients may have a range of symptoms from subjective feelings of laxity with overhead activities to complete dislocations.

Caution should be used in the treatment of voluntary instability of the shoulder. Patients who are able to consciously subluxate or dislocate their shoulders may respond poorly to both surgical and nonsurgical treatment.[3,49,50] A full psychiatric history should also be obtained.

Physical Examination

Examination of the MDI shoulder involves the same tests as anterior instability. Apprehension, anterior and posterior drawer testing, relocation test, and sulcus sign should all be evaluated in both shoulders. The sulcus sign appears when downward traction is applied to the arm and a dimple appears between the humeral head and acromion, and is common in MDI.[33] Any signs of Sprengel deformity or scapular motion dysfunction should be noted. Patients with voluntary instability may also be able to dislocate or subluxate the shoulder on command. Testing for ligamentous laxity should also be performed by testing for hyperextension of the elbow and knee, thumb opposition to the forearm, and ability to place the palms flat on the floor with the knees extended.

Treatment

Most cases of MDI are treated with modification of activities and physical therapy. Therapy focusing on strengthening and stabilization of the rotator cuff and periscapular muscles is the centerpiece of treatment. Providing increased dynamic stability counteracts the deficiencies of the static stabilizers.

Overall good results have been reported with nonoperative treatment. One large cohort of patients with either anterior instability or MDI showed excellent results in 80% of patients with a diagnosis of MDI.[51] Kuroda and colleagues[52] followed 573 shoulders in 341 patients and found that there was a higher rate of spontaneous resolution in patients who were younger and who avoided overhead sports. They recommended avoidance of surgical treatment; however, no specific recommendations were made regarding physical therapy. In general, most patients who are treated with physical therapy report improvement in their symptoms; however, continued pain and instability are a common finding.[53]

For patients who continue to have pain and instability associated with MDI after nonoperative treatment, surgical stabilization is an option. Many practitioners advise a waiting period of 6 months of physical therapy and activity modification before surgery is recommended.[3]

Traditional methods of stabilization relied on open techniques that included an inferior capsular shift. Good results were reported with regard to elimination of instability symptoms and return to sports.[54]

Arthroscopic techniques of stabilization of MDI have increased in popularity as the rate of shoulder arthroscopy in general has increased. Advantages of arthroscopic treatment compared with open procedures include the ability to treat both anterior and posterior disorders as well as decreased surgical morbidity. Early arthroscopic techniques relied on capsular shift.[55] More recent advances in arthroscopic treatment have involved plication of the capsule with sutures through the labrum or tied to the capsule (Fig. 5).[56,57]

Results of arthroscopic treatment have been encouraging. Recurrence rates of instability have been reported from 2% to 12%. Return to sports, range of motion, and pain scores have also been good to excellent for most patients.[58]

TRAUMATIC INJURIES OF THE SHOULDER
Introduction
Many of the injuries of the shoulder in children and adolescents are acute fractures. Fractures of the proximal humerus in adolescents often involve the physis, but may also involve the metaphysis only. Most physeal injuries are Salter-Harris type I injuries, although type II or III injuries may also occur. Because of the large amount of humeral length arising from the proximal physis, remodeling potential is great. These injuries have traditionally been treated nonoperatively, but surgery may be indicated for severely displaced fractures, especially in older patients approaching skeletal maturity. The biceps tendon may be interposed between the fracture fragments, preventing adequate healing.[59] Injuries to the axillary and radial nerves have also been reported, but usually resolve spontaneously.[35]

The clavicle fracture is one of the most common fractures encountered in pediatric orthopaedics, accounting for 5% to 15% of all pediatric fractures.[60,61] Despite the commonality of pediatric clavicle fractures, most of the current literature cited is extrapolated from studies involving adult or older adolescent clavicle fracture.

Injuries involving the sternoclavicular (SC) and acromioclavicular (AC) joint are also seen in adolescents participating in high-energy activities such as football or motocross. AC injuries in children are often avulsion fractures wherein the distal clavicle separates from the periosteal sleeve, which remains attached to the acromion. True AC and SC dislocations are also seen, usually in more skeletally mature adolescents. Posterior SC dislocations are often from high-energy mechanisms and can present as a surgical emergency.

PROXIMAL HUMERUS FRACTURES

Proximal humerus fractures may occur because of falls, collisions, or acute fracture of a previously stressed proximal humeral physis.[59] Patients are likely to present similarly to a shoulder dislocation, with internal rotation and adduction of the arm. A complete neurovascular examination should be performed to rule out axillary nerve or brachial plexus injury. Any previous history of arm pain from pitching should be elucidated.

Patients can usually expect good outcomes with treatment in a sling or hanging-arm cast. A hanging-arm cast is often recommended if there is angulation or shortening of a fracture (Fig. 6). Operative treatment may be indicated for open fractures or fractures with unacceptable angulation in older children, often caused by biceps entrapment.[59] Treatment options include percutaneous screw fixation, pin fixation, and retrograde flexible nails[62] (Fig. 7).

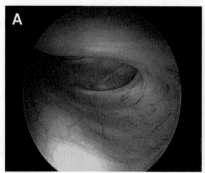
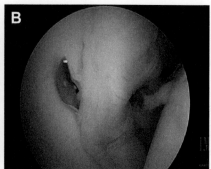

Fig. 5. (A) Patulous capsule with large inferior humeral recess in a 15-year-old softball player with symptoms of MDI. (B) Suture passer in anterior capsule and labrum. Additional sutures were placed posteriorly and inferiorly.

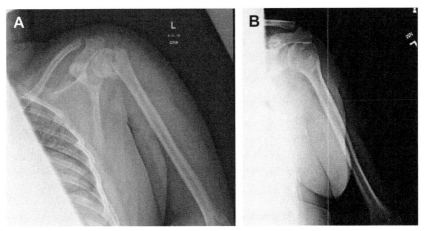

Fig. 6. (A) A 16-year-old boy with Salter-Harris II fracture of proximal humerus who fell while playing basketball. (B) Appearance of shoulder after 3 months of conservative treatment, including hanging-arm cast. Function was normal at final follow-up.

CLAVICLE FRACTURES

School-aged children often sustain fractures from a fall involving a lateral compression force to the shoulder, as opposed to a fall on an outstretched hand.[63] Typical activities include fall from bicycles, sporting activities, or playgrounds. Treatment is typically nonoperative, with immobilization for 4 to 6 weeks. Immobilization is typically performed in a sling, with little benefit seen with braces (Fig. 8).[64]

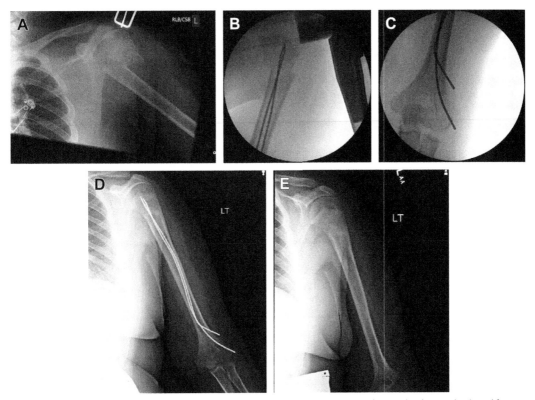

Fig. 7. (A) A 13-year-old boy with shoulder pain after a fall during motocross. Radiographs show a displaced fracture of the proximal humeral metaphysis. (B) Fluoroscopic image of the proximal humerus taken during closed reduction and elastic nail fixation. (C) Appearance of the elbow during elastic nail placement. (D, E) Appearance of the proximal humerus at 6 months and after nail removal. The patient had regained full function and returned to sport.

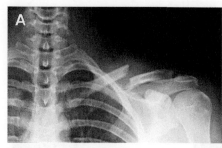
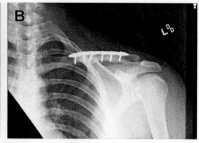

Fig. 8. (A) A 17-year-old boy with left clavicle fracture from football. Radiographs show a 100% displaced and minimally shortened fracture. After discussion with family, he elected operative fixation. (B) Appearance of clavicle fracture 3 months after plate fixation.

Adolescents sustain clavicle fractures from injuries that involve similar mechanics to those in school-aged children, as well as high-energy mechanisms such as motor vehicle and all-terrain vehicle accidents or competitive sports. Although less common, stress fracture can also be incurred secondary to repetitive, high-intensity training in sporting activity such as rowing or gymnastics.[65]

For acute, traumatic fracture with no or mild displacement, nonoperative management is typically the recommended treatment, with previous studies reporting union rates from 95% to 100%.[66,67] Most nondisplaced fractures have significant union by 6 to 8 weeks, with displaced fractures taking longer, reported at 10 to 12 weeks.[66] Historically, nonoperative treatment has been the preferred treatment modality with the expectation of bony union without adverse effects from a functional standpoint.[68,69] There is a risk of refracture after nonoperative treatment, reported at 18%.[70]

Absolute indications for operative treatment include open fractures and significant skin tenting/compromise. Over the last 10 years there has been an overall increase in operative management for displaced midshaft clavicle fractures, specifically in the 15 to 19 years age group (see Fig. 8).[71] Recent studies published have suggested that open reduction and internal fixation (ORIF) for displaced fractures in skeletally immature patients is safe and effective,[72,73] including a randomized clinical trial that favored operative treatment (ORIF) for acute, displaced clavicle fractures.[74] Other studies have concluded that nonoperative treatment can be safely used for midshaft fractures in pediatric patients without risk of clinically meaningful loss of shoulder range of motion or strength.[75,76] The studies showing successful nonoperative management with good outcomes suggest that favoring operative fixation may lead to over-treatment and excessive cost.[67,77,78]

DISTAL CLAVICLE AND ACROMIOCLAVICULAR INJURIES

The distal aspect of the clavicle articulates with the scapula via the AC joint. Ligamentous attachments include the AC and coracoclavicular ligaments, both of which are firmly attached the clavicle's thick periosteal sleeve. True AC injuries are rare during skeletal immaturity compared with fractures of the distal clavicle (Fig. 9). Often the clavicle displaces out of the periosteal sleeve, leaving the periosteum attached to the coracoclavicular and AC ligaments, leading to high remodeling potential (Fig. 10).[5,79,80]

Physical examination should include notation of any deformity, swelling, ecchymosis, or skin tenting. Palpation over the AC joint should elicit significant discomfort. A thorough neurologic examination to assess for brachial plexus or cervical spine injury should also be performed.

Initial imaging should include anteroposterior and axillary lateral views of the shoulder to help determine diagnosis. A Zanca view is also recommended as part of the initial radiographs

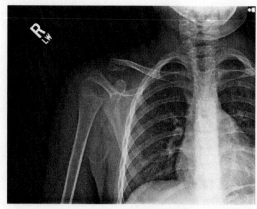

Fig. 9. An 11-year-old boy after a fall in gymnastics. Radiographs at presentation show fracture of the distal clavicle with elevation of the proximal fragment.

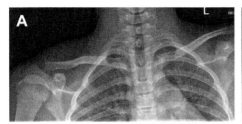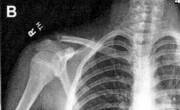

Fig. 10. (A) A 12-year-old boy with a distal clavicle fracture from a fall during soccer. (B) Appearance of the clavicle 2 months later with abundant fracture callus.

when AC dislocation is suspected.[5] The Zanca view is obtained with the patient upright, the injured arm hanging with gravity, and the x-ray beam 10° to 15° cephalad.

Many of these injuries are treated nonoperatively with a sling and rest. Although some investigators recommend nonoperative treatment of all pediatric AC injuries, operative management is frequently advocated for athletes or patients with more severe injuries.[5,80,81]

STERNOCLAVICULAR INJURIES

SC joint injuries are uncommon, representing less than 5% of all shoulder girdle injuries.[80,82,83] Dislocation/fractures are classified based on the direction of displacement (anterior or posterior) and the chronicity of the injury (acute or chronic). Most cases of anterior SC instability are atraumatic and associated with ligamentous laxity.[5]

The SC joint is well stabilized by the numerous ligamentous and muscular attachments, typically requiring a significant amount of force to disrupt it. Adolescents landing on their lateral shoulder during football or other sports may cause a posterior SC dislocation.[84]

On physical examination there may be significant swelling and ecchymosis present, sometimes making determination of the direction of dislocation more challenging. Careful evaluation

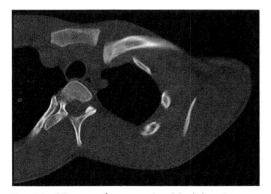

Fig. 11. CT scan of a posterior SC dislocation sustained from a fall during an equestrian event.

for concomitant injury such as rib fractures, brachial plexopathy, or associated chest wall injuries should be performed.

Plain radiographs are the preferred initial imaging modality. The serendipity view described by Wirth and Rockwood[83] is performed by angling the x-ray beam 40° cephalad while it is centered on the sternum, providing a view of both SC joints. In the serendipity view, the affected side appears superiorly displaced in cases of anterior dislocation; conversely the affected side appears inferiorly displaced in cases of posterior dislocation. The easiest method to evaluate the SC joint in cases of suspected fracture or dislocation remains CT (Fig. 11).

It is recommended that atraumatic anterior dislocation be treated nonoperatively.[5] Nonoperative management of a nondisplaced injury typically consists of sling immobilization for 3 to 4 weeks followed by gradual return to activities. A closed reduction of an anterior dislocation can be performed; however, recurrent instability is common. Posterior fracture-dislocations are usually treated operatively, with some investigators advocating performing closed reduction maneuver because of potential stability of reduction and remodeling of the medial clavicle.[5,83,84]

SUMMARY

Pediatric and adolescent athletes are at risk for both chronic and acute injuries to the shoulder and surrounding structures. Overuse injuries are the most common injuries in overhead athletes, with potential consequences to the physis and developing structures of the glenohumeral joint. Most overuse injuries may be treated with a period of rest and rehabilitation, with gradual return to activities. Patients who have sustained anterior dislocations of the shoulder during sports may require operative stabilization. Patients with MDI are often treated nonoperatively, but may require surgery if symptoms persist. Although falls may occur with any activity, children and adolescents participating in high-energy sports such as football, rugby, and motocross are at higher risk of fractures of the osseous structures of the shoulder. Treatment of these injuries is usually patient and fracture dependent.

REFERENCES

1. Robinson TW, Corlette J, Collins CL, et al. Shoulder injuries among US high school athletes, 2005/2006-2011/2012. Pediatrics 2014;133(2):272–9.
2. Mariscalco MW, Saluan P. Upper extremity injuries in the adolescent athlete. Sports Med Arthrosc 2011;19(1):17–26.
3. Milewski MD, Nissen CW. Pediatric and adolescent shoulder instability. Clin Sports Med 2013;32(4):761–79.
4. Gardner E. The embryology of the clavicle. Clin Orthop 1968;58:9–16.
5. Abzug JM, Waters PM, Flynn JM, et al. Clavicle and scapula fractures: Acromioclavicular and sternoclavicular injuries. In: Flynn JM, Skaggs DL, Waters PM, editors. Rockwood and Wilkin's fractures in children. 8th edition. Philadelphia: Lippincott Williams & Wilkins; 2015. p. 807–42.
6. Stracciolini A, Casciano R, Friedman HL, et al. A closer look at overuse injuries in the pediatric athlete. Clin J Sport Med 2015;25(1):30–5.
7. American College of Sports Medicine. Current comment from the American College of Sports Medicine: the prevention of sport injuries of children and adolescents. Med Sci Sports Exerc 1993; 25(8 Suppl):1–7.
8. Loud KJ, Gordon CM, Micheli LJ, et al. Correlates of stress fractures among preadolescent and adolescent girls. Pediatrics 2005;115(4):e399–406.
9. Lyman S, Fleisig GS, Waterbor JW, et al. Longitudinal study of elbow and shoulder pain in youth baseball pitchers. Med Sci Sports Exerc 2001;33(11):1803–10.
10. Olsen SJ 2nd, Fleisig GS, Dun S, et al. Risk factors for shoulder and elbow injuries in adolescent baseball pitchers. Am J Sports Med 2006;34(6):905–12.
11. Lyman S, Fleisig GS, Andrews JR, et al. Effect of pitch type, pitch count, and pitching mechanics on risk of elbow and shoulder pain in youth baseball players. Am J Sports Med 2002;30(4):463–8.
12. Shanley E, Rauh MJ, Michener LA, et al. Incidence of injuries in high school softball and baseball players. J Athl Train 2011;46(6):648–54.
13. Nissen CW, Westwell M, Ounpuu S, et al. A biomechanical comparison of the fastball and curveball in adolescent baseball pitchers. Am J Sports Med 2009;37(8):1492–8.
14. Zaremski JL, Krabak BJ. Shoulder injuries in the skeletally immature baseball pitcher and recommendations for the prevention of injury. PM R 2012;4(7):509–16.
15. Carson WG, Gasser SL. Little Leaguer's shoulder: a report of 23 cases. Am J Sports Med 1998;26:575–80.
16. Osbahr DC, Kim HJ, Dugas JR. Little league shoulder. Curr Opin Pediatr 2010;22(1):35–40.
17. Han KJ, Kim YK, Lim SK, et al. The effect of physical characteristics and field position on the shoulder and elbow injuries of 490 baseball players: confirmation of diagnosis by magnetic resonance imaging. Clin J Sport Med 2009;19(4):271–6.
18. Rauck RC, LaMont LE, Doyle SM. Pediatric upper extremity stress injuries. Curr Opin Pediatr 2013; 25(1):40–5.
19. Shanley E, Rauh MJ, Michener LA, et al. Shoulder range of motion measures as risk factors for shoulder and elbow injuries in high school softball and baseball players. Am J Sports Med 2011;39(9):1997–2006.
20. Chen FS, Diaz VA, Loebenberg M, et al. Shoulder and elbow injuries in the skeletally immature athlete. J Am Acad Orthop Surg 2005;13(3):172–85.
21. Johnson L. Patterns of shoulder flexibility among college baseball players. J Athl Train 1992;27(1):44–9.
22. Levine WN, Brandon ML, Stein BS, et al. Shoulder adaptive changes in youth baseball players. J Shoulder Elbow Surg 2006;15(5):562–6.
23. Murachovsky J, Ikemoto RY, Nascimento LG, et al. Does the presence of proximal humerus growth plate changes in young baseball pitchers happen only in symptomatic athletes? An x ray evaluation of 21 young baseball pitchers. Br J Sports Med 2010;44(2):90–4.
24. Simonet WT, Melton LJ 3rd, Cofield RH, et al. Incidence of anterior shoulder dislocation in Olmsted County, Minnesota. Clin Orthop Relat Res 1984;(186):186–91.
25. Cleeman E, Flatow EL. Shoulder dislocations in the young patient. Orthop Clin North Am 2000;31(2):217–29.
26. Postacchini F, Gumina S, Cinotti G. Anterior shoulder dislocation in adolescents. J Shoulder Elbow Surg 2000;9(6):470–4.
27. Owens BD, Agel J, Mountcastle SB, et al. Incidence of glenohumeral instability in collegiate athletics. Am J Sports Med 2009;37(9):1750–4.
28. Wagner KT Jr, Lyne ED. Adolescent traumatic dislocations of the shoulder with open epiphyses. J Pediatr Orthop 1983;3(1):61–2.
29. Shymon SJ, Roocroft J, Edmonds EW. Traumatic anterior instability of the pediatric shoulder: a comparison of arthroscopic and open Bankart repairs. J Pediatr Orthop 2015;35(1):1–6.
30. Lawton RL, Choudhury S, Mansat P, et al. Pediatric shoulder instability: presentation, findings, treatment, and outcomes. J Pediatr Orthop 2002;22(1):52–61.
31. Rowe CR. Prognosis in dislocations of the shoulder. J Bone Joint Surg Am 1956;38-A(5):957–77.
32. Curtis RJ, Dameron TB, Rockwood CA Jr. Fractures and dislocations of the shoulder in children. In:

Wilkins KE, King RE, Rockwood CA Jr, editors. Fractures in children. Philadelphia: JB Lippincott; 1991.

33. Marshall KW, Marshall DL, Busch MT. Shoulder pain in the adolescent athlete: a multidisciplinary diagnostic approach from the medical, surgical, and imaging perspective. Pediatr Radiol 2010;40: 453–60.

34. Ellis HB Jr, Seiter M, Wise K, et al. Glenoid bone loss in traumatic glenohumeral instability in the adolescent population. J Pediatr Orthop 2015. [Epub ahead of print].

35. Flynn JM, Waters PM, Skaggs DL. Humeral shaft and proximal humerus, shoulder dislocation. Rockwood and Wilkins' fractures in children. Lippincott Williams & Wilkins.

36. Itoi E, Hatakeyama Y, Sato T, et al. Immobilization in external rotation after shoulder dislocation reduces the risk of recurrence. A randomized controlled trial. J Bone Joint Surg Am 2007;89(10): 2124–31.

37. Liavaag S, Brox JI, Pripp AH, et al. Immobilization in external rotation after primary shoulder dislocation did not reduce the risk of recurrence: a randomized controlled trial. J Bone Joint Surg Am 2011;93(10): 897–904.

38. Finestone A, Milgrom C, Radeva-Petrova DR, et al. Bracing in external rotation for traumatic anterior dislocation of the shoulder. J Bone Joint Surg Br 2009;91(7):918–21.

39. Robinson CM, Howes J, Murdoch H, et al. Functional outcome and risk of recurrent instability after primary traumatic anterior shoulder dislocation in young patients. J Bone Joint Surg Am 2006; 88(11):2326–36.

40. Taylor DC, Krasinski KL. Adolescent shoulder injuries: consensus and controversies. J Bone Joint Surg Am 2009;91(2):462–73.

41. Safran O, Milgrom C, Radeva-Petrova DR, et al. Accuracy of the anterior apprehension test as a predictor of risk for redislocation after a first traumatic shoulder dislocation. Am J Sports Med 2010;38(5):972–5.

42. Marans HJ, Angel KR, Schemitsch EH, et al. The fate of traumatic anterior dislocation of the shoulder in children. J Bone Joint Surg Am 1992;74(8): 1242–4.

43. Jones KJ, Wiesel B, Ganley TJ, et al. Functional outcomes of early arthroscopic Bankart repair in adolescents aged 11 to 18 years. J Pediatr Orthop 2007;27(2):209–13.

44. Castagna A, Delle Rose G, Borroni M, et al. Arthroscopic stabilization of the shoulder in adolescent athletes participating in overhead or contact sports. Arthroscopy 2012;28(3):309–15.

45. Gerber C, Nyffeler RW. Classification of glenohumeral joint instability. Clin Orthop Relat Res 2002;(400):65–76.

46. Heyworth BE, Kocher MS. Shoulder instability in the young athlete. Instr Course Lect 2013;62:435–44.

47. Emery RJ, Mullaji AB. Glenohumeral joint instability in normal adolescents. Incidence and significance. J Bone Joint Surg Br 1991;73(3):406–8.

48. Bak K, Fauno P. Clinical findings in competitive swimmers with shoulder pain. Am J Sports Med 1997;25(2):254–60.

49. Rowe CR, Pierce DS, Clark JG. Voluntary dislocation of the shoulder. A preliminary report on a clinical, electromyographic, and psychiatric study of twenty-six patients. J Bone Joint Surg Am 1973; 55(3):445–60.

50. Hattrup SJ, Cofield RH, Weaver AL. Anterior shoulder reconstruction: prognostic variables. J Shoulder Elbow Surg 2001;10(6):508–13.

51. Burkhead WZ Jr, Rockwood CA Jr. Treatment of instability of the shoulder with an exercise program. J Bone Joint Surg Am 1992;74(6):890–6.

52. Kuroda S, Sumiyoshi T, Moriishi J, et al. The natural course of atraumatic shoulder instability. J Shoulder Elbow Surg 2001;10(2):100–4.

53. Misamore GW, Sallay PI, Didelot W. A longitudinal study of patients with multidirectional instability of the shoulder with seven- to ten-year follow-up. J Shoulder Elbow Surg 2005; 14(5):466–70.

54. Neer CS 2nd, Foster CR. Inferior capsular shift for involuntary inferior and multidirectional instability of the shoulder. A preliminary report. J Bone Joint Surg Am 1980;62(6):897–908.

55. Pollock RG, Owens JM, Flatow EL, et al. Operative results of the inferior capsular shift procedure for multidirectional instability of the shoulder. J Bone Joint Surg Am 2000;82-A(7):919–28.

56. Caprise PA Jr, Sekiya JK. Open and arthroscopic treatment of multidirectional instability of the shoulder. Arthroscopy 2006;22(10):1126–31.

57. Wiley WB, Goradia VK, Pearson SE. Arthroscopic capsular plication-shift. Arthroscopy 2005;21: 119–21.

58. Baker CL 3rd, Mascarenhas R, Kline AJ, et al. Arthroscopic treatment of multidirectional shoulder instability in athletes: a retrospective analysis of 2- to 5-year clinical outcomes. Am J Sports Med 2009;37(9):1712–20.

59. Dobbs MB, Luhmann SL, Gordon JE, et al. Severely displaced proximal humeral epiphyseal fractures. J Pediatr Orthop 2003;23(2):208–15.

60. Nordvist A, Petersson C. The incidence of fractures of the clavicle. Clin Orthop Relat Res 1994; 300:127–32.

61. Robinson CM. Fractures of the clavicle in the adult. Epidemiology and classification. J Bone Joint Surg Br 1998;80:476–84.

62. Shore BJ, Hedequist DJ, Miller PE, et al. Surgical management for displaced pediatric proximal

humeral fractures: a cost analysis. J Child Orthop 2015;9(1):55–64.

63. Stanley D, Trowbridge EA, Norris SH. The mechanism of clavicular fracture: a clinical and biomechanical analysis. J Bone Joint Surg Br 1988;70:461–4.

64. Ersen A, Atalar AC, Birisik F, et al. Comparison of simple arm sling and figure of eight clavicular bandage for midshaft clavicular fractures: a randomised controlled study. Bone Joint J 2015;97-B(11):1562–5.

65. Abbot AE, Hannafin JA. Stress fracture of the clavicle in a female lightweight rower. A case report and review of the literature. Am J Sports Med 2001;29:370–2.

66. Vander Have KL, Perdue AM, Caird MS, et al. Operative versus nonoperative treatment of midshaft clavicle fractures in adolescents. J Pediatr Orthop 2010;30:307–12.

67. Khan LA, Bradnock TJ, Scott C, et al. Fractures of the clavicle. J Bone Joint Surg Am 2009;91:447–60.

68. Stanley D, Norris SH. Recovery following fractures of the clavicle treated conservatively. Injury 1988;19:162–4.

69. Robinson CM, Court-Brown CM, McQueen MM, et al. Estimating the risk of nonunion following nonoperative treatment of a clavicular fracture. J Bone Joint Surg Am 2004;86-A:1359–65.

70. Masnovi ME, Mehlman CT, Eismann EA, et al. Pediatric refracture rates after angulated and completely displaced clavicle shaft fractures. J Orthop Trauma 2014;28(11):648–52.

71. Yang S, Werner B, Gwathmey F. Treatment trends in adolescent clavicle fractures. J Pediatr Orthop 2015;35(3):229–33.

72. Mehlman CT, Yihua G, Bochang C, et al. Operative treatment of completely displaced clavicle shaft fractures in children. J Pediatr Orthop 2009;29:851–5.

73. Namdari S, Ganley TJ, Baldwin K, et al. Fixation of displaced midshaft clavicle fractures in skeletally immature patients. J Pediatr Orthop 2011;31:507–11.

74. Canadian Orthopedic Trauma Society. Nonoperative treatment compared with plate fixation of displaced midshaft clavicular fractures. A multicenter, randomized clinical trial. J Bone Joint Surg Am 2007;89:1–10.

75. Bae DS, Shah AS, Kalish LA, et al. Shoulder motion, strength, and functional outcomes in children with established malunion of the clavicle. J Pediatr Orthop 2013;33(5):544–9.

76. Robinson L, Gargoum R, Auer R, et al. Sports participation and radiographic findings of adolescents treated nonoperatively for displaced clavicle fractures. Injury 2015;46:1372–6.

77. McKee MD, Wild LM, Schemitsch EH. Midshaft malunions of the clavicle. J Bone Joint Surg Am 2003;85-A:790–7.

78. Robinson CM, Goudie EB, Murray IR, et al. Open reduction and plate fixation versus nonoperative treatment for displaced midshaft clavicular fractures: a multicenter, randomized, controlled trial. J Bone Joint Surg Am 2013;95(17):1576–84.

79. Havránek P. Injuries of distal clavicular physis in children. J Pediatr Orthop 1989;9(2):213–5.

80. Kocher MS, Waters PM, Micheli LJ. Upper extremity injuries in the pediatric athlete. Sports Med 2000;30:117–35.

81. Gstettner C, Tauber M, Hitzl W, et al. Rockwood type III acromioclavicular dislocation: surgical versus conservative treatment. J Shoulder Elbow Surg 2008;17:220–5.

82. Nettles JL, Linscheid RL. Sternoclavicular dislocations. J Trauma 1968;8:158–64.

83. Wirth MA, Rockwood CA. Acute and chronic traumatic injuries of the sternoclavicular joint. J Am Acad Orthop Surg 1996;4:268–78.

84. Chaudhry S. Pediatric posterior sternoclavicular joint injuries. J Am Acad Orthop Surg 2015;23(8):468–75.

Pediatric Knee Osteochondritis Dissecans Lesions

Aristides I. Cruz Jr, MD[a],[*], Kevin G. Shea, MD[b],
Theodore J. Ganley, MD[c]

KEYWORDS

- Cartilage • Chondral • Knee pain • Knee swelling • Sports medicine

KEY POINTS

- Osteochondritis dissecans (OCD) lesion of the knee is a relatively common cause of knee pain in pediatric patients.
- Most pediatric OCD lesions of the knee will heal with nonoperative treatment, which includes a period of rest or activity modification with or without immoblization.
- Surgical treatment is indicated for patients with closed physes or unstable or unsalvageable lesions.
- The goals of surgical treatment include maintenance of articular cartilage congruity, rigid fixation of unstable fragments, and repair of osteochondral defects with cells or tissue that can adequately replace lost or deficient cartilage.
- High-quality evidence for the optimal evaluation and management of pediatric OCD lesions remains sparse, and continued research is needed.

INTRODUCTION

Osteochondritis dissecans (OCD) of the knee can be a source of pain and dysfunction in pediatric patients. The estimated incidence of OCD ranges from 9.5 to 29 cases per 100,000 population.[1-3] Boys have an approximately fourfold increased incidence of OCD of the knee compared with girls.[3] Most lesions are found within the distal femur, and the most common site is the lateral aspect of the medial femoral condyle.[3,4] OCD is an acquired condition of articular cartilage and subchondral bone that initially manifests itself as a softening of the overlying cartilage (Fig. 1). Without treatment, this can progress to articular cartilage fissuring, separation, partial detachment, and eventually, osteochondral separation.[5-9] OCD of the knee can be subcategorized based on the status of the distal femoral physis. Juvenile OCD occurs in patients with open physes and has a much better prognosis than adult OCD. Greater than 50% of juvenile OCD cases will show healing within 6 to 18 months with nonoperative treatment, whereas patients with adult OCD frequently require operative intervention.[10]

HISTORY AND ETIOLOGY

The etiology of OCD remains unclear, and no theory regarding its cause is universally accepted.[11] Theories on etiology include inflammation, ischemia, ossification abnormalities, genetic factors, and repetitive microtrauma.[11-14] In 1887, König suggested an inflammatory etiology, coining the term "osteochondritis dissecans."[15]

Disclosure Statement: The authors have no relevant disclosures.
[a] Department of Orthopaedic Surgery, Hasbro Children's Hospital, The Warren Alpert Medical School of Brown University, 2 Dudley Street, Suite 200, Providence, RI 02906, USA; [b] St. Luke's Children's Hospital, Boise, ID 83702, USA; [c] Department of Orthopaedic Surgery, The Children's Hospital of Philadelphia, Philadelphia, PA 19104, USA
* Corresponding author.
E-mail address: aristides_cruz@brown.edu

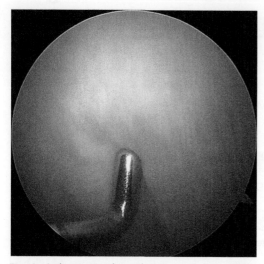

Fig. 1. Arthroscopic photo showing articular cartilage softening found in OCD lesions. (*Courtesy of* Theodore J. Ganley, MD, Philadelphia, PA.)

Further study, however, did not support inflammation as the primary cause of OCD. Ribbing attributed abnormalities in ossification within the distal femoral epiphysis as a cause.[16] A possible vascular etiology has been proposed, with relative ischemia and subsequent necrosis being important components in the development of OCD.[17,18] Other studies, however, have failed to definitively identify avascular necrosis of the OCD fragment or find a relative ischemic watershed area of the lateral aspect of the medial femoral condyle (the most common location of OCD lesions).[19–22] More recent research in the development of OCD lesions in animals has focused on the role that vascular architecture may play in the development of OCD.[23–25] Both pigs and people develop OCD lesions in similar anatomic regions, and the vascular anatomy in both species demonstrates that both species have similar vascular architecture, which may predispose them to the development of OCD of the femoral condyles.[23] This research suggests that vascularity may play a role in the development of OCD in people.

A genetic predisposition for the development of OCD has also been proposed. Several cases of monozygotic twins with OCD lesions have been described,[26–31] as well as large reports of OCD lesions within the same family.[13,14,32] Additionally, there are several genetic diseases that are associated with the development of OCD lesions. Patients with Stickler syndrome have been found to have multiple OCD lesions.[30] OCD lesions are also commonly reported in association with dwarfism.[33–37]

Mechanical factors such as malalignment[38] or repetitive microtrauma[39] have also been implicated in the development of OCD. The frequent occurrence of OCD lesions in patients who are involved in activities and sports with repetitive impact as well as the association with abnormal meniscal anatomy help support the concept of altered knee biomechanics as a cause of OCD.[40–42] This theory holds that OCD occurs as a result of an initial stress reaction, which may then progress to a stress fracture of the underlying subchondral bone. With progressive repetitive loading, the stress fracture fails to heal, and the subchondral bone becomes necrotic,[12] causing the fragment to eventually dissect and separate from the fracture bed.

Although the precise etiology of OCD is unclear, it is known that if these lesions are left untreated and fail to heal appropriately, they have a high potential of contributing to the development of future osteoarthritis.[43,44]

BIOLOGY OF ARTICULAR CARTILAGE AND SUBCHONDRAL BONE

Understanding the anatomy and morphology of subchondral bone is important to adequately evaluate and manage conditions that affect the subchondral bone such as OCD.[45–47] The subchondral zone or the subchondral bone plate refers to the cortical endplate lying adjacent to the calcified zone of the articular cartilage with its accompanying subarticular spongiosa (**Fig. 2**). The cement line separates the calcified zone from the subchondral bone plate, with the thickness of the subchondral bone plate varying depending on the joint.

The architecture of the subchondral bone plate consists of 2 mineralized layers, which together form a single unit, separating the articular cartilage from the bone marrow. There is a discrete band of calcified cartilage on the articular side of the subchondral bone plate. This band appears as the tidemark on hematoxylin and eosin histologic staining. The tidemark is a complex 3-dimensional structure. The tidemark is significant, because it represents the mineralization front and is a transition zone between 2 dissimilar regions of cartilage[45] (see **Fig. 2**). The tidemark separates the type II collagen fibrils of the articular cartilage from the type I collagen found deeper (away from the joint surface). The tidemark has significant biomechanical functions and changes in response to microinjury. There is evidence that collagen fibrils cross the tidemark, resulting in a strong link

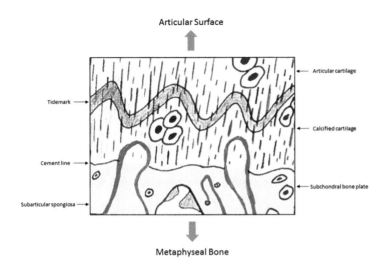

Articular Surface

Tidemark

Cement line

Subarticular spongiosa

Metaphyseal Bone

Articular cartilage

Calcified cartilage

Subchondral bone plate

Fig. 2. Schematic drawing depicting the anatomy and architecture of subchondral bone. Note collagen fibrils (depicted as *dark, vertical lines*) crossing tidemark, extending from the articular cartilage into calcified cartilage. No collagen fibrils connect the calcified cartilage to the subchondral bone plate. Blood vessels from subchondral region can extend into overlying calcified cartilage through canals in subchondral bone plate. (*Adapted from* Madry H, van Dijk CN, Mueller-Gerbl M. The basic science of subchondral bone. Knee Surg Sports Traumatol Arthrosc 2010;18(4):422. Original Figure 3; with permission.)

between these 2 zones.[46] This is clinically relevant, because meticulous removal of all calcified cartilage during articular cartilage repair procedures is important to allow for good attachment of any repair tissue to the subchondral bone plate.

The calcified cartilage extends further toward the marrow cavity, where it is remodeled and replaced by woven or lamellar bone, taking on the appearance of the supporting trabeculae. The dense cancellous bone underlying the calcified cartilage has a honeycomb appearance that looks like a solid mass of bone fenestrated by intercommunicating spaces. Deeper away from the articular cartilage surface is the subarticular spongiosa. No collagen fibers transverse the area between the calcified cartilage and the cortical endplate, making the osteochondral junction an area of regional weakness. This is in contrast to the tidemark that separates the calcified cartilage from the articular cartilage, which is crossed by collagen fibrils.

There are a high number of arterial and venous vessels as well as nerves, sending small branches into the calcified cartilage layer. The subchondral plate is fenestrated by hollow spaces, which may provide a direct connection between the unmineralized cartilage and the marrow cavity of the subarticular spongiosa. Blood vessels have the potential of reaching the overlying articular cartilage directly, such as during microfracture procedures, in which the calcified zone of cartilage is removed prior to surgically penetrating through to the subchondral bone plate into the subarticular spongiosa.

EVALUATION AND DIAGNOSIS
Clinical Presentation
The initial presentation in most children with knee OCD is relatively nonspecific. In stable lesions, knee aching and activity-related pain are the most common complaints. Symptoms may mimic patellofemoral pain due to chondromalacia patella or subtle patellofemoral malalignment. Knee instability or mechanical symptoms are unusual. On physical examination, children with stable lesions may walk with a slight limp. Palpation through varying degrees of knee flexion often reveals a point of maximal tenderness over the involved femoral condyle, typically the lateral aspect of the medial femoral condyle. In long-standing symptomatic lesions, quadriceps dysfunction may be noted. Knee effusion and crepitus are unusual in stable lesions; however, unstable lesions more commonly present with mechanical symptoms, effusion, limping, and crepitus, as the knee is taken through a range of motion.[11] In younger patients with significant growth remaining, unstable lesions and associated mechanical symptoms are rare. Some stable lesions may develop symptomatic plica bands or synovial folds, which can produce some mechanical symptoms. Symptoms and examination of the contralateral knee should also be assessed, since lesions may be bilateral in 20% to 25% of cases.[40]

Imaging
The ideal imaging modality for the evaluation of OCD lesions should be reliable, reproducible, and provide prognostic information on the lesion's ability to heal with nonoperative management. Imaging begins with plain radiography

and should include anterior-posterior (AP), lateral, and tunnel or notch views of the knee (Fig. 3). A sunrise or Merchant view should also be obtained if there is suspicion for a trochlear or patellar lesion. Full-length, bilateral, lower extremity standing alignment films are useful to assess patients' mechanical axis, particularly in those with uncommon lesion locations (ie, lateral femoral condyle lesions) (Fig. 4). Plain radiography is useful to characterize lesion location, rule out other bony pathology, and evaluate skeletal maturity, which is prognostic of healing potential. Plain radiographs can also be used to longitudinally monitor lesion healing. In younger patients (typically <7 years old), the distal femoral epiphyseal ossification center may appear irregular and mimic the appearance of an OCD,[48] making correlation with clinical findings important. Contralateral knee radiographs may also be considered to assess ossification irregularities as well as potential asymptomatic lesions. Important characteristics that can be noted on plain radiographs include lesion size, location, shape/contour, radiodensity, and fragmentation.[49]

MRI has become a routine part of the evaluation of OCD lesions and is useful for determining lesion size, cartilage morphology, and condition of the underlying subchondral bone.[50,51] MRI has also been shown to correlate well with histopathologic findings in juvenile OCD lesions[52]

and can be used to assess areas of increased T2 signal deep to the osteochondral fragment as well as the presence of loose bodies. De Smet and colleagues[53] described MRI findings found on T2-weighted sequences that could be used to predict lesion stability (Table 1). The authors found that a high signal line deep to the OCD fragment was most predictive of an unstable lesion (Fig. 5). This high signal line may indicate the presence of either healing vascular granulation tissue or synovial fluid beneath the subchondral bone implying a break in the articular surface (when interpreted in conjunction with a breach in the articular surface as seen on T1-weighted images).[54–56] It has been shown that patients with this finding on MRI are less likely to heal with nonoperative treatment.[57] Additionally, lesion size as assessed on MRI has been shown to be predictive of healing potential.[58] Despite the widespread use of MRI in the evaluation of pediatric OCD lesions, appearance on MRI does not always correlate with lesion stability. Kijowski and colleagues[59] showed that although the sensitivity of MRI for diagnosing an unstable lesion in pediatric patients is 100%, the specificity was only 11% in their series. Heywood and colleagues[56] had similar findings when correlating MRI findings with arthroscopy. Table 2 summarizes the MRI classification of OCD lesions. Based on current

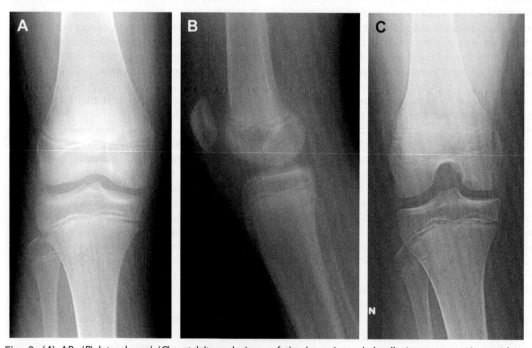

Fig. 3. (A) AP, (B) lateral, and (C) notch/tunnel views of the knee in a skeletally immature patient with an OCD lesion of the lateral aspect of the medial femoral condyle. Lesions are often best seen on notch/tunnel view. (*Courtesy of* Theodore J. Ganley, MD, Philadelphia, PA.)

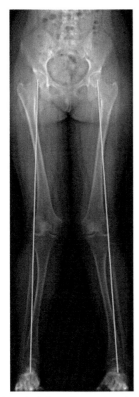

Fig. 4. Full-length, bilateral, standing lower extremity radiographs to assess mechanical alignment. Note significant genu valgum in this patient with bilateral, lateral femoral condyle OCD lesions. (*Courtesy of* Theodore J. Ganley, MD, Philadelphia, PA.)

literature, smaller lesions with intact cartilage are more likely to heal with nonoperative management alone, especially in skeletally immature patients.

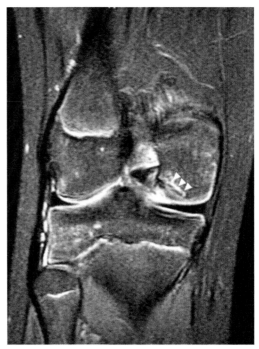

Fig. 5. High signal line (*arrow heads*) on, T2-weighted imaging deep to OCD lesion suggestive of unstable lesion. (*Courtesy of* Theodore J. Ganley, MD, Philadelphia, PA.)

Arthroscopic Appearance

Recently, the Research on Osteochondritis Dissecans of the Knee (ROCK) Study Group developed a knee arthroscopy classification system of OCD lesions.[60] In this classification system, lesions are divided into 2 groups based on

Table 1
De Smet MRI criteria for fragment stability

	Description
1	Thin line of high signal intensity 5 mm or more in length at the interface between the OCD and underlying bone
2	Discrete, round area of homogenous high signal intensity 5 mm or more in diameter beneath the lesion
3	Focal defect with a width of 5 mm or more in the articular surface of the lesion
4	High signal intensity line traversing the articular cartilage and subchondral bone plate into the lesion

Adapted from Heywood CS, Benke MT, Brindle K, et al. Correlation of magnetic resonance imaging to arthroscopic findings of stability in juvenile osteochondritis dissecans. Arthroscopy 2011;27(2):195; with permission.

Table 2
MRI classification of osteochondritis dissecans lesions

Stage	MRI Findings
I	Small change of signal without clear margins of fragment
II	Osteochondral fragment with clear margins but without fluid between fragment and underlying bone
III	Fluid is visible partially between fragment and underlying bone
IV	Fluid is completely surrounding the fragment, but the fragment remains in situ
V	Fragment is completely detached and displaced (loose body)

From Hefti F, Beguiristain J, Krauspe R, et al. Osteochondritis dissecans: a multicenter study of the European Pediatric Orthopedic Society. J Pediatr Orthop B 1999;8(4):234.

diagnostic arthroscopy: immobile or mobile. These groups are further subdivided into 3 categories within each group describing specific lesion characteristics (Fig. 6). Intraclass correlation coefficients were used to measure intra- and inter-rater reliability during the development of the classification system, and very good to excellent reliability was found among orthopedic surgeon members of the ROCK group. This classification system will be useful for future radiograph and MRI validation studies and for facilitating multicenter OCD research.

TREATMENT

In 2010, the American Academy of Orthopaedic Surgeons released clinical practice guidelines regarding the evaluation and treatment of OCD lesions.[61] At the time, there was noted to be a lack of high-quality evidence to support many recommendations; however, the guidelines offer a concise outline for future research on OCD of the knee. Fig. 7 summarizes the authors' preferred treatment algorithm for pediatric OCD lesions.

NONOPERATIVE MANAGEMENT

Nonoperative management is the treatment of choice in skeletally immature children because of the favorable natural history of OCD lesions in those with open physes.[62] There is controversy regarding the use of immobilization for nonoperative treatment,[61] with proponents for or against

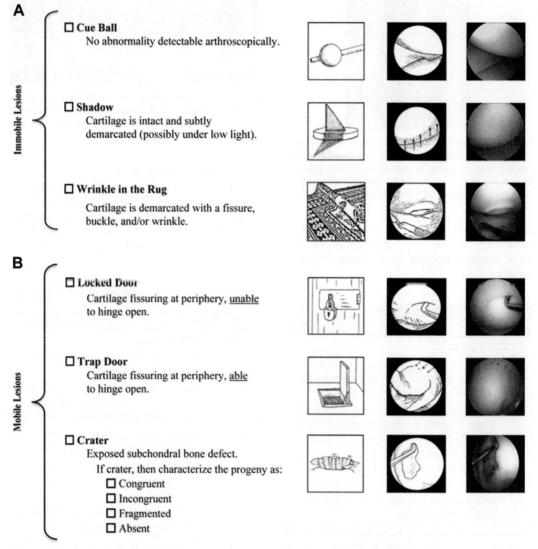

A

Immobile Lesions

☐ **Cue Ball**
No abnormality detectable arthroscopically.

☐ **Shadow**
Cartilage is intact and subtly demarcated (possibly under low light).

☐ **Wrinkle in the Rug**
Cartilage is demarcated with a fissure, buckle, and/or wrinkle.

B

Mobile Lesions

☐ **Locked Door**
Cartilage fissuring at periphery, <u>unable</u> to hinge open.

☐ **Trap Door**
Cartilage fissuring at periphery, <u>able</u> to hinge open.

☐ **Crater**
Exposed subchondral bone defect.
    If crater, then characterize the progeny as:
        ☐ Congruent
        ☐ Incongruent
        ☐ Fragmented
        ☐ Absent

Fig. 6. (*A*) ROCK Group arthroscopic classification and description of immobile OCD lesions. (*B*) Classification and description of mobile OCD lesions. (*Courtesy of* Theodore J. Ganley, MD, Philadelphia, PA.)

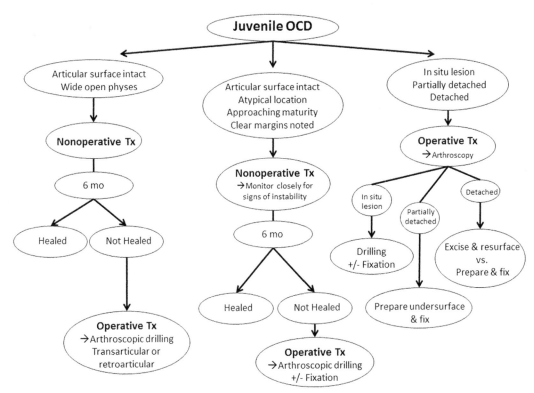

Fig. 7. Authors' preferred treatment algorithm for pediatric OCD lesions of the knee. (*Courtesy of* Theodore J. Ganley, MD, Philadelphia, PA.)

immobilization generally falling into 2 schools of thought. Those who consider OCD primarily a disease of articular cartilage encourage motion to maintain chondral health, while those who consider OCD primarily a disease of subchondral bone advocate immobilization to allow for bony healing. In either scenario, nonoperative treatment centers on relative rest and activity modification; sports and activities that require high-impact, repetitive loading are avoided.

Immobilization can be achieved in a cast, brace, or knee immobilizer. Some authors prefer partial weight bearing in a cylinder cast in slight flexion to potentially allow some compressive forces across the lesion while minimizing shear stress. While bracing may be easier to allow for activities of daily living, compliance with brace or immobilizer use can be challenging in the pediatric patient. Some authors recommend an unloader type brace specific to the location of the lesion. Further study is needed to determine the optimal immobilization protocol. Table 3 represents the authors' preferred nonoperative treatment regimen.

Several authors have attempted to describe clinical and radiographic predictors of successful nonoperative treatment. Wall and colleagues[58] retrospectively reviewed 47 skeletally immature

patients with stable OCD lesions to determine potential predictors of healing after nonoperative treatment. After logistic regression analysis, failure of lesions to progress to healing after 6 months of nonoperative treatment were associated with increased size and associated swelling and/or mechanical symptoms compared with healed lesions. Based on their findings, the authors developed a nomogram to predict the likelihood of OCD healing based on the quantitative size and qualitative symptoms (mechanical symptoms vs pain only) of lesions (Fig. 8). Krause and colleagues[63] retrospectively examined 62 skeletally immature patients (76 stable OCD lesions) who were treated nonoperatively. After 6 months of treatment, 67% of lesions showed no progression towards healing. After multivariable logistic regression analysis, the authors found that normalized lesion width, patient age, and the size of cyst-like lesions deep to the OCD as measured on MRI were most predictive of lesion healing.

OPERATIVE MANAGEMENT

In skeletally mature patients or patients with open physes in which no healing has been demonstrated after 3 to 6 months of nonoperative

Table 3
Nonoperative treatment protocol for pediatric osteochondritis dissecans of the knee

Phase[a]	Wk	Treatment	Follow-up Imaging
1	0–6	• Knee immobilization[b] • Crutch-protected partial weight bearing	Radiograph
2	6–12	• Immobilization discontinued • Progressive weight bearing • Rehabilitation program: emphasize knee range of motion, quadriceps/hamstring strengthening	Radiograph
3	>12-healing	• Supervised initiation of running, jumping, cutting activities • High-impact and shear activities restricted until pain free with low-impact conditioning and MRI documents healing	MRI

[a] Criteria for protocol advancement: resolution of pain and swelling. At any phase, if symptoms return or radiographs show lesion progression, repeat immobilization is considered.
[b] Cylinder cast versus knee immobilizer individualized to patient/family preference/tolerance.

treatment, surgical treatment is considered. Surgery should also be considered for patients with detached or unstable lesions as assessed on imaging or during diagnostic arthroscopy. The goals of surgical treatment include maintenance of articular cartilage congruity, rigid fixation of unstable fragments, and repair of osteochondral defects with cells or tissue that can adequately replace lost or deficient articular cartilage.[64]

The optimal surgical treatment provides a stable construct of subchondral bone, calcified tidemark, as well as cartilage with the viability and biomechanical properties similar to native hyaline cartilage.

Intact Lesions

Lesions with intact cartilage that remain contained within the femoral subchondral bone

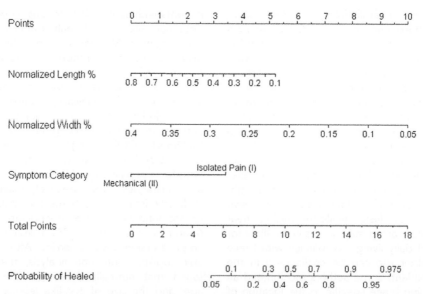

Fig. 8. Nomogram developed from regression analysis used to predict outcome of pediatric OCD lesions based on normalized width, normalized length, and symptoms. To use the nomogram, one places a straight edge vertically so that it touches the designated variable on the axis for each predictor. The value that each of the 3 predictors provides the points axis at the top of the diagram. All of the recorded points are then summed, and this value is located on the total points line with a straight edge. A vertical line drawn down from the total points line to the probability of healed line will identify the probability that the patient will demonstrate healing or progression towards healing after 6 months of conservative treatment based on the predictive variables. (*From* Wall EJ, Vourazeris J, Myer GD, et al. The healing potential of stable juvenile osteochondritis dissecans knee lesions. J Bone Joint Surg Am 2008;90(12):2659. Original Figure 3; with permission.)

bed are amenable to arthroscopic drilling with or without fixation, depending on lesion stability as assessed on diagnostic arthroscopy.[65–67] Several drilling techniques have been described including retroarticular, transarticular, and intercondylar notch drilling[68] (Fig. 9). Retroarticular drilling avoids articular cartilage penetration; however, it may be more technically challenging to obtain accurate drilling of the lesion. Transarticular drilling may be less technically challenging; however, there is cartilage surface penetration, and it may be more challenging to identify the lesion based solely on the gross appearance of the overlying articular cartilage. Intercondylar notch drilling involves accessing the OCD lesion via the intercondylar notch and offers the advantage of avoiding violation of the articular cartilage (Fig. 10).[68] Although this technique may be suitable for the most common location of OCD lesions (lateral aspect, medial femoral condyle), not all lesion locations may be accessible to this drilling technique.

Unstable Lesions

Unstable lesions should be evaluated arthroscopically and rigidly fixed, provided that the progeny bone remains reasonably congruent with the parent bone defect, and that there is adequate subchondral bone attached to the unstable lesion to afford stable fixation. Complete debridement of fibrous tissue from the underlying subchondral bone bed prior to lesion reduction and fixation is important for successful treatment. Congruency of the articular surface is also important, and any subchondral bone loss should be bone grafted prior to lesion fixation to help prevent subsidence of the lesion.

Fixation options include metal or bioabsorbable pins and screws, primarily based on surgeon preference. The advantage of bioabsorbable implants is the avoidance of a second surgery to remove them; however, these implants have been associated with synovitis, chronic effusion, and osteolysis of the surrounding bone.[69] When using metal screws, the authors prefer small diameter screws, which are buried deep to the articular surface, fully within the subchondral bone (Fig. 11). Good results have been reported after treatment of unstable OCD lesions irrespective of implant choice.[70–72]

Salvage Procedures

Long-term results after excision of loose OCD lesions in skeletally mature patients can be poor, and this has led some authors to recommend more aggressive attempts to preserve articular cartilage and avoid excision of fragments.[73–75] However, some lesions may be unsalvageable, and other treatment options aside from OCD fragment retention can be utilized. Several salvage procedures have been described to replace or resurface the defect left behind by the OCD lesion. Drilling, abrasion arthroplasty, and microfracture can be used to stimulate fibrocartilage formation within the parent bone defect by recruiting pluripotent stem cells from underlying marrow elements. This method is most effective in small (<2 cm^2) osteochondral lesions.[76–78] In cases of significant subchondral bone loss, however, use of microfracture may be limited in its ability to address the bone defect.

Because fibrocartilage does not have the same biomechanical characteristics and durability as hyaline cartilage, alternative techniques

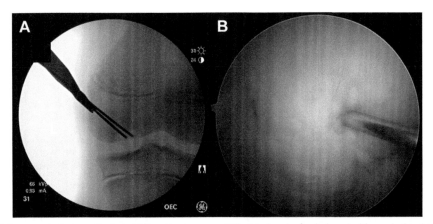

Fig. 9. (A) Antegrade (retroarticular) drilling. K-wires are drilled to level of subchondral bone behind OCD lesion using fluoroscopy to guide K-wire placement. (B) Retrograde (transarticular drilling). Small diameter K-wire is drilled directly through overlying articular cartilage overlying OCD lesion into subchondral bone. (*Courtesy of* Theodore J. Ganley, MD, Philadelphia, PA.)

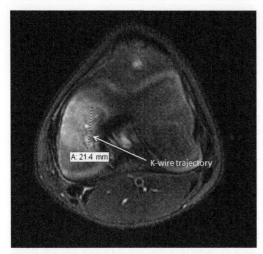

Fig. 10. Schematic depicting the K-wire trajectory for intercondylar notch drilling of medial femoral condyle OCD lesion. (*Courtesy of* Theodore J. Ganley, MD, Philadelphia, PA.)

to replace cartilage defects can be employed. Autologous osteochondral plugs obtained from nonweight-bearing portions of the knee (ie, lateral superior edge of the femoral trochlea or intercondylar notch) can be transplanted to replace the defect. This technique has been shown to have good clinical results in patients younger than 18 years with OCD.[77] However, it can be technically challenging to match the autograft to the defect and may also result in donor site morbidity. In patients with larger defects, in which the osteochondral donor site would be unacceptably large, fresh-frozen osteochondral allograft transplantation can be

considered (Fig. 12).[79,80] This technique can be used for patients who have large defects not amenable to other techniques, as well as in those who have failed prior procedures. Fresh osteochondral allograft transplantation has recently been shown to be effective in patients younger than 18 years.[80]

Autologous chondrocyte implantation (ACI) is another technique that can be used to treat unsalvageable OCD lesions.[81] ACI attempts to regenerate hyaline or hyaline-like cartilage within the osteochondral defect by the harvesting patient's own chondral tissue. The harvested tissue is then replicated in vitro and reimplanted into the defect during a second procedure. The ideal indication for ACI is similar to osteochondral transplantation and may be considered in patients with a normal mechanical axis who have large (>2 cm^2), isolated, contained, full-thickness, chondral lesions within the femoral condyles or trochlea. Outcomes following ACI are similar to those following osteochondral transplantation.[81] A major concern about the use of ACI for treating OCD lesions is the loss of subchondral bone, or poorly vascularized progeny bone, which may compromise the integration of ACI tissue. Techniques to address this concern are under development.

No single salvage technique for the treatment of OCD has been proven to be superior to others over the long term. When treating OCD lesions of the knee, the treating surgeon should

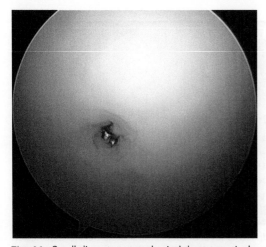

Fig. 11. Small-diameter screw buried deep to articular cartilage surface fixing unstable OCD lesion. (*Courtesy of* Theodore J. Ganley, MD, Philadelphia, PA.)

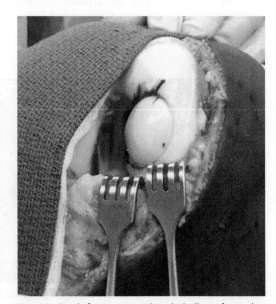

Fig. 12. Fresh-frozen osteochondral allograft used to fill defect left by large, unsalvageable OCD lesion. (*Courtesy of* Theodore J. Ganley, MD, Philadelphia, PA.)

be aware of the various techniques in order to implement lesion specific treatment based on lesion size and morphology, as well as patient- and surgeon-related factors.

SUMMARY

OCD of the knee may be a source of knee pain in pediatric patients. Although the exact etiology remains unknown, the end result is a disorder of articular cartilage and subchondral bone. Timely recognition is essential, as most stable lesions with an intact articular surface will heal with nonoperative treatment. Lesions in skeletally mature patients, large lesions, and lesions that show radiographic signs of instability are less likely to heal without surgical intervention. The overall goals of surgery are to stimulate OCD healing, maintain lesion stability, and prevent the development of osteochondral defects and secondary osteoarthritis in young patients. In unsalvageable lesions, several surgical options can be utilized to help provide a sufficient substitute for the native hyaline cartilage-bearing surface of the knee.

ACKNOWLEDGMENT

The authors would like to acknowledge Michaela Procaccini, NP for her assistance in the preparation of this manuscript.

REFERENCES

1. Hughston JC, Hergenroeder PT, Courtenay BG. Osteochondritis dissecans of the femoral condyles. J Bone Joint Surg Am 1984;66(9):1340–8.
2. Linden B. The incidence of osteochondritis dissecans in the condyles of the femur. Acta Orthop Scand 1976;47(6):664–7.
3. Kessler JI, Nikizad H, Shea KG, et al. The demographics and epidemiology of osteochondritis dissecans of the knee in children and adolescents. Am J Sports Med 2014;42(2):320–6.
4. Hefti F, Beguiristain J, Krauspe R, et al. Osteochondritis dissecans: a multicenter study of the European Pediatric Orthopedic Society. J Pediatr Orthop B 1999;8(4):231–45.
5. Aichroth P. Osteochondritis dissecans of the knee. A clinical survey. J Bone Joint Surg Br 1971;53(3):440–7.
6. Cahill BR. Osteochondritis Dissecans of the Knee: Treatment of Juvenile and Adult Forms. J Am Acad Orthop Surg 1995;3(4):237–47.
7. Clanton TO, DeLee JC. Osteochondritis dissecans. History, pathophysiology and current treatment concepts. Clin Orthop Relat Res 1982;(167):50–64.
8. Glancy GL. Juvenile osteochondritis dissecans. Am J Knee Surg 1999;12(2):120–4.
9. Kocher MS, Micheli LJ. The pediatric knee: evaluation and treatment. In: Insall JN, Scott WN, editors. Surgery of the knee. 3rd edition. New York: Churchill Livingstone; 2001. p. 1356–97.
10. Ganley TJ, Flynn JM. Osteochondritis dissecans. In: Scott WN, editor. Insall & scott surgery of the knee, vol. 2, 4th edition. Philadelphia: Elsevier; 2006. p. 1234–41.
11. Crawford DC, Safran MR. Osteochondritis dissecans of the knee. J Am Acad Orthop Surg 2006; 14(2):90–100.
12. Shea KG, Jacobs JC Jr, Carey JL, et al. Osteochondritis dissecans knee histology studies have variable findings and theories of etiology. Clin Orthop Relat Res 2013;471(4):1127–36.
13. Mubarak SJ, Carroll NC. Familial osteochondritis dissecans of the knee. Clin Orthop Relat Res 1979;(140):131–6.
14. Stougaard J. Familial Occurrence of Osteochondritis Dissecans. J Bone Joint Surg Br 1964;46:542–3.
15. König F. Ueber freie Körper in den Gelenken. Dtsch Z Chir 1887;27:90–109.
16. Ribbing S. The hereditary multiple epiphyseal disturbance and its consequences for the aetiogenesis of local malacias–particularly the osteochondrosis dissecans. Acta Orthop Scand 1955;24(4):286–99.
17. Green WT, Banks HH. Osteochondritis dissecans in children. J Bone Joint Surg Am 1953;35-A(1):26–47. passim.
18. Linden B, Telhag H. Osteochondritis dissecans. A histologic and autoradiographic study in man. Acta Orthop Scand 1977;48(6):682–6.
19. Chiroff RT, Cooke CP 3rd. Osteochondritis dissecans: a histologic and microradiographic analysis of surgically excised lesions. J Trauma 1975;15(8):689–96.
20. Koch S, Kampen WU, Laprell H. Cartilage and bone morphology in osteochondritis dissecans. Knee Surg Sports Traumatol Arthrosc 1997;5(1):42–5.
21. Reddy AS, Frederick RW. Evaluation of the intraosseous and extraosseous blood supply to the distal femoral condyles. Am J Sports Med 1998;26(3):415–9.
22. Rogers WM, Gladstone H. Vascular foramina and arterial supply of the distal end of the femur. J Bone Joint Surg Am 1950;32(A:4):867–74.
23. Toth F, Nissi MJ, Ellermann JM, et al. Novel application of magnetic resonance imaging demonstrates characteristic differences in vasculature at predilection sites of osteochondritis dissecans. Am J Sports Med 2015;43(10):2522–7.
24. Olstad K, Hendrickson EH, Carlson CS, et al. Transection of vessels in epiphyseal cartilage canals leads to osteochondrosis and osteochondrosis

dissecans in the femoro-patellar joint of foals; a potential model of juvenile osteochondritis dissecans. Osteoarthritis Cartilage 2013;21(5):730–8.

25. Martel G, Kiss S, Gilbert G, et al. Differences in the vascular tree of the femoral trochlear growth cartilage at osteochondrosis-susceptible sites in foals revealed by SWI 3T MRI. J Orthop Res 2016. [Epub ahead of print].

26. Gans I, Sarkissian EJ, Grant SF, et al. Identical osteochondritis dissecans lesions of the knee in sets of monozygotic twins. Orthopedics 2013; 36(12):e1559–62.

27. Hammett RB, Saxby TS. Osteochondral lesion of the talus in homozygous twins—the question of heredity. Foot Ankle Surg 2010;16(3):e55–6.

28. Kenniston JA, Beredjiklian PK, Bozentka DJ. Osteochondritis dissecans of the capitellum in fraternal twins: case report. J Hand Surg Am 2008;33(8):1380–3.

29. Mackie T, Wilkins RM. Case report: Osteochondritis dissecans in twins: treatment with fresh osteochondral grafts. Clin Orthop Relat Res 2010; 468(3):893–7.

30. Mei-Dan O, Mann G, Steinbacher G, et al. Bilateral osteochondritis dissecans of the knees in monozygotic twins: the genetic factor and review of the etiology. Am J Orthop (Belle Mead NJ) 2009;38(9): E152–5.

31. Woods K, Harris I. Osteochondritis dissecans of the talus in identical twins. J Bone Joint Surg Br 1995; 77(2):331.

32. Fonseca AS, Keret D, MacEwen GD. Familial osteochondritis dissecans. Orthopedics 1990;13(11): 1259–62.

33. Fraser WNC. Familial Osteochondritis Dissecans. J Bone Joint Surg Br 1966;48-B(3):598.

34. Pick MP. Familial osteochondritis dissecans. J Bone Joint Surg Br 1955;37-B(1):142–5.

35. Roberts N, Hughes R. Osteochondritis dissecans of the elbow joint; a clinical study. J Bone Joint Surg Br 1950;32-B(3):348–60.

36. White J. Osteochondritis dissecans in association with dwarfism. J Bone Joint Surg Br 1957;39-B(2): 261–7.

37. Zellweger H, Ebnother M. A familial skeletal disorder with multilocular, aseptic bone necrosis, and with osteochondritis dissecans in particular. Helv Paediatr Acta 1951;6(2):95–111 [in Undetermined Language].

38. Jacobi M, Wahl P, Bouaicha S, et al. Association between mechanical axis of the leg and osteochondritis dissecans of the knee: radiographic study on 103 knees. Am J Sports Med 2010;38(7):1425–8.

39. Fairbank HAT. Osteochondritis dissecans. Br J Surg 1933;21:67–82.

40. Flynn JM, Kocher MS, Ganley TJ. Osteochondritis dissecans of the knee. J Pediatr Orthop 2004; 24(4):434–43.

41. Hashimoto Y, Yoshida G, Tomihara T, et al. Bilateral osteochondritis dissecans of the lateral femoral condyle following bilateral total removal of lateral discoid meniscus: a case report. Arch Orthop Trauma Surg 2008;128(11):1265–8.

42. Deie M, Ochi M, Sumen Y, et al. Relationship between osteochondritis dissecans of the lateral femoral condyle and lateral menisci types. J Pediatr Orthop 2006;26(1):79–82.

43. Twyman RS, Desai K, Aichroth PM. Osteochondritis dissecans of the knee. A long-term study. J Bone Joint Surg Br 1991;73(3):461–4.

44. Linden B. Osteochondritis dissecans of the femoral condyles: a long-term follow-up study. J Bone Joint Surg Am 1977;59(6):769–76.

45. Madry H, van Dijk CN, Mueller-Gerbl M. The basic science of the subchondral bone. Knee Surg Sports Traumatol Arthrosc 2010;18(4):419–33.

46. Madry H. The subchondral bone: a new frontier in articular cartilage repair. Knee Surg Sports Traumatol Arthrosc 2010;18(4):417–8.

47. Pape D, Filardo G, Kon E, et al. Disease-specific clinical problems associated with the subchondral bone. Knee Surg Sports Traumatol Arthrosc 2010; 18(4):448–62.

48. Milgram JW. Radiological and pathological manifestations of osteochondritis dissecans of the distal femur. A study of 50 cases. Radiology 1978;126(2): 305–11.

49. Wall EJ, Polousky JD, Shea KG, et al. Novel radiographic feature classification of knee osteochondritis dissecans: a multicenter reliability study. Am J Sports Med 2015;43(2):303–9.

50. Kocher MS, DiCanzio J, Zurakowski D, et al. Diagnostic performance of clinical examination and selective magnetic resonance imaging in the evaluation of intraarticular knee disorders in children and adolescents. Am J Sports Med 2001;29(3):292–6.

51. Samora WP, Chevillet J, Adler B, et al. Juvenile osteochondritis dissecans of the knee: predictors of lesion stability. J Pediatr Orthop 2012;32(1):1–4.

52. Zbojniewicz AM, Stringer KF, Laor T, et al. Juvenile Osteochondritis Dissecans: Correlation Between Histopathology and MRI. AJR Am J Roentgenology 2015;205(1):W114–23.

53. De Smet AA, Ilahi OA, Graf BK. Untreated osteochondritis dissecans of the femoral condyles: prediction of patient outcome using radiographic and MR findings. Skeletal Radiol 1997; 26(8):463–7.

54. Bohndorf K. Osteochondritis (osteochondrosis) dissecans: a review and new MRI classification. Eur Radiol 1998;8(1):103–12.

55. O'Connor MA, Palaniappan M, Khan N, et al. Osteochondritis dissecans of the knee in children. A comparison of MRI and arthroscopic findings. J Bone Joint Surg Br 2002;84(2):258–62.

56. Heywood CS, Benke MT, Brindle K, et al. Correlation of magnetic resonance imaging to arthroscopic findings of stability in juvenile osteochondritis dissecans. Arthroscopy 2011;27(2):194–9.

57. Pill SG, Ganley TJ, Milam RA, et al. Role of magnetic resonance imaging and clinical criteria in predicting successful nonoperative treatment of osteochondritis dissecans in children. J Pediatr Orthop 2003;23(1):102–8.

58. Wall EJ, Vourazeris J, Myer GD, et al. The healing potential of stable juvenile osteochondritis dissecans knee lesions. J Bone Joint Surg Am 2008; 90(12):2655–64.

59. Kijowski R, Blankenbaker DG, Shinki K, et al. Juvenile versus adult osteochondritis dissecans of the knee: appropriate MR imaging criteria for instability. Radiology 2008;248(2):571–8.

60. Carey JL, Wall EJ, Shea KG, et al. Reliability of the ROCK osteochondritis dissecans knee arthroscopy classification system–multicenter validation study. POSNA Annual Conferece. Toronto (ON), May 1–4, 2013.

61. Chambers HG, Shea KG, Anderson AF, et al. American Academy of Orthopaedic Surgeons clinical practice guideline on: the diagnosis and treatment of osteochondritis dissecans. J Bone Joint Surg Am 2012;94(14):1322–4.

62. Van Demark RE. Osteochondritis dissecans with spontaneous healing. J Bone Joint Surg Am 1952; 34:143–8.

63. Krause M, Hapfelmeier A, Moller M, et al. Healing predictors of stable juvenile osteochondritis dissecans knee lesions after 6 and 12 months of nonoperative treatment. Am J Sports Med 2013;41(10): 2384–91.

64. Smillie IS. Treatment of osteochondritis dissecans. J Bone Joint Surg Br 1957;39-B(2):248–60.

65. Kocher MS, Tucker R, Ganley TJ, et al. Management of osteochondritis dissecans of the knee: current concepts review. Am J Sports Med 2006;34(7):1181–91.

66. Ganley TJ, Gaugler RL, Kocher MS, et al. Osteochondritis dissecans of the knee. Oper Tech Sports Med 2006;14:147–58.

67. Beck NA, Patel NM, Ganley TJ. The pediatric knee: current concepts in sports medicine. J Pediatr Orthop B 2014;23(1):59–66.

68. Kawasaki K, Uchio Y, Adachi N, et al. Drilling from the intercondylar area for treatment of osteochondritis dissecans of the knee joint. Knee 2003;10(3): 257–63.

69. Friederichs MG, Greis PE, Burks RT. Pitfalls associated with fixation of osteochondritis dissecans fragments using bioabsorbable screws. Arthroscopy 2001;17(5):542–5.

70. Tabaddor RR, Banffy MB, Andersen JS, et al. Fixation of juvenile osteochondritis dissecans lesions of the knee using poly 96L/4D-lactide copolymer bioabsorbable implants. J Pediatr Orthop 2010; 30(1):14–20.

71. Kocher MS, Czarnecki JJ, Andersen JS, et al. Internal fixation of juvenile osteochondritis dissecans lesions of the knee. Am J Sports Med 2007;35(5):712–8.

72. Adachi N, Deie M, Nakamae A, et al. Functional and radiographic outcomes of unstable juvenile osteochondritis dissecans of the knee treated with lesion fixation using bioabsorbable pins. J Pediatr Orthop 2015;35(1):82–8.

73. Wright RW, McLean M, Matava MJ, et al. Osteochondritis dissecans of the knee: long-term results of excision of the fragment. Clin Orthop Relat Res 2004;(424):239–43.

74. Anderson AF, Pagnani MJ. Osteochondritis dissecans of the femoral condyles. Long-term results of excision of the fragment. Am J Sports Med 1997; 25(6):830–4.

75. Murray JR, Chitnavis J, Dixon P, et al. Osteochondritis dissecans of the knee; long-term clinical outcome following arthroscopic debridement. Knee 2007;14(2):94–8.

76. Steadman JR, Briggs KK, Rodrigo JJ, et al. Outcomes of microfracture for traumatic chondral defects of the knee: average 11-year follow-up. Arthroscopy 2003;19(5):477–84.

77. Gudas R, Simonaityte R, Cekanauskas E, et al. A prospective, randomized clinical study of osteochondral autologous transplantation versus microfracture for the treatment of osteochondritis dissecans in the knee joint in children. J Pediatr Orthop 2009;29(7):741–8.

78. Richter DL, Schenck RC Jr, Wascher DC, et al. Knee articular cartilage repair and restoration techniques: a review of the literature. Sports Health 2015;8(2):153–60.

79. Briggs DT, Sadr KN, Pulido PA, et al. The Use of Osteochondral Allograft Transplantation for Primary Treatment of Cartilage Lesions in the Knee. Cartilage 2015;6(4):203–7.

80. Murphy RT, Pennock AT, Bugbee WD. Osteochondral allograft transplantation of the knee in the pediatric and adolescent population. Am J Sports Med 2014;42(3):635–40.

81. Harris JD, Siston RA, Pan X, et al. Autologous chondrocyte implantation: a systematic review. J Bone Joint Surg Am 2010;92(12):2220–33.

Anterior Cruciate Ligament Injuries in Children and Adolescents

Peter D. Fabricant, MD, MPH[a],
Mininder S. Kocher, MD, MPH[b],*

KEYWORDS

- ACL • Anterior cruciate ligament • Youth athlete • Young athlete • Pediatric sports
- Iliotibial band • Hamstring

KEY POINTS

- Youth and adolescent athletes comprise the largest demographic of anterior cruciate ligament (ACL) tears, and the incidence is increasing.
- Growth disturbance is a common concern for those who treat ACL injuries in skeletally immature athletes.
- Nonoperative management leads to high rates of sport dropout; continued instability can result in progressive meniscal and cartilage damage as well as arthritic changes.
- Several physeal-respecting ACL reconstruction techniques exist for use in skeletally immature patients to minimize risk of growth disturbance.

INTRODUCTION

Tears of the anterior cruciate ligament (ACL) were once considered rare in skeletally immature athletes; however, they are now observed with increasing frequency. A dramatic increase in youth competitive athletic activity, early sport specialization, and year-round training and competition, along with increased awareness of ACL injuries in children, have led to a commensurate increase in the frequency of ACL tears in the skeletally immature. A recent epidemiologic analysis of a New York State administrative database revealed that the rate of ACL reconstruction in children less than 20 years of age had increased nearly 3-fold over a 20-year period from 1990 to 2009, and indicated that adolescents and teenagers represent the largest per capita demographic of ACL reconstructions.[1]

Although, historically, nonoperative management until skeletal maturity followed by traditional ACL reconstruction was a popular treatment strategy, recent understanding of the risks of nonoperative treatment and surgical delay have supported a trend toward early operative treatment.[2–7] In light of this, along with the increasing frequency and awareness of ACL injuries in children, surgical methods and instrumentation have evolved, in order to accommodate the unique anatomy of skeletally immature patients.

This article discusses the anatomy of the skeletally immature knee, ACL imaging and physical examination that is unique to children, and treatment strategies for ACL injuries in children and adolescents, including both nonoperative and surgical. The authors also offer their preferred treatment strategy for skeletally immature youth athletes with ACL tears.

ANATOMY

The physes about the knee remain the greatest anatomic concern of surgeons who treat skeletally immature patients with ACL tears.

[a] Pediatric Orthopaedic Surgery Service, Hospital for Special Surgery, Weill Cornell Medical College, 535 East 70th Street, New York, NY 10021, USA; [b] Division of Sports Medicine, Department of Orthopedic Surgery, Boston Children's Hospital, Harvard Medical School, 300 Longwood Avenue, Boston, MA 02115, USA
* Corresponding author.
E-mail address: mininder.kocher@childrens.harvard.edu

Orthop Clin N Am 47 (2016) 777–788
http://dx.doi.org/10.1016/j.ocl.2016.05.004
0030-5898/16/$ – see front matter © 2016 Elsevier Inc. All rights reserved.

Significant damage to the tibial or femoral physis may lead to growth disturbance and subsequent length or angular deformity of the lower limb. An understanding of this unique anatomy is vital when planning surgery for youth with ACL injuries.

The tibial and femoral physes are the greatest contributors to overall lower limb longitudinal growth. The distal femoral physis contributes 70% of the femoral length and 37% of the overall limb length over the course of skeletal development at an average rate of 10 mm/y. The distance of the femoral physeal plate and perichondral ring from the femoral origin of the ACL remains unchanged from gestational age, and is 3 mm from the over-the-top-position.[8] The proximal tibial physis contributes approximately 55% of the tibial length and 25% of the overall limb length over the course of skeletal development at a rate of 6 mm/y, on average. Furthermore, the tibial tubercle apophysis is subject to injury and can result in recurvatum deformity.[9] Although skeletal maturity occurs around age 14 years in girls and age 16 years in boys, negligible (<1 cm in each limb segment) growth remains around the knee after age 12 to 13 years in girls and 14 years in boys.[10] Until these ages, ACL reconstruction strategies must respect the growing physes. To date, only small case series have reported on growth disturbance after ACL reconstruction,[11–17] so the precise incidence is not known. Experienced surgeons from the Herodicus Society and the ACL Study Group revealed 15 cases of postoperative deformity caused by physeal injury, including distal femoral valgus deformity, tibial recurvatum, genu valgum, and significant leg length discrepancy.[9] More recent case reports and imaging studies show the potential for growth disturbance after transphyseal ACL reconstruction,[18] physeal-sparing all-epiphyseal ACL reconstruction,[19,20] and partial transphyseal reconstruction.[16]

PATIENT EVALUATION AND DIAGNOSIS

Every evaluation should begin with a thorough history and physical examination, as well as ruling out concurrent injury. In adolescents presenting with acute traumatic hemarthrosis, ACL injuries can be present in up to 65% of cases.[21] Reliable physical examination maneuvers to detect ACL insufficiency are similar to those in adult patients and include the Lachman test, anterior drawer test, and the pivot shift. However, pain and swelling can increase guarding and affect patient compliance and subsequent accuracy of these tests; the pivot shift test has been shown to be 98% positive in anesthetized patients compared with only 35% positive in patients who are awake during the examination. It is important to evaluate baseline clinical limb alignment as well as leg length discrepancy. This discrepancy is typically measured with a tape measure (anterior superior iliac spine to medial malleolus), as well as using blocks under the clinically short leg to correct pelvic obliquity and measure functional limb length discrepancy.

MRI is the principal imaging modality used to evaluate for internal derangement of the knee, and is 95% sensitive and 88% specific in detecting ACL tears in children.[22] MRI also allows further evaluation for common associated injuries, including meniscus tears, chondral lesions, and combined ligamentous injury. Traumatic chondral lesions have been observed in up to half of high school athletes with ACL injuries, so careful examination of all cartilage surfaces is important.[23] Identification of these associated injuries may be important in guiding treatment options.

In addition to the standard radiographic evaluation (anteroposterior [AP], lateral, notch, Merchant), surgeons can consider obtaining 130-cm (51-inch) standing AP hip-to-ankle radiographs to quantify any baseline leg length discrepancy and angular deformity noted during the physical examination.[11,24] Skeletal age should be determined for children and adolescents with open physes, and is most frequently assessed using a posteroanterior left hand radiograph[25–27]; however, alternative methods based on pelvis, elbow, and calcaneal radiographs have also been described.[28–31] Clinically, timing of peak growth velocity may be estimated from Tanner staging as well as onset of menses in female patients.[32] A thorough understanding of preexisting length and angular deformities as well as remaining growth allows surgeons to both document preexisting deformity and consider realignment using an osteotomy or implant-mediated guided growth in more extreme cases.

NONOPERATIVE AND DELAYED SURGICAL TREATMENT

Nonoperative or delayed surgical management were historically appealing options given the increased healing potential of children and the risk of physeal damage with surgical reconstruction.[33] However, subsequent reports have indicated that nonoperative management leads to high rates of sport dropout (up to 94% unable to participate at preinjury level of activity and up to 50% unable to participate at all) because of recurrent knee instability.[34–36] Furthermore, continued instability can result in progressive meniscal and cartilage damage, as well as arthritic changes in 61% of knees.[35,37,38] This finding is particularly true in children and adolescents because they are not frequently compliant in modifying their postinjury activity levels. Delaying reconstruction until skeletal maturity also has significant drawbacks; several studies have shown increasing frequency of cartilage and meniscus damage with instability episodes[39] and treatment delay.[4–7,40–42] Moksnes and colleagues[36] performed a large, prospective, MRI-based study that advocated against the routine reconstruction of ACL tears in skeletally immature patients. However, the investigators noted that during the 4 years postinjury, 1 in 3 patients required ACL reconstruction for persistent instability and 1 in 5 sustained a new meniscal disorder requiring treatment. Recent meta-analysis of existing data favored early stabilization to decrease instability, pathologic laxity, and return to activity.[43]

Despite this, routine ACL reconstruction may not be necessary for every ACL injury. In one series, 1 in 3 children (mean age, 13.7 years) with partial ACL tears treated nonoperatively with a hinged knee brace, partial weight bearing for 6 to 8 weeks, and a progressive ACL rehabilitation protocol ultimately required surgical reconstruction for persistent instability. Nonoperative management of ACL injury had greater success in children and adolescents of that cohort who sustained tears less than half of the thickness of the ACL, tears of the anteromedial bundle only, less than a grade B pivot shift examination, and those with a skeletal age younger than 14 years.[44] It may be reasonable to consider a trial of nonoperative treatment in patients who meet those criteria, with the understanding that recurrent instability may inevitably persist.

OPERATIVE TREATMENT AND TECHNIQUES

Given the perils of nonoperative treatment of complete ACL tears in children outlined earlier, and the understanding of respecting the physis during skeletal growth and development, contemporary surgical instrumentation and techniques allow a variety of reconstruction options. These options may be broadly classified into 3 categories: physeal sparing, partial transphyseal, and transphyseal.

In prepubescent children (Tanner stage 1–2; skeletal age ≤11 years in girls, ≤12 years in boys), a Modified MacIntosh combined intra-articular and extra-articular iliotibial (IT)

band reconstruction described by Micheli and Kocher[45,46] may be performed. During this reconstruction, the central portion of the IT band is harvested proximally and left attached to Gerdy's tubercle distally. The graft is brought through the knee in an over-the-top-position posteriorly and passed under the intermeniscal ligament anteriorly within an epiphyseal groove on the tibia. The graft is fixed with suture to the intermuscular septum and periosteum on the femur and periosteum on the tibia. This technique has the advantages of avoiding the physes, improving the ease of revision surgery (no previous tunnels and all other autograft sources remain intact), and providing an additional extra-articular limb similar to anterolateral ligament reconstruction.[46–49] Although some opponents of this technique cite its nonanatomic configuration, biomechanics studies have shown restoration of kinematic constraint[50] and good clinical outcomes with low revision rates at a mean of 5.3 years postoperatively.[46] More recently, techniques using hamstring autograft and all-epiphyseal tunnels with epiphyseal fixation have been described,[20,51–54] but midterm to long-term outcomes data for this technique in large clinical series are lacking. In small series, graft rupture rates of 11% to 17% have been reported,[19,20] and MRI investigation has noted physeal compromise in 10 of 15 tibiae (67%) and 1 of 23 femora (4%), with no clinical growth disturbances at 1 year.[55]

In older children and adolescents with some growth remaining (Tanner stage ≥3; skeletal age ≥12 years in girls, ≥13 years in boys), several physeal-respecting reconstruction options are available that either attempt to avoid the physes or remove an acceptable amount of physeal tissue and use soft tissue grafts without transphyseal fixation hardware.[24,56] Although the precise amount of acceptable physeal violation in humans is unknown, animal studies indicate that removing greater than 7% of the area of the physeal plate is associated with an increased risk of growth disturbance.[57–59] These include all-epiphyseal reconstructions,[20,51–54] partial transphyseal reconstructions (all-epiphyseal femoral tunnel or over-the-top femoral positioning and transphyseal tibial tunnel), and complete transphyseal reconstructions[60,61] with more vertical tunnels to minimize cross-sectional area of physeal damage and subsequent risk of growth arrest.[57] Because no technique has shown universal superiority, multiple instrumentation sets and fixation options are available depending on surgeon preference. Biomechanical studies have indicated restoration of many knee kinematic parameters,[50,62] but long-term comparative outcomes studies are lacking. Lack of careful attention during tunnel drilling may lead to physeal damage and resultant limb length or angular deformity. Furthermore, revision surgery may only use allograft or remaining autograft tissue and must take previously created tunnels into consideration.

In older adolescents nearing skeletal maturity, adult reconstruction techniques may be used. In the absence of collagen abnormalities, many clinicians advocate the use of autograft tissue for primary ACL reconstruction in youth,[63,64] because large, multicenter studies have shown significantly higher rates of failure with allograft tissue in young athletes.[65]

AUTHOR'S PREFERRED TREATMENT

In the senior author's practice, youth athletes are evaluated for ACL tears as outlined above. In the event a tear is diagnosed, operative management is frequently recommended. However, if the athlete has a skeletal age younger than 14 years, the injury is a partial tear less than half of the thickness of the ACL (particularly of the anteromedial bundle only), and the examination shows less than a grade B pivot shift examination, a patient-centered dialogue with the athlete and family is conducted as to the expectations of a trial of nonoperative management. If nonoperative management is elected, we treat the athlete with a hinged knee brace, partial weight bearing for 6 to 8 weeks, a progressive ACL rehabilitation protocol, activity restriction from pivoting or contact sports, and close follow-up to assess for knee instability or subsequent chondral or meniscal injury.

For operative candidates, a course of pre-reconstruction physical therapy is prescribed focusing on reducing pain, swelling, and effusion; regaining normal gait mechanics; and maximizing quadriceps and hamstring strength preoperatively. This delay of approximately 4 weeks helps to minimize postoperative arthrofibrosis.[66] In the event of an urgent meniscal (eg, locked bucket-handle tear) or osteochondral injury, the reconstructive surgery can either be staged or performed earlier after appropriate counseling of the risks, benefits, and requirements involved in either approach. Our treatment algorithm is outlined in Fig. 1.

Prepubescent Patients with Significant Growth Remaining (Tanner Stage 1–2; Skeletal Age ≤11 Years [Girls] or ≤12 Years [Boys])

In prepubescent patients with significant growth remaining (Tanner stage 1–2; skeletal age ≤11 years in girls or ≤12 years in boys), we perform

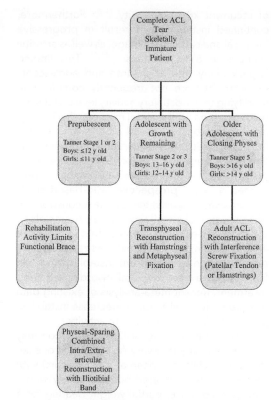

Fig. 1. Authors' preferred treatment algorithm for ACL tears in youth athletes.

a physeal-sparing ACL reconstruction with IT band autograft (Fig. 2).[45,46] After an examination under anesthesia, surgery begins with IT band harvest through a longitudinal-oblique 4.5-cm incision from the lateral joint line (a point equidistant from Gerdy's tubercle and the lateral epicondyle) to the superior border of the IT band. A Cobb elevator is used to elevate the subcutaneous tissue off the superficial surface of the IT band 15 cm or more up the thigh. The anterior and posterior borders of the IT band are identified. Anteriorly, the IT band is confluent with the fascia of the vastus lateralis. The transition point is noted where the dense and opaque IT band tissue transitions to a more transparent vastus fascia. Posteriorly, the IT band blends into the posterior intermuscular septum. Once these borders are identified, the IT band is incised near either border leaving a few millimeters of intact IT band on either side. The cuts are continued proximally with curved meniscotomes for a distance of at least 15 cm. The graft is truncated proximally with a curved meniscotome or an open-ended tendon harvester with cutting mechanism. After harvest, the free end is tubularized with a nonabsorbable suture. The graft is further freed distally from the

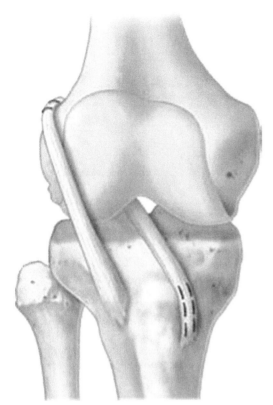

Fig. 2. Modified MacIntosh IT band ACL reconstruction.

lateral joint capsule but leaving it attached to the Gerdy tubercle (Fig. 3). The graft is then placed back in the wound to prevent desiccation during arthroscopy.

Diagnostic arthroscopy is performed through standard anterolateral and anteromedial portals and any meniscal or chondral work is performed at this point. The medial portal is widened and a large curved clamp is introduced into the over-the-top position. The clamp is placed through the soft tissue remnants at the posterior aspect of the over-the-top position to allow for a sling, pushed through the posterolateral capsule of the knee and into the IT band defect on the lateral knee. The suture attached to the free end of the graft is placed in the clamps and brought back into the knee (Fig. 4).

Next, a longitudinal incision is made medial to the tibial tubercle and distal to the tibial epiphysis just proximal to the pes anserinus tendon insertion. Dissection is carried down to, but not through, the periosteum and then blunt dissection is directed proximally with a curved clamp up into the knee underneath the intermeniscal ligament. This passageway is then dilated to aid with tibial preparation and graft passage. A curved rat-tail rasp is used to create a groove in the tibial ACL footprint in order to create an exposed bony bed to facilitate intra-articular healing of the graft as well as to posteriorize the tibial footprint to a more anatomic position that minimizes the chance of impingement in extension. The clamp is then reintroduced in the knee and the intra-articular sutures are grasped and brought out through the tibial incision, advancing the graft to its final intra-articular position (Fig. 5). With tension on the graft, the knee is flexed and extended to confirm impingement-free range of motion.

The arthroscope is removed and the knee is allowed to hang in 90° of relaxed flexion with neutral foot rotation in order to prevent overconstraining the knee.[50] With tension on the graft, the graft is sewn into the periosteum of the lateral femoral condyle and the intermuscular septum (Fig. 6) with a heavy nonabsorbable suture.

After completion of the tenodesis, the leg is placed in extension. The periosteum in the tibial

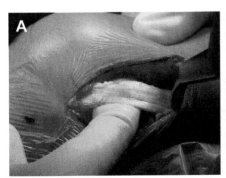
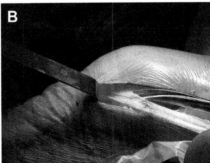

Fig. 3. IT band graft harvest. Isolation of the midportion of the IT band (A) is followed by proximal detachment and dissection distally to the Gerdy tubercle (B). The graft is then tubularized proximally with sutures that are used to pass the graft. (From Kocher MS, Garg S, Micheli LJ. Physeal sparing reconstruction of the anterior cruciate ligament in skeletally immature prepubescent children and adolescents. J Bone Joint Surg Am 2005;87(11):2373; with permission.)

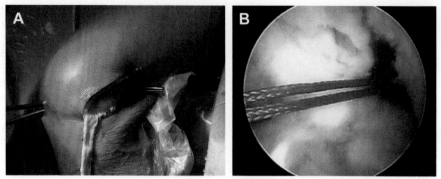

Fig. 4. IT band graft passage is performed by using a curved clamp in the over-the-top position (A). The sutures are then passed intra-articularly (B). (*From* Kocher MS, Garg S, Micheli LJ. Physeal sparing reconstruction of the anterior cruciate ligament in skeletally immature prepubescent children and adolescents. J Bone Joint Surg Am 2005;87(11):2374; with permission.)

incision is incised and elevated with a periosteal elevator. The bone is decorticated, and 3 to 4 sutures are then placed through the periosteal flaps and graft. Once all sutures are placed they are tied sequentially with firm tension on the graft and a posterior drawer on the tibia. The knee is checked to confirm a negative Lachman examination.

Pubescent Patients with Growth Remaining and Skeletally Mature Patients (Tanner Stage ≥3; Skeletal Age ≥12 Years [Girls] or ≥13 Years [Boys])

In pubescent patients with growth remaining (Tanner stage ≥3; skeletal age ≥12 years in girls or ≥13 years in boys), the authors perform a transphyseal ACL reconstruction with hamstring

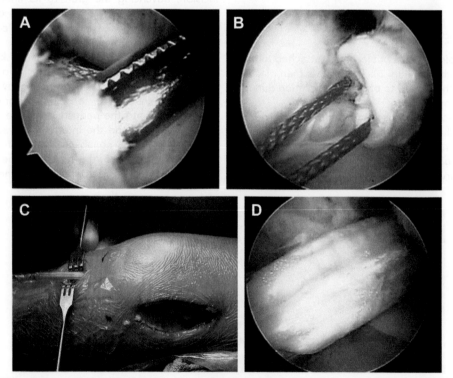

Fig. 5. IT band graft passage to final position. A tonsil clamp is used to grasp the passing sutures underneath the intermeniscal ligament (A) and the graft is pulled out through the tibial incision (B, C), resulting in positioning of the graft in its anatomic position (D). (*From* [A, C, D] Kocher MS, Garg S, Micheli LJ. Physeal sparing reconstruction of the anterior cruciate ligament in skeletally immature prepubescent children and adolescents. J Bone Joint Surg Am 2005;87(11):2371–9; with permission.)

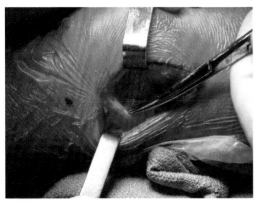

Fig. 6. With tension on the graft, the graft is sewn into the periosteum of the lateral femoral condyle and the intermuscular septum (identified here with clamp) with a heavy nonabsorbable suture using at least 2 figure-of-eight stitches to achieve an extra-articular tenodesis.

autograft and metaphyseal fixation (Fig. 7). The semitendinosus and gracilis tendons are harvested through a longitudinal incision centered on the pes anserinus. They are each doubled to produce a quadrupled graft and sized using standard instruments. The quadrupled graft is

then placed on a 15-mm fixed-loop suspensory cortical fixation device and pre-tensioned on a graft preparation board.

Diagnostic arthroscopy and any meniscal and/ or chondral work is performed through standard anterolateral and anteromedial portals. A notch-plasty can be performed if necessary taking care to avoid vigorous resection deep in the notch given the proximity of the distal femoral growth plate.

Bone tunnel drilling is typically done using a transtibial technique in order to obtain a central tunnel across the physis. The tibial guide is set to 55° to ensure a long metaphyseal tunnel distal to the physis. To ensure that the tibial tunnel does not violate the tibial tubercle apophysis, the guide pin is inserted medially at the tibial cortex, anterior to the medial collateral ligament fibers. This location is typically 1 cm anterior to the posteromedial border of the tibia. The guide pin is placed in the posterior-central portion of the tibial ACL footprint to allow easy access to the over-the-top position (Fig. 8). The tibial tunnel is reamed over the guide pin with the appropriate-sized tibial reamer to match the size of the hamstring graft. An over-the-top femoral guide is selected based on the formula 0.5 × graft diameter + 1 to allow a 1-mm to 1.5-mm back wall and is positioned through the tibial tunnel. The femoral tunnel is reamed over a guidewire in preparation to support the suspensory fixation construct, taking into account the length of tunnel required for the fixed loop and flipping the cortical button. Passing sutures are used for graft passage using the Beath pin (Fig. 9A). The button is flipped and security is assessed by sequentially pulling tension (toggling) the passing sutures as well as pulling firm tension on the graft distally. Fluoroscopy

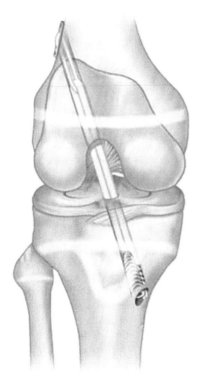

Fig. 7. Transphyseal ACL reconstruction with hamstring autograft and metaphyseal fixation.

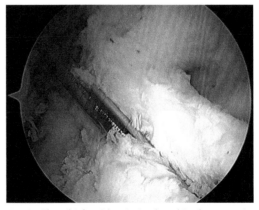

Fig. 8. The tibial guide pin is placed in the posterior portion of the tibial ACL footprint to allow easy access to the over-the-top position.

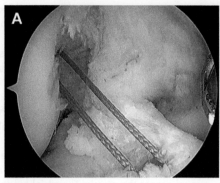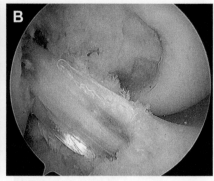

Fig. 9. During transphyseal ACL reconstruction with hamstring autograft, graft passage is facilitated by passing sutures (A). Final graft position is anatomic (B).

may also be used to confirm appropriate button placement. The graft is visualized arthroscopically to confirm appropriate position and impingement-free motion (Fig. 9B). Tibial fixation is performed at 20° to 30° of knee flexion. With the transtibial technique, a 20-mm to 25-mm interference screw is usually sufficient to be completely placed and still be distal to the physis. The screw diameter should either match the tunnel and graft diameter or be oversized by 1 mm in softer bone.

REHABILITATION

At present, few youth-specific ACL rehabilitation protocols have been described, and many have been designed based on a combination of the adult literature and clinical expertise.[24,51,53,67,68] In the senior author's practice, rehabilitation is largely similar for both IT band ACL reconstructions and for transphyseal hamstring autograft reconstructions, with the main difference being weight bearing and range of motion in the first 6 weeks postoperatively. Patients who undergo IT band ACL reconstruction maintain touch-down weight bearing (20% of body weight) for 6 weeks postoperatively with range of motion limited to 0° to 30° for 2 weeks followed by 0° to 90° through week 6. This schedule allows for adequate protection of implant-free periosteal fixation of the IT band autograft. Patients who undergo transphyseal ACL reconstruction with hamstring autograft remain partial weight bearing (50% of body weight) for 2 weeks and are then progressed to weight bearing as tolerated, with 0° to 90° of motion allowed immediately postoperatively. After 6 weeks, rehabilitation is identical and consists of regaining full range of motion, working on closed-chain strengthening, with straight-line jogging initiated 10 weeks postoperatively. Running

and agility training are started at 12 weeks and progressed toward sport-specific training and jump-landing. Patients are evaluated with an ACL return-to-play (RTP) assessment at 6 months, including range of motion, strength, thigh girth, balance, and functional testing. Any identified deficits are targeted. RTP is gradual and initiated at 6 to 9 months depending on RTP assessment. Patients wear a hinged knee brace postoperatively until week 6, when quadriceps control returns, at which point they are converted to functional ACL brace for use during exercise and sports out to 2 years postoperatively. Two years after surgery, bracing becomes optional but is encouraged for younger, prepubescent patients and those who compete in high-risk sports.

SURGICAL OUTCOMES

Outcomes after ACL reconstruction using IT band autograft in 44 patients (mean chronologic age, 10.3 years) with minimum 2-year follow-up (mean 5.3 years' follow-up) resulted in a retear rate of 4.5%; in the remaining patients the International Knee Documentation Committee (IKDC) subjective knee score was 96.7 ± 6.0 and the Lysholm knee score was 95.7 ± 6.7.[46] No growth disturbances were observed either clinically or radiographically. These results have been maintained in the longer term as well with a subsequent study of 237 patients at an average of 6.2 years postoperatively showing a 5.8% revision rate, 2% arthrofibrosis rate, less than 0.5% rate of septic arthritis, and no limb length or angular deformities. Pedi-IKDC and Lysholm scores averaged 93 points each (Kocher MS, Heyworth BE, Tepolt F, Fabricant PD, Micheli LJ. Outcomes of physeal-sparing ACL reconstruction with IT band in skeletally immature children, unpublished data, 2016). Clinical success has been replicated in other series as well: 22 knees at an average follow-up of 3.0 years had mean Pedi-IKDC and Lysholm scores of 96.5 and 95 points, respectively, with high mean patient satisfaction, no limb length or angular deformities, and 3 knees (14%) requiring revision ACL surgery.[69]

With regard to transphyseal ACL reconstructions, a series of 61 knees in 59 skeletally immature pubescent adolescents (Tanner stage 3) evaluated at a mean of 3.6 years postoperatively resulted in a 3% revision rate; in the remaining patients the IKDC subjective knee score was 90 and the Lysholm knee score was 91. No limb length or angular deformities arose.[70] This finding is in line with other reports of complete transphyseal reconstructions.[12,61,70–77] When leg length discrepancy occurs, it is frequently clinically insignificant (mean, 1.2–6.2 mm), but in some studies it has occurred in up to 30% of patients.[12,61,72] At a mean follow-up of 2 to 4 years, IKDC and Lysholm scores in the 90s have been reported,[61,70,72–74] with durable results as long as 6 to 10 years postoperatively.[76,77] Arthrofibrosis[66,70] and superficial infections[74] are rare complications, but may occur in up to 5% of patients. There is typically a low rate of revision surgery (0%–13%), which is often required because of reinjury after return to full sports participation.[60,70,74–77] ACL injury prevention programs can be used as part of RTP readiness training, and may reduce the risk of reinjury as well as contralateral ACL injury.[78–81]

SUMMARY

Although ACL tears were historically considered rare injuries in skeletally immature athletes they are now observed with increasing frequency due in part to a dramatic increase in youth competitive athletic activity, early sport specialization, and year-round training and competition. Recent epidemiologic data have shown that the greatest number of ACL reconstructions per capita are being performed in adolescents and teenagers, including skeletally immature patients. In light of the increasing frequency and awareness of ACL injuries in children, diagnostic and treatment strategies have evolved and now cater to the unique anatomy of skeletally immature patients. Current literature supports the trend toward early operative treatment to restore knee stability and prevent progressive meniscal and/or chondral damage, whereas a small subset of patients may attempt nonoperative management with reasonable success. Future research should focus on widespread implementation of ACL injury prevention programs and optimizing surgical technique and postoperative rehabilitation protocols using youth-validated patient-reported outcomes.[82,83]

REFERENCES

1. Dodwell ER, Lamont LE, Green DW, et al. 20 years of pediatric anterior cruciate ligament reconstruction in New York State. Am J Sports Med 2014; 42(3):675–80.
2. Fabricant PD, Lakomkin N, Cruz AI, et al. ACL reconstruction in youth athletes results in an improved rate of return to athletic activity when compared with non-operative treatment: a systematic review of the literature. JISAKOS 2016; 1(2):62–9.
3. Fabricant PD, Lakomkin N, Cruz AI, et al. Early ACL reconstruction in children leads to less meniscal and articular cartilage damage when compared with conservative or delayed treatment. JISAKOS 2016;1(1):10–5.
4. Newman JT, Carry PM, Terhune EB, et al. Factors predictive of concomitant injuries among children and adolescents undergoing anterior cruciate ligament surgery. Am J Sports Med 2015;43(2):282–8.
5. Anderson AF, Anderson CN. Correlation of meniscal and articular cartilage injuries in children and adolescents with timing of anterior cruciate ligament reconstruction. Am J Sports Med 2015;43(2): 275–81.
6. Lawrence JT, Argawal N, Ganley TJ. Degeneration of the knee joint in skeletally immature patients with a diagnosis of an anterior cruciate ligament tear: is there harm in delay of treatment? Am J Sports Med 2011;39(12):2582–7.
7. Dumont GD, Hogue GD, Padalecki JR, et al. Meniscal and chondral injuries associated with pediatric anterior cruciate ligament tears: relationship of treatment time and patient-specific factors. Am J Sports Med 2012;40(9):2128–33.
8. Behr CT, Potter HG, Paletta GA Jr. The relationship of the femoral origin of the anterior cruciate ligament and the distal femoral physeal plate in the skeletally immature knee. an anatomic study. Am J Sports Med 2001;29(6):781–7.
9. Kocher MS, Saxon HS, Hovis WD, et al. Management and complications of anterior cruciate ligament injuries in skeletally immature patients: survey of the Herodicus Society and the ACL Study Group. J Pediatr Orthop 2002;22(4):452–7.
10. Kelly PM, Dimeglio A. Lower-limb growth: how predictable are predictions? J Child Orthop 2008;2(6): 407–15.
11. Shifflett GD, Green DW, Widmann RF, et al. Growth arrest following ACL reconstruction with hamstring

autograft in skeletally immature patients: a review of 4 cases. J Pediatr Orthop 2016;36(4):355–61.

12. Lipscomb AB, Anderson AF. Tears of the anterior cruciate ligament in adolescents. J Bone Joint Surg Am 1986;68(1):19–28.

13. Chotel F, Henry J, Seil R, et al. Growth disturbances without growth arrest after ACL reconstruction in children. Knee Surg Sports Traumatol Arthrosc 2010;18(11):1496–500.

14. Higuchi T, Hara K, Tsuji Y, et al. Transepiphyseal reconstruction of the anterior cruciate ligament in skeletally immature athletes: an MRI evaluation for epiphyseal narrowing. J Pediatr Orthop B 2009; 18(6):330–4.

15. Koman JD, Sanders JO. Valgus deformity after reconstruction of the anterior cruciate ligament in a skeletally immature patient. A case report. J Bone Joint Surg Am 1999;81(5):711–5.

16. Lawrence JT, West RL, Garrett WE. Growth disturbance following ACL reconstruction with use of an epiphyseal femoral tunnel: a case report. J Bone Joint Surg Am 2011;93(8):e39.

17. Robert HE, Casin C. Valgus and flexion deformity after reconstruction of the anterior cruciate ligament in a skeletally immature patient. Knee Surg Sports Traumatol Arthrosc 2010;18(10):1369–73.

18. Yoo WJ, Kocher MS, Micheli LJ. Growth plate disturbance after transphyseal reconstruction of the anterior cruciate ligament in skeletally immature adolescent patients: an MR imaging study. J Pediatr Orthop 2011;31(6):691–6.

19. Koch PP, Fucentese SF, Blatter SC. Complications after epiphyseal reconstruction of the anterior cruciate ligament in prepubescent children. Knee Surg Sports Traumatol Arthrosc 2014. [Epub ahead of print].

20. Cruz AI Jr, Fabricant PD, McGraw M, et al. All-epiphyseal ACL reconstruction in children: review of safety and early complications. J Pediatr Orthop 2015. [Epub ahead of print].

21. Stanitski CL, Harvell JC, Fu F. Observations on acute knee hemarthrosis in children and adolescents. J Pediatr Orthop 1993;13(4):506–10.

22. Lee K, Siegel MJ, Lau DM, et al. Anterior cruciate ligament tears: MR imaging-based diagnosis in a pediatric population. Radiology 1999;213(3):697–704.

23. Piasecki DP, Spindler KP, Warren TA, et al. Intraarticular injuries associated with anterior cruciate ligament tear: findings at ligament reconstruction in high school and recreational athletes. An analysis of sex-based differences. Am J Sports Med 2003; 31(4):601–5.

24. Fabricant PD, Jones KJ, Delos D, et al. Reconstruction of the anterior cruciate ligament in the skeletally immature athlete: a review of current concepts: AAOS exhibit selection. J Bone Joint Surg Am 2013;95(5):e28.

25. Zerin JM, Hernandez RJ. Approach to skeletal maturation. Hand Clin 1991;7(1):53–62.

26. Acheson RM, Fowler G, Fry EI, et al. Studies in the reliability of assessing skeletal maturity from X-rays. I. Greulich-Pyle atlas. Hum Biol 1963;35: 317–49.

27. Heyworth BE, Osei DA, Fabricant PD, et al. The shorthand bone age assessment: a simpler alternative to current methods. J Pediatr Orthop 2013; 33(5):569–74.

28. Dimeglio A, Charles YP, Daures JP, et al. Accuracy of the Sauvegrain method in determining skeletal age during puberty. J Bone Joint Surg Am 2005; 87(8):1689–96.

29. Hans SD, Sanders JO, Cooperman DR. Using the Sauvegrain method to predict peak height velocity in boys and girls. J Pediatr Orthop 2008; 28(8):836–9.

30. Nicholson AD, Liu RW, Sanders JO, et al. Relationship of calcaneal and iliac apophyseal ossification to peak height velocity timing in children. J Bone Joint Surg Am 2015;97(2):147–54.

31. Sitoula P, Verma K, Holmes L Jr, et al. Prediction of curve progression in idiopathic scoliosis: validation of the sanders skeletal maturity staging system. Spine (Phila Pa 1976) 2015;40(13):1006–13.

32. Granados A, Gebremariam A, Lee JM. Relationship between timing of peak height velocity and pubertal staging in boys and girls. J Clin Res Pediatr Endocrinol 2015;7(3):235–7.

33. Woods GW, O'Connor DP. Delayed anterior cruciate ligament reconstruction in adolescents with open physes. Am J Sports Med 2004; 32(1):201–10.

34. McCarroll JR, Rettig AC, Shelbourne KD. Anterior cruciate ligament injuries in the young athlete with open physes. Am J Sports Med 1988;16(1): 44–7.

35. Mizuta H, Kubota K, Shiraishi M, et al. The conservative treatment of complete tears of the anterior cruciate ligament in skeletally immature patients. J Bone Joint Surg Br 1995;77(6):890–4.

36. Moksnes H, Engebretsen L, Risberg MA. Prevalence and incidence of new meniscus and cartilage injuries after a nonoperative treatment algorithm for ACL tears in skeletally immature children: a prospective MRI study. Am J Sports Med 2013;41(8): 1771–9.

37. Graf BK, Lange RH, Fujisaki CK, et al. Anterior cruciate ligament tears in skeletally immature patients: meniscal pathology at presentation and after attempted conservative treatment. Arthroscopy 1992;8(2):229–33.

38. Aichroth PM, Patel DV, Zorrilla P. The natural history and treatment of rupture of the anterior cruciate ligament in children and adolescents. A prospective review. J Bone Joint Surg Br 2002;84(1):38–41.

39. Funahashi KM, Moksnes H, Maletis GB, et al. Anterior cruciate ligament injuries in adolescents with open physis: effect of recurrent injury and surgical delay on meniscal and cartilage injuries. Am J Sports Med 2014;42(5):1068–73.

40. Henry J, Chotel F, Chouteau J, et al. Rupture of the anterior cruciate ligament in children: early reconstruction with open physes or delayed reconstruction to skeletal maturity? Knee Surg Sports Traumatol Arthrosc 2009;17(7):748–55.

41. Millett PJ, Willis AA, Warren RF. Associated injuries in pediatric and adolescent anterior cruciate ligament tears: does a delay in treatment increase the risk of meniscal tear? Arthroscopy 2002;18(9): 955–9.

42. Vavken P, Murray MM. Treating anterior cruciate ligament tears in skeletally immature patients. Arthroscopy 2011;27(5):704–16.

43. Ramski DE, Kanj WW, Franklin CC, et al. Anterior cruciate ligament tears in children and adolescents: a meta-analysis of nonoperative versus operative treatment. Am J Sports Med 2014;42(11):2769–76.

44. Kocher MS, Micheli LJ, Zurakowski D, et al. Partial tears of the anterior cruciate ligament in children and adolescents. Am J Sports Med 2002;30(5): 697–703.

45. Micheli LJ, Rask B, Gerberg L. Anterior cruciate ligament reconstruction in patients who are prepubescent. Clin Orthop Relat Res 1999;(364):40–7.

46. Kocher MS, Garg S, Micheli LJ. Physeal sparing reconstruction of the anterior cruciate ligament in skeletally immature prepubescent children and adolescents. J Bone Joint Surg Am 2005;87(11):2371–9.

47. Vincent JP, Magnussen RA, Gezmez F, et al. The anterolateral ligament of the human knee: an anatomic and histologic study. Knee Surg Sports Traumatol Arthrosc 2012;20(1):147–52.

48. Parsons EM, Gee AO, Spiekerman C, et al. The biomechanical function of the anterolateral ligament of the knee. Am J Sports Med 2015;43(3): 669–74.

49. Claes S, Vereecke E, Maes M, et al. Anatomy of the anterolateral ligament of the knee. J Anat 2013; 223(4):321–8.

50. Kennedy A, Coughlin DG, Metzger MF, et al. Biomechanical evaluation of pediatric anterior cruciate ligament reconstruction techniques. Am J Sports Med 2011;39(5):964–71.

51. Fabricant PD, McCarthy MM, Cordasco FA, et al. All-inside, all-epiphyseal autograft reconstruction of the anterior cruciate ligament in the skeletally immature athlete. JBJS Essential Surgical Techniques 2013;3(2):e9.

52. Lawrence JT, Bowers AL, Belding J, et al. All-epiphyseal anterior cruciate ligament reconstruction in skeletally immature patients. Clin Orthop Relat Res 2010;468(7):1971–7.

53. McCarthy MM, Graziano J, Green DW, et al. All-epiphyseal, all-inside anterior cruciate ligament reconstruction technique for skeletally immature patients. Arthrosc Tech 2012;1(2):e231–9.

54. Anderson AF. Transepiphyseal replacement of the anterior cruciate ligament using quadruple hamstring grafts in skeletally immature patients. J Bone Joint Surg Am 2004;86-A Suppl 1(Pt 2):201–9.

55. Nawabi DH, Jones KJ, Lurie B, et al. All-inside, physeal-sparing anterior cruciate ligament reconstruction does not significantly compromise the physis in skeletally immature athletes: a postoperative physeal magnetic resonance imaging analysis. Am J Sports Med 2014;42(12):2933–40.

56. Gausden EB, Calcei JG, Fabricant PD, et al. Surgical options for anterior cruciate ligament reconstruction in the young child. Curr Opin Pediatr 2015;27(1):82–91.

57. Makela EA, Vainionpaa S, Vihtonen K, et al. The effect of trauma to the lower femoral epiphyseal plate. an experimental study in rabbits. J Bone Joint Surg Br 1988;70(2):187–91.

58. Janarv PM, Wikstrom B, Hirsch G. The influence of transphyseal drilling and tendon grafting on bone growth: an experimental study in the rabbit. J Pediatr Orthop 1998;18(2):149–54.

59. Stadelmaier DM, Arnoczky SP, Dodds J, et al. The effect of drilling and soft tissue grafting across open growth plates. A histologic study. Am J Sports Med 1995;23(4):431–5.

60. Lemaitre G, Salle de Chou E, Pineau V, et al. ACL reconstruction in children: a transphyseal technique. Orthop Traumatol Surg Res 2014; 100(4 Suppl):S261–5.

61. Cohen M, Ferretti M, Quarteiro M, et al. Transphyseal anterior cruciate ligament reconstruction in patients with open physes. Arthroscopy 2009; 25(8):831–8.

62. McCarthy MM, Tucker S, Nguyen JT, et al. Contact stress and kinematic analysis of all-epiphyseal and over-the-top pediatric reconstruction techniques for the anterior cruciate ligament. Am J Sports Med 2013;41(6):1330–9.

63. Engelman GH, Carry PM, Hitt KG, et al. Comparison of allograft versus autograft anterior cruciate ligament reconstruction graft survival in an active adolescent cohort. Am J Sports Med 2014;42(10): 2311–8.

64. Ellis HB, Matheny LM, Briggs KK, et al. Outcomes and revision rate after bone-patellar tendon-bone allograft versus autograft anterior cruciate ligament reconstruction in patients aged 18 years or younger with closed physes. Arthroscopy 2012; 28(12):1819–25.

65. Kaeding CC, Aros B, Pedroza A, et al. Allograft versus autograft anterior cruciate ligament reconstruction. predictors of failure from a MOON

prospective longitudinal cohort. Sports Health 2011;3(1):73–81.

66. Nwachukwu BU, McFeely ED, Nasreddine A, et al. Arthrofibrosis after anterior cruciate ligament reconstruction in children and adolescents. J Pediatr Orthop 2011;31(8):811–7.

67. Akinleye SD, Sewick A, Wells L. All-epiphyseal ACL reconstruction: a three-year follow-up. Int J Sports Phys Ther 2013;8(3):300–10.

68. Greenberg EM, Albaugh J, Ganley TJ, et al. Rehabilitation considerations for all epiphyseal ACL reconstruction. Int J Sports Phys Ther 2012;7(2): 185–96.

69. Willimon SC, Jones CR, Herzog MM, et al. Micheli anterior cruciate ligament reconstruction in skeletally immature youths: a retrospective case series with a mean 3-year follow-up. Am J Sports Med 2015;43(12):2974–81.

70. Kocher MS, Smith JT, Zoric BJ, et al. Transphyseal anterior cruciate ligament reconstruction in skeletally immature pubescent adolescents. J Bone Joint Surg Am 2007;89(12):2632–9.

71. Courvoisier A, Grimaldi M, Plaweski S. Good surgical outcome of transphyseal ACL reconstruction in skeletally immature patients using four-strand hamstring graft. Knee Surg Sports Traumatol Arthrosc 2011; 19(4):588–91.

72. McIntosh AL, Dahm DL, Stuart MJ. Anterior cruciate ligament reconstruction in the skeletally immature patient. Arthroscopy 2006;22(12):1325–30.

73. Aronowitz ER, Ganley TJ, Goode JR, et al. Anterior cruciate ligament reconstruction in adolescents with open physes. Am J Sports Med 2000;28(2): 168–75.

74. Liddle AD, Imbuldeniya AM, Hunt DM. Transphyseal reconstruction of the anterior cruciate ligament in prepubescent children. J Bone Joint Surg Br 2008;90(10):1317–22.

75. Hui C, Roe J, Ferguson D, et al. Outcome of anatomic transphyseal anterior cruciate ligament reconstruction in tanner stage 1 and 2 patients with open physes. Am J Sports Med 2012;40(5): 1093–8.

76. Calvo R, Figueroa D, Gili F, et al. Transphyseal anterior cruciate ligament reconstruction in patients with open physes: 10-year follow-up study. Am J Sports Med 2015;43(2):289–94.

77. Kumar S, Ahearne D, Hunt DM. Transphyseal anterior cruciate ligament reconstruction in the skeletally immature: follow-up to a minimum of sixteen years of age. J Bone Joint Surg Am 2013;95(1):e1.

78. Swart E, Redler L, Fabricant PD, et al. Prevention and screening programs for anterior cruciate ligament injuries in young athletes: a cost-effectiveness analysis. J Bone Joint Surg Am 2014;96(9):705–11.

79. Mandelbaum BR, Silvers HJ, Watanabe DS, et al. Effectiveness of a neuromuscular and proprioceptive training program in preventing anterior cruciate ligament injuries in female athletes: 2-year follow-up. Am J Sports Med 2005;33(7):1003–10.

80. Hewett TE, Ford KR, Myer GD. Anterior cruciate ligament injuries in female athletes: part 2, a meta-analysis of neuromuscular interventions aimed at injury prevention. Am J Sports Med 2006;34(3): 490–8.

81. Hewett TE, Myer GD, Ford KR, et al. Biomechanical measures of neuromuscular control and valgus loading of the knee predict anterior cruciate ligament injury risk in female athletes: a prospective study. Am J Sports Med 2005;33(4):492–501.

82. Fabricant PD, Robles A, Downey-Zayas T, et al. Development and validation of a pediatric sports activity rating scale: the hospital for special surgery pediatric functional activity brief scale (HSS pedi-FABS). Am J Sports Med 2013;41(10):2421–9.

83. Kocher MS, Smith JT, Iversen MD, et al. Reliability, validity, and responsiveness of a modified international knee documentation committee subjective knee form (Pedi-IKDC) in children with knee disorders. Am J Sports Med 2011;39(5):933–9.

Upper Extremity

Ulnar-Sided Wrist Pain in the Athlete

Chance J. Henderson, MD[a],*, Ky M. Kobayashi, MD[b]

KEYWORDS

- Ulnar-sided wrist pain • Triangular fibrocartilage complex • Hamate fracture • Pisiform
- Hypothenar hammer • Ulnocarpal impaction syndrome • Lunotriquetral ligament tear
- Extensor carpi ulnaris tendinitis

KEY POINTS

- The athlete can present an interesting clinical challenge due to the overlap between acute injury and susceptibility to overuse phenomena from repetitive activities experienced during athletic pursuit.
- Although most of the entities described in this section are found among all patient groups, their treatment may differ in an athlete due to sport-specific considerations, temporal restraints, and outside influences on the athlete (coaching staff/trainers/recruiters).
- Thoughtful consideration of all of these factors will lead to a more satisfying outcome for the athlete with a goal of a safe and expedient return to sports activities.

INTRODUCTION

Management of hand and wrist injuries in the athlete can be a challenge and requires a good assessment of sport-specific athletic demands and the degree of impairment incurred by the athlete. Conservative management consisting of splints, medications, and therapy is beneficial in many cases; however, more definitive intervention is sometimes necessary to alleviate pain and preserve athletic function. The focus of this section is common ulnar-sided wrist conditions and injuries sustained in athletes. Many of the conditions outlined in this article can present as a result of participation in a variety of sports and occupational pursuits and as a normal consequence of physical training. Successful management often requires a thoughtful blending of treatment modalities for this unique class of patients.

HOOK OF HAMATE FRACTURES

Although hamate hook fractures represent only 2% to 4% of all carpal fractures, they are frequently seen in racket sports as well as golf, baseball, and hockey.[1–3] Hamate hook fractures are thought to be caused from a direct blow sometimes seen after grounding a golf club or during a check swing in baseball (Fig. 1). These fractures can be further subdivided by identifying them as tip, waist, or body fractures. Hamate fractures are notoriously poor healers with waist and tip fractures progressing to nonunion most commonly secondary to poor vascularity.[4,5] Because these injuries may be difficult to diagnose, hamate hook fractures must be suspected in athletes with ulnar-sided wrist pain competing in racquet or club sports.

Examination Findings
Patients may complain of pain over the hypothenar eminence and hamate hook and pain with resisted flexion of ring and small finger. In chronic cases, ulnar nerve dysfunction or crepitus with ring and small finer motion may be detected.

Imaging
Radiographic visualization of a hamate hook fracture can be difficult even with oblique and carpal tunnel views. Computed tomography

[a] Hand Surgery, USAF Academy, 4102 Pinion Drive, USAFA, CO 80840, USA; [b] Colorado Center of Orthopaedic Excellence, 2446 Research Parkway, Suite 200, Colorado Springs, CO 80920, USA
* Corresponding author.
E-mail address: chance.henderson@us.af.mil

Orthop Clin N Am 47 (2016) 789–798
http://dx.doi.org/10.1016/j.ocl.2016.05.017
0030-5898/16/$ – see front matter Published by Elsevier Inc.

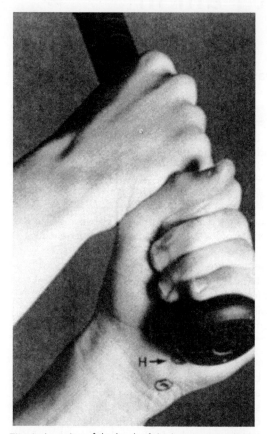

Fig. 1. Location of the hook of the hamate (H) relative to a bat end in the nondominant left hand of a right-handed hitter. (*From* Walsh JJ IV, Bishop AT. Diagnosis and management of hamate hook fractures. Hand Clin 2000;16(3):397–403; with permission.)

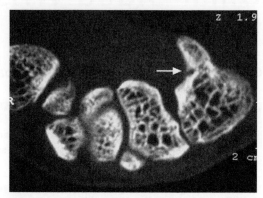

Fig. 2. CT scan visualization of fracture at the base of the hook of hamate with a large fracture fragment (*arrow*). (*From* Woon CYL, Lee JYL, Teoh LC. Attritional rupture of the small finger flexor tendons following local steroid injections of a hook of hamate fracture. Injury Extra 2007;38:200; with permission.)

an avulsion fracture from a sudden contraction of the flexor carpi ulnaris, which surrounds the pisiform.[2,8] Pisiform fractures make up about 2% of carpal fractures and are usually described as parasagittal, transverse, comminuted, and pisiform-triquetral impaction fractures.

Examination Findings
Presenting symptoms usually include pain directly over the pisiform or hypothenar eminence along with occasional ulnar nerve irritation.

Imaging
Visualizing the fracture on plain radiographs is difficult, but a 30° supinated view, 45° supinated oblique view, carpal tunnel view, or a CT scan may be necessary[2,8] (Fig. 3).

(CT) is the image modality of choice when a hamate hook fracture is suspected[1] (Fig. 2).

Treatment
Although acute nondisplaced fractures can be managed with cast immobilization, athletes should be counseled regarding the poor healing rate and prolonged immobilization, and that even after lengthy immobilization, they may still require surgery. Most investigators recommend fracture excision for displaced or nonunited fractures. Excision has been shown to have no adverse effect on grip strength or wrist range of motion.[2,4–7] Complications of hook of hamate fractures can include ulnar neuritis, flexor tendon irritation and rupture, ulnar artery thrombosis, and most commonly, symptomatic nonunion.[2]

PISIFORM FRACTURES

In athletes, pisiform fractures commonly occur from a direct blow. A more rare mechanism is

Treatment
Nondisplaced fractures typically heal with cast immobilization. Displaced and comminuted fractures are typically treated with pisiform excision with reliable pain relief and no loss of motion.

HYPOTHENAR HAMMER SYNDROME

Hypothenar hammer syndrome (HHS) is a vascular phenomenon that results typically from repetitive blunt trauma to the hypothenar hand where the relatively unprotected ulnar artery remains superficial as it exits Guyon canal. Although HHS has classically been described in the dominant hand of middle-aged male workers who habitually use the ulnar palm as a tool to hammer objects, it has also been reported in athletes participating in a variety of sports, including baseball, golf, tennis, biking,

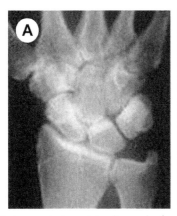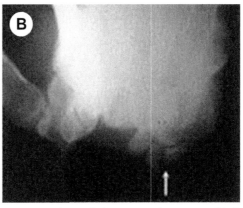

Fig. 3. (A) Anteroposterior wrist radiograph of a patient with ulnar-sided wrist pain shows a possible fracture of the pisiform. (B) Carpal tunnel view clearly shows a displaced parasagittal pisiform fracture (arrow). (From Shah MA, Viegas SF. Fractures of the carpal bones excluding the scaphoid. J Am Soc Surg Hand 2002;2:134; with permission.)

and lifting. The pathophysiology of HHS is related to trauma to the ulnar artery as it travels around the hook of the hamate, with the hook acting as an "anvil" upon which the artery may be impacted.[9–11] It is accepted that HHS symptoms occur secondarily as a result of thrombosis with or without embolic events.

Examination Findings
Ischemia in the ulnar digits of the hand associated with hypothenar callus, cold sensitivity, paresthesias, and pain are common findings. Other findings may include hamate hook fracture and ulnar tunnel syndrome. The Allen test and Doppler ultrasound are clinically useful to evaluate the patency of the ulnar artery and superficial palmar arch.

Imaging
Imaging may be accomplished with ultrasound; however, angiography is the accepted standard for definitively establishing the diagnosis of HHS and localizing the site of occlusion or aneurysm[9] (Fig. 4).

Treatment
Nonsurgical treatment is aimed at avoiding repetitive insults in episodically symptomatic patients. Calcium channel blockers and oral sympatholytics have been shown to be equally effective in this subset of patients.[9,10] Thrombolysis can also be attempted if the onset is acute enough for a chance of success. Recombinant tissue plasminogen activator is commonly used for this purpose via intra-arterial administration.[12] Surgery is the only treatment that will prevent recurrence of emboli and decompresses the adjacent neurologic structures. Surgical options include ligation of the ulnar artery if a

complete radial arch exists. Excision of the damaged artery and reconstruction with an interposition vein graft is more common.[9,10] Because there appears to be a subset of the population that is inherently susceptible to developing HHS, prevention is accomplished by ensuring athletes wear proper protective equipment and are taught proper grip techniques.

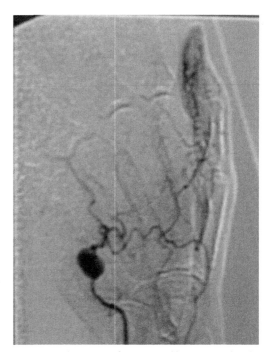

Fig. 4. In this case of HHS, initial angiography demonstrated ulnar artery occlusion and additional scattered, distal small-vessel embolic lesions. (From Iannuzzi NP, Higgins JP. Acute arterial thrombosis of the hand. J Hand Surg 2015;40:2099–116; with permission.)

TRIANGULAR FIBROCARTILAGE COMPLEX INJURIES

Triangular fibrocartilage complex (TFCC) injuries are common in athletes and may result from repetitive load bearing and rotational stresses seen in sports such as tennis, golf, hockey (from impact with the boards in slap shots, resulting in hypersupination), lacrosse, gymnastics, golf, boxing, waterskiing (from traction injury), and pole vaulting.[13] The TFCC is an important stabilizer of the distal radioulnar joint (DRUJ) and load absorber of the wrist. The TFCC is composed of a central articular portion that is avascular and a peripheral ligamentous portion that is a stabilizer of the DRUJ. This peripheral portion is more vascular and has a healing capacity[14] (Fig. 5).

Examination Findings
Ulnar-sided wrist pain in the athlete may be vague and associated with tenderness in the foveal area along with occasional clicks and pops.

Imaging
Imaging studies should include posteroanterior (PA) zero rotation view (with the shoulder abducted 90° and elbow flexed 90°), clenched fist pronation PA view, and contralateral views to assess ulnar variance and which may impact treatment decisions if ulnocarpal abutment is suspected. Although MRI arthrography is the definitive imaging modality of choice, it is associated with interpretative difficulty, and findings must be viewed in context of the clinical history and physical examination.[15–17]

Treatment
If the DRUJ is unstable, early intervention with arthroscopy and peripheral TFCC repair is indicated. If the DRUJ is stable with continued symptoms for 2 to 3 weeks, arthroscopy may be indicated.[1]

TFCC tears are broadly classified as either traumatic (class 1) or degenerative (class 2).[18] Traumatic tears from a fall on the outstretched hand are most commonly noted in young athletes. These tears are generally amendable to arthroscopic debridement (central tears) or repair (peripheral tears). Arthroscopic central debridement is associated with 90% good-to-excellent results and allows early return to activity in 1 to 2 months (Figs. 6 and 7).[18–20]

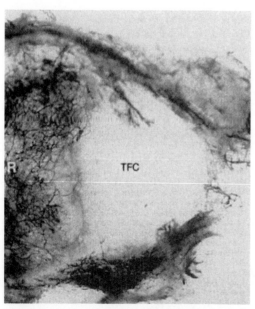

Fig. 5. End-on view of the distal radius (R) and TFC after India ink injection. The radioulnar ligaments and peripheral 15% to 20% of the articular disc are well vascularized. No vessels have been identified in the central area of the articular disc. (*From* Dailey SW, Palmer AK. The role of arthroscopy in the evaluation and treatment of triangular fibrocartilage complex injuries in athletes. Hand Clin 2000;16:461–76; with permission.)

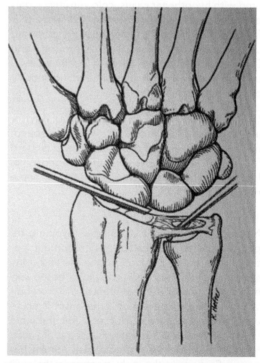

Fig. 6. Arthroscopic burr placed in 6-R portal for performing wafer procedure. (*From* Loftus JB. Arthroscopic wafer for ulnar impaction syndrome. Tech Hand Up Extrem Surg 2000;4:182–8; with permission.)

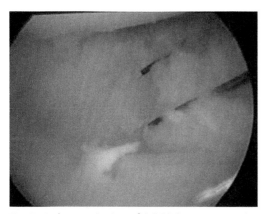

Fig. 7. Arthroscopic view of 2-0 PDS sutures securing peripheral TFCC tear. (*From* Sachar K. Ulnar-sided wrist pain: evaluation and treatment of triangular fibrocartilage complex tears, ulnocarpal impaction syndrome, and lunotriquetral ligament tears. J Hand Surg Am 2012;37:1489–500; with permission.)

Peripheral repairs are performed via several different effective techniques and protected in a Muenster cast for at least 6 weeks followed by therapy and strengthening. Return to sport occurs in 3 to 4 months with 90% good-to-excellent results.[21–23]

ULNOCARPAL IMPACTION SYNDROME

Palmer and Werner[24] have demonstrated that axial load transmission across the TFCC and ulna is approximately 18% of total load in an ulnar neutral wrist. This 18% total load has been shown to increase to 42% when ulnar length is increased 2.5 mm. Conversely, the ulnar carpus absorbs only 4.3% of axial load when the ulnar variance is decreased 2.5 mm.[19]

Examination Findings
As compared with TFC injuries, patients with ulnocarpal impaction syndrome present with more insidious onset of pain over the ulnar wrist. Athletes may complain the pain is worse with heavy grip or in pronation and ulnar deviation. Typically, the pain can be re-created in the clinic with ulnar stress testing, although this is not a specific test.[25,26] The ulnar stress test is performed by placing the wrist in maximum ulnar deviation while axially loading the wrist and taking the forearm through pronation and supination.[27]

Imaging
Radiographs will usually demonstrate ulnar-positive variance; however, a pronated grip view may be needed to show relative

lengthening of the ulna.[27] Dynamic fluoroscopy can also show relative lengthening of the ulna with power grip. Characteristic findings on radiographs include "kissing" lesions of the lunate, triquetrum, and ulnar head with subchondral cysts and sclerosis[27] (**Fig. 8**). MRI can help confirm the diagnosis showing subchondral bone marrow edema, which may be evident before radiographic findings in the ulnar lunate, radial triquetrum, and the radial aspect of the ulnar head.[27]

Treatment
Nonoperative treatment of ulnocarpal impaction syndrome includes immobilization, nonsteroidal anti-inflammatory medications (NSAIDs), avoidance of provocative activities, and corticosteroid injections. Pain relief with corticosteroid injection may help confirm the diagnosis.[27]

The goal of surgery is to shorten the ulna relative to the distal radius. This shortening can be accomplished via an open osteotomy or arthroscopically at the distal ulna. So long as the ulna-positive variance is 5 mm or less, the authors prefer arthroscopic wafer resection as described by Feldon and colleagues[28] because there is no risk of nonunion and no need for hardware removal. Comparison between arthroscopic wafer resection and osteotomy shows similar results.[25,29]

An arthroscopic resection of the distal ulna or a formal open ulnar shortening osteotomy can be considered for ulnar-positive or neutral variance.[30] Arthroscopic debridement alone in

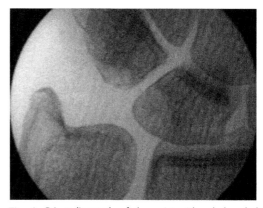

Fig. 8. PA radiograph of the wrist with subchondral lucency in the proximal ulnar corner of the lunate and the proximal corner of the triquetrum due to ulnar-positive variance and ulnar impaction. (*From* Bickel KD. Arthroscopic treatment of ulnar impaction syndrome. J Hand Surg Am 2008;33:1420–3; with permission.)

ulnar-positive wrists is associated with a 13% to 60% failure rate.[25,31,32]

Careful attention to associated injuries and ulnar variance will help guide treatment and postoperative course. The treatment goal is to return the competitive athlete to play in a timely and safe fashion. Early wrist arthroscopy is an excellent diagnostic and therapeutic tool that can help treat these sometimes challenging injuries.

LUNOTRIQUETRAL LIGAMENT TEARS

Isolated lunotriquetral (LT) ligament tears can occur from a fall on an outstretched hand or a direct blow.

Examination Findings

Athletes may present with tenderness and swelling to the ulnar side of the wrist over the LT articulation. This articulation can be palpated between the fourth and fifth extensor compartments. Provocative examination maneuvers include the ballottement test forcing the triquetrum radially into the lunate. The Regan "shuck" test is done by moving the lunate volar-dorsal and the triquetrum (with the pisiform) in the opposite direction.[27]

Imaging

Radiographs may demonstrate carpal instability with flexion of the lunate or carpal instability. MRI arthrogram may show dye extravasation through the torn LT ligament. Recent studies show a 3-T MRI has sensitivity and specificity for lunotriquetral interosseous ligament (LTIL) tears of 50% to 82% and 94% to 100%, respectively.[33] Also noted, the presence of a stepoff between the lunate and triquetrum calls for closer scrutiny of the LT ligament[34] (Fig. 9).

Treatment

Treatment options for LT ligament tears without instability include immobilization for acute, isolated tears and corticosteroid injections for more chronic presentations.

Arthroscopy is a valid option for those who fail nonoperative management. Arthroscopic treatment can be guided using the Geissler classification system (Table 1), which grades instability using both the radiocarpal and the midcarpal portals.[35,36] Arthroscopic options progress from debridement alone to debridement with pinning of the LT joint to the addition of a dorsal reinforcement procedure to the debridement and pinning. Excellent results

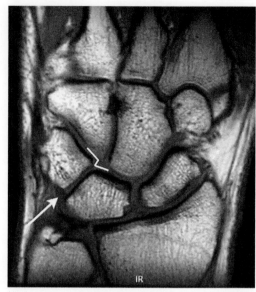

Fig. 9. Secondary sign of an LTIL tear. In this patient with a normal MRI appearance of the LTIL, the lunotriquetral stepoff (*arrow*) seen on the coronal T1-weighted fast spin echo MRI was the only evidence of the surgically confirmed LTIL tear. (*From* Ringler MD. MRI of wrist ligaments. J Hand Surg Am 2013;38:2034–46; with permission.)

have been reported with debridement alone.[35,36] Others have reported less compelling results with 4 of 5 patients reporting poor results.[37] In more unstable wrists (Geissler III/IV), arthroscopic debridement and pinning of the LT articulation can be considered. Osterman and Seidman[38] reported 80% complete pain relief with this technique. Open options for LT instability include direct repair of the LT ligament, LT ligament reconstruction, and LT fusion, although the results or LT fusion are not encouraging.[39]

EXTENSOR CARPI ULNARIS TENDINITIS

Extensor carpi ulnaris (ECU) tendinitis is an overuse injury and is seen in racquet sports and rowers.[40] Underlying wrist abnormality such as TFCC injury may lead to ECU tendinitis.[38,40]

Examination Findings

The ECU tendon sheath lies just dorsal to the TFCC and can easily be palpated along its length.[27] The synergy test has been described as a way to differentiate ECU tendinitis from other abnormality. It is performed with the subject's elbow flexed 90° with the elbow resting

Table 1 Geissler classification			
Grade	Definition	Arthroscopic Findings	Management
I	Attenuation hemorrhage of interosseous ligaments seen from the radiocarpal joint. No incongruency noted in the midcarpal space.	There is a loss of the normal concave appearance between the carpal bones and the interosseous ligament attenuates and becomes convex as seen from the radiocarpal space. In the midcarpal space, the interval between the carpal bones will still be tight with no stepoff.	Immobilization
II	Attenuation hemorrhage of interosseous ligaments seen from the radiocarpal joint. Incongruency/stepoff as seen from the midcarpal space. A slight gap between the carpal bones may be noted.	A slight gap (less than the width of a probe) between the carpal bones may be present. The interosseous ligament continues to become attenuated and is convex as seen from the radial carpal space. In the midcarpal space, the interval between the involved carpal bones is no longer congruent and a stepoff is present. In LT instability, increased translation between the triquetrum and lunate will be seen when palpated with a probe.	Arthroscopic reduction and pinning
III	Incongruency/stepoff of carpal alignment is seen in both the radiocarpal and the midcarpal spaces.	The interosseous ligament has started to tear and a gap is visualized between the carpal bones in the radiocarpal space. A 2-mm probe may be placed between the carpal bones and twisted in the midcarpal space.	Arthroscopic/open reduction and pinning
IV	Incongruency/stepoff of carpal alignment is seen in both the radiocarpal and the midcarpal spaces. Gross instability with manipulation is noted.	A 2.7-mm arthroscope may be passed through the gap between the carpal bones (the "drive-through" sign) from the radiocarpal space into the midcarpal space. The interosseous ligament is completely detached between the involved carpal bones.	Open reduction and repair

on a table. The forearm is in full supination, and the examiner then resists radial abduction of the athlete's thumb while applying a counter-force to the middle finger as shown in Fig. 10. If the patient's pain is re-created, this is considered a positive test.

Treatment

Treatment options for ECU tendinitis include rest, splinting, NSAIDs, as well as corticosteroid injection. Failure to improve should illicit serial examination and consideration of MRI.

SUBLUXATION OF THE EXTENSOR CARPI ULNARIS

Subluxation of the ECU results from either rupture or attenuation of the ECU subsheath and may be seen in tennis players, golfers, weight-lifters, and rough stock rodeo cowboys.[40–43]

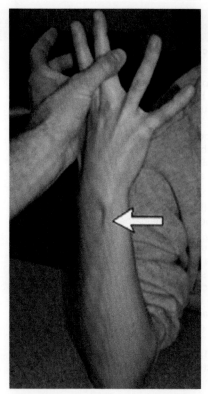

Fig. 10. The ECU synergy test is performed by having the patient radially deviate the thumb against resistance. Note that the ECU tendon bowstrings against the skin (arrow). (From Ruland RT, Hogan CJ. The ECU synergy test: an aid to diagnose ECU tendonitis. J Hand Surg Am 2008;33:1777–82; with permission.)

Examination Findings

Physical examination involves observation of the ECU subluxing with active ulnar deviation in maximum supination (Fig. 11).

Treatment

Conservative treatment options for acute injuries include casting with the wrist pronated and dorsiflexed.[44,45] Some investigators advocate early repair with early aggressive therapy for acute tears.[43] Refractory chronic injures are addressed with reconstruction or tightening of the subsheath with good-to-excellent results with average return to sports in 3 months.[40]

SUMMARY

The athlete can present an interesting clinical challenge because of the overlap between acute injury and susceptibility to overuse phenomena from repetitive activities experienced during athletic pursuit. Although most of the entities described in this section are found among all patient groups, their treatment may differ in an athlete because of sport-specific considerations, temporal restraints, and outside influences on the athlete (coaching staff/trainers/recruiters). Thoughtful consideration of all of these factors will lead to a more satisfying outcome for the athlete with a goal of a safe and expedient return to sports activities.

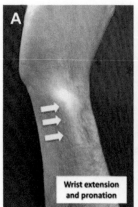
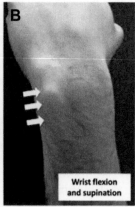
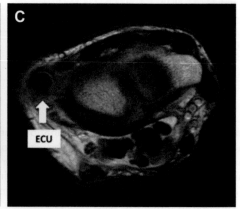

Fig. 11. (A, B) Clinical photographs demonstrating subluxation of the ECU tendon (arrows) in and out of the groove during wrist motion. (A) During wrist extension and pronation (backswing), the ECU tendon remains within the groove; however, following impact with the ball (B), the wrist moves into flexion and supination (follow through), and the ECU tendon subluxates out of the groove. (C) A T1-weighted MRI scan showing marked inflammatory changes around the ECU tendon (arrow) with complete disruption of the ECU sheath. (From Ek ET, Suh N, Weiland AJ. Hand and wrist injuries in golf. J Hand Surg Am 2013;38(10) 2029–33; with permission.)

REFERENCES

1. Rettig AC. Athletic injuries of the wrist and hand part I: traumatic injuries of the wrist. Am J Sports Med 2003;31:1038–48.
2. Suh N, Ek ET, Wolfe SW. Carpal fractures. J Hand Surg Am 2014;39(4):785–91.
3. Ek ET, Suh N, Weiland AJ. Hand and wrist injuries in golf. J Hand Surg Am 2013;38(10):2029–33.
4. Carroll RE, Lakin JF. Fracture of the hook of the hamate: acute treatment. J Trauma 1993;34(6):803–5.
5. Failla JM. Hook of hamate vascularity: vulnerability to osteonecrosis and nonunion. J Hand Surg Am 1993;18(6):1075–9.
6. Stark HH, Chao EK, Zemel NP, et al. Fracture of the hook of the hamate. J Bone Joint Surg Am. 1989; 71(8):1202–7.
7. Devers BN, Douglas KC, Naik RD, et al. Outcomes of hook of hamate fracture excision in high-level amateur athletes. J Hand Surg Am 2013;38(1):72–6.
8. O'Shea K, Weiland AJ. Fractures of the hamate and pisiform bones. Hand Clin 2012;28(3):287–300, viii.
9. Ablett CT, Hackett LA. Hypothenar hammer syndrome: case reports and brief review. Clin Med Res 2008;1:3–8.
10. Stuart JJ, Joe KJ, Kobayashi KM. Surgical management of ulnar artery thrombosis. Poster presentation, Society of Military Orthopaedic Surgeons. 2007.
11. Wong GB, Whetzel TP. Hypothenar hammer syndrome: review and case report. Vasc Surg 2001; 35:163–6.
12. Iannuzzi NP, Higgins JP. Acute arterial thrombosis of the hand. J Hand Surg Am 2015;40:2099–116.
13. Palmer AK, Werner FW. The triangular fibrocartilage complex of the wrist: anatomy and function. J Hand Surg Am 1981;6:153–62.
14. Dailey SW, Palmer AK. The role of arthroscopy in the evaluation and treatment of triangular fibrocartilage complex injuries in athletes. Hand Clin 2000; 16:461–76.
15. Potter HG, Asnis-Ernberg L, Weiland AJ, et al. The utility of high-resolution magnetic resonance imaging in the evaluation of the triangular fibrocartilage complex of the wrist. J Bone Joint Surg Am. 1997; 79(11):1675–84.
16. Iordache SD, Rowan R, Gavin G, et al. Prevalence of triangular fibrocartilage complex abnormality on MRI scans of asymptomatic wrists. J Hand Surg Am 2012;37:98–103.
17. Faber KJ, Iordache SD, Grewal R. Magnetic resonance imaging for ulnar wrist pain. J Hand Surg Am 2010;35(2):303–7.
18. Palmer AK. Triangular fibrocartilage complex lesions: a classification. J Hand Surg 1989;14(11):2236–42.
19. Friedman SL, Palmer AK. The ulnar impaction syndrome. Hand Clin 1991;7:295–310.
20. Bednar JM, Osterman AL. The role of arthroscopy in the treatment of traumatic triangular fibrocartilage injuries. Hand Clin 1994;10:605–14.
21. Shinohara T, Tatebe M, Okui N, et al. Arthroscopically assisted repair of triangular fibrocartilage complex foveal tears. J Hand Surg 2013;38A:271–7.
22. Bednar MS, Arnoczky SP, Weiland AJ. The microvasculature of the triangular fibrocartilage complex: its clinical significance. J Hand Surg Am 1991;16:1101–5.
23. Corso SJ, Savoie FH, Geissler WB, et al. Arthroscopic repair of peripheral avulsions of the triangular fibrocartilage complex of the wrist: a multicenter study. Arthroscopy 1997;13:78–84.
24. Palmer AK, Werner FW. Biomechanics of the distal radioulnar joint. Clin Orthop 1984;187:26–35.
25. Bernstein MA, Nagle DJ, Martinez A, et al. A comparison of combined arthroscopic triangular fibrocartilage complex debridement and arthroscopic wafer distal ulna resection versus arthroscopic triangular fibrocartilage complex debridement and ulnar shortening osteotomy for ulnocarpal abutment syndrome. Arthroscopy 2004;20:392–401.
26. Nakamura R, Horii E, Imaeda T, et al. The ulnocarpal stress test in the diagnosis of ulnar-sided wrist pain. J Hand Surg Am 1997;22:719–23.
27. Sachar K. Ulnar-sided wrist pain: evaluation and treatment of triangular fibrocartilage complex tears, ulnocarpal impaction syndrome, and lunotriquetral ligament tears. J Hand Surg Am 2012;37:1489–500.
28. Tomaino MM, Elfar J. Ulnar impaction syndrome. Hand Clin 2005;21:567–75.
29. Constantine KJ, Tomaino MM, Herndon JH, et al. Comparison of ulnar shortening osteotomy and the wafer resection procedure as treatment for ulnar impaction syndrome. J Hand Surg Am 2000;25:55–60.
30. Feldon P, Terrono AL, Belsky MR. Wafer distal ulna resection for triangular fibrocartilage tears and/or ulna impaction syndrome. J Hand Surg Am 1992; 17:731–7.
31. Minami A, Ishikawa I, Suenaga N, et al. Clinical results of treatment of triangular fibrocartilage complex tears by arthroscopic debridement. J Hand Surg Am 1996;21:406–11.
32. Hulsizer D, Weiss AP, Akelman E. Ulna shortening osteotomy after failed arthroscopic debridement of the failed arthroscopic debridement of the triangular fibrocartilage complex. J Hand Surg Am 1997;22:694–8.
33. Magee T. Comparison of 3-T MRI and arthroscopy of intrinsic wrist ligament and TFCC tears. AJR Am J Roentgenol 2009;192(1):80–5.
34. Ringler MD. MRI of wrist ligaments. J Hand Surg Am 2013;38:2034–46.
35. Chloros GD, Wiesler ER, Poehling GG. Current concepts in wrist arthroscopy. Arthroscopy 2008; 24:343–54.

36. Geissler WB, Freeland AE, Savoie FH, et al. Intra-carpal soft-tissue lesions associated with an intra-articular fracture of the distal end of the radius. J Bone Joint Surg Am 1996;78:357–65.

37. Westkaemper JG, Mitsionis G, Giannakopoulos PN, et al. Wrist arthroscopy for the treatment of ligament and triangular fibrocartilage complex injuries. Arthroscopy 1998;14:479–83.

38. Osterman AL, Seidman GD. The role of arthroscopy in the treatment of lunatotriquetral ligament injuries. Hand Clin 1995;11:41–50.

39. Shin AY, Weinstein LP, Berger RA, et al. Treatment of isolated injuries of the lunotriquetral ligament. A comparison of arthrodesis, ligament reconstruction and ligament repair. J Bone Joint Surg Br 2001;83:1023–8.

40. Rettig AC. Athletic injuries of the wrist and hand part II: overuse injuries of the wrist and traumatic injuries to the hand. Am J Sports Med 2003;32:262–73.

41. Melone CP. Complex joint injuries of the hand, in American Academy of Orthopaedic Surgeons Symposium on Upper Extremity Injuries in Athletes. St Louis (MO): CV Mosby; 1986. p. 142–69.

42. Pitner M. Pathophysiology of overuse injuries in the hand and wrist. J Hand Clin 1990;6:355–64.

43. Rowland SA. Acute traumatic subluxation of the extensor carpi ulnaris tendon at the wrist. J Hand Surg Am 1986;11(6):809.

44. Taleisnik J. The ligaments of the wrist. In: Taleisnik J, editor. The wrist. New York: Churchill Livingstone; 1985. p. 13–38.

45. Burkhart S, Wood M, Linscheid RL. Post-traumatic recurrent subluxation of the extensor carpi ulnaris tendon. J Hand Surg 1982;7:1.

Thumb Ligament Injuries in the Athlete

F. Patterson Owings, MD, James H. Calandruccio, MD*, Benjamin M. Mauck, MD

KEYWORDS

- Thumb • Ligament injuries • Ulnar collateral ligament • Radial collateral ligament
- Carpometacarpal joint • Metacarpophalangeal joint • Trauma

KEY POINTS

- Injuries to the hand account for up to 15% of all sports injuries and are common in contact sports and in sports with a high risk of falling.
- Ligamentous injuries to the thumb include thumb carpometacarpal dislocations, thumb metacarpophalangeal dislocations, and collateral ligament injuries and interphalangeal dislocations.
- Management requires knowledge of the type of injury, demands of the sport, competitive level, future athletic expectations, and the role of rehabilitation and protective splints for return to play.

INTRODUCTION

Injuries to the hand account for up to 15% of all sports injuries and are common in contact sports such as football and in sports with a high risk of falling such as skiing, biking, in-line skating and gymnastics.[1–3] In many sports, the thumb is one of the most frequently injured areas.[1] Appropriate management requires knowledge of the type of injury, demands of the specific sport and position played, competitive level of the athlete, future athletic demands and expectations, and the role of rehabilitation and protective splints for return to play. In contrast with the nonathlete, management of the athlete often requires more aggressive and expedient diagnostic intervention and treatment to minimize time away from sport while also ensuring safe return to competition. This paper describes ligamentous injuries to the thumb including thumb carpometacarpal dislocations, thumb metacarpophalangeal dislocations, collateral ligament injuries and interphalangeal (IP) dislocations, their evaluation, treatment and outcomes.

THUMB CARPOMETACARPAL JOINT DISLOCATION

The thumb trapeziometacarpal joint consists of the concavoconvex articular surfaces of the thumb metacarpal base and the trapezium oriented in opposition to one another with perpendicular axes similar to 2 reciprocally opposed saddles. The joint is stabilized by its capsule and the palmar oblique, intermetacarpal, dorsal–radial, and dorsal oblique ligaments. The primary restraints to dorsal subluxation and dislocation are the palmar oblique ligament and dorsoradial ligament.[4]

Injuries to the thumb carpometacarpal joint may be complete or partial. Partial injuries are far more common and result in varying degrees of joint subluxation. Complete injuries with dislocation of the thumb carpometacarpal joint are relatively rare and occur when a flexed metacarpal is loaded axially. Dislocations are invariably dorsal and result in tearing of the dorsal radial ligament and volar oblique ligament.[4] Physical examination typically reveals an adducted thumb with dorsal subluxation

Disclosures: The authors have nothing to disclose.
Department of Orthopaedic Surgery and Biomechanical Engineering, Campbell Clinic, University of Tennessee, 1211 Union Avenue, Suite 520, Memphis, TN 38104, USA
* Corresponding author.
E-mail address: jcalandruccio@campbellclinic.com

that reduces with a palmar directed force or thumb extension. Evaluation with standard posteroanterior and true lateral radiographs must be performed to evaluate for associated fractures (ie, Bennett fracture–dislocation) and may show dorsoradial subluxation of the metacarpal. Evaluation of the thumb carpometacarpal joint is best obtained with a Robert view in which the forearm is fully pronated with the dorsum of the thumb on the cassette and the x-ray beam angled 15° from distal to proximal (Figs. 1 and 2). Posteroanterior stress radiographs with the radial aspect of the distal phalanges pressed firmly together are often helpful to access for instability and allow comparison with the contralateral uninjured joint (Fig. 3).

Treatment should consist of immediate reduction and assessment of joint stability. If the joint is well-reduced and stable after reduction, immobilization in a thumb spica cast for 4 to 6 weeks may be sufficient to maintain reduction and prevent long-term instability. Frequently, however, the joint remains unstable and open reduction, repair of the dorsoradial ligament and K-wire fixation of the joint is indicated. If reduction is delayed beyond 3 weeks or there is persistent instability, ligament reconstruction with a strip of the flexor carpi radialis as described by Eaton and colleagues is advised.[5]

A dorsoradial incision is made along the proximal half of the first metacarpal curving ulnarward proximally around the base of the thenar eminence parallel with the distal flexor crease

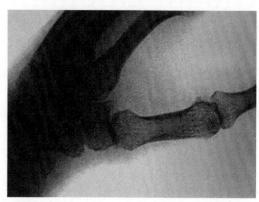

Fig. 2. Anteroposterior view of the first carpometacarpal joint (Robert's view). (*From* Blake M, Isaacs JE. Diagnosis, evaluation, and conservative treatment of posttraumatic arthritis and osteoarthritis of the wrist. In: Chhabra AB, Isaacs JE, editors. Arthritis and arthroplasty: the hand, wrist and elbow. 1st edition. Philadelphia: Elsevier; 2009; with permission.)

of the wrist. The carpometacarpal joint of the thumb is exposed subperiosteally and the distal part of the flexor carpi radialis is isolated. A 6-cm distally based strip of the flexor carpi radialis is harvested from the radial side of the tendon and freed proximally, ensuring that it remains attached to the base of the second metacarpal distally. The thumb metacarpal is then reduced on the trapezium and secured with a K-wire ensuring that its path will not interfere with the site through which the tendon transfer will eventually pass. A hole is drilled transversely through the base of the thumb metacarpal ulnar to the extensor pollicis brevis tendon exiting near the volar beak. The harvested tendon strip is passed through this tunnel deep to the abductor pollicis longus tendon and sutured to the periosteum near its exit. It is then looped around the flexor

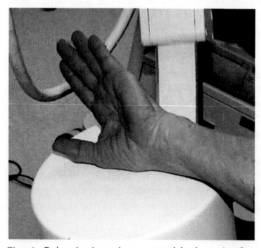

Fig. 1. Robert's view gives a good look at the first carpometacarpal joint. (*From* Blake M, Isaacs JE. Diagnosis, evaluation, and conservative treatment of posttraumatic arthritis and osteoarthritis of the wrist. In: Chhabra AB, Isaacs JE, editors. Arthritis and arthroplasty: the hand, wrist and elbow. 1st edition. Philadelphia: Elsevier; 2009; with permission.)

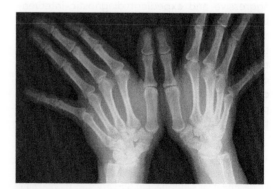

Fig. 3. Stress view of the carpometacarpal joint. (*From* Wolf JM, Oren TW, Ferguson B, et al. The carpometacarpal stress view radiograph in the evaluation of trapeziometacarpal joint laxity. J Hand Surg 2009;34A:1405; with permission.)

carpi radialis near its insertion and sutured to the base of the thumb metacarpal (Fig. 4).

Postoperatively, the thumb is immobilized for 4 weeks in extension and abduction. Treatment of traumatic dislocations of the thumb carpometacarpal joint when instability is present remains a subject of debate. Simonian and Trumble[6] retrospectively compared closed reduction and percutaneous pinning with early ligamentous reconstruction. One-half of the patients (4/8) initially treated with closed reduction and percutaneous pinning were noted to have unsatisfactory results secondary to recurrent instability and degenerative arthritis and were converted to early (within an average of 7 days of injury) ligamentous reconstruction as described. At follow-up, these patients were noted to have good pain relief and well-preserved grip strength and range of motion (ROM). Other studies have demonstrated favorable results with good pain relief, stability, and improvements in pinch strength[7,8] after ligamentous reconstruction in the setting of persistent instability.

THUMB METACARPOPHALANGEAL JOINT DISLOCATION

The soft tissue stabilizers of the thumb metacarpophalangeal joint include paired collateral ligaments and the volar plate. The collateral ligament complex is composed of a proper and accessory collateral ligament. The proper collateral ligament arises from the lateral condyles and inserts on the volar aspect of the proximal phalanx. The accessory collateral ligaments arise more volarly and insert on the volar plate and sesamoids.

Thumb metacarpophalangeal dislocations are typically dorsal and occur secondary to a

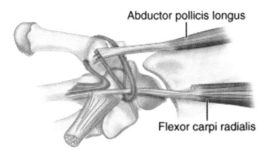

Fig. 4. Volar and radial ligament reconstruction with strip from tendon of flexor carpi radialis, which is left attached at its insertion at base of second metacarpal. Course of tendon strip creates reinforcement of volar, dorsal, and radial aspects of joint. (*From* Calandruccio JH. Fractures, dislocations, and ligamentous injuries. In: Canale ST, Beaty JH, editors. Campbell's operative orthopaedics. 12th edition. Philadelphia: Elsevier; 2013; with permission.)

hyperextension injury with associated injuries to the collateral ligaments, volar plate, and capsule. Dislocations are classified as simple (reducible with closed techniques) or complex (irreducible with closed techniques) and present with a hyperextension deformity and metacarpal adduction. Complex dislocations often present with puckering of the palmar skin overlying the metacarpal head and imply interposed soft tissue, most often the volar plate, which has avulsed proximally, or the flexor pollicis longus.[9,10] Radiographic evaluation should include standard posteroanterior and true lateral radiographs to evaluate for associated fracture–dislocation.

Reduction is accomplished under local anesthetic block with wrist flexion to relax the flexor tendons, gentle recreation of the deformity (ie, hyperextension), and a palmar-directed force on the proximal phalanx to reduce it onto the metacarpal head. Longitudinal traction should be avoided because displacement of the flexor pollicis longus to the ulnar side of the metacarpal head, in conjunction with the radial sided adductor musculature, can produce a "noose" around the metacarpal head. Longitudinal traction serves to tighten this noose converting a reducible dislocation into an irreducible one.

Dislocations that cannot be reduced by closed means require open reduction, most commonly via a dorsal or volar approach. The dorsal approach uses the interval between the extensor pollicis brevis and longus and offers the advantage of minimal risk to the neurovascular bundles whereas the volar approach with a Bruner incision has the advantage of allowing direct visualization of structures that may be impeding reduction (ie, volar plate, sesamoids, and flexor pollicis longus). Either approach may be used based on surgeon preference. After reduction the thumb is immobilized in a dorsal block splint with the metacarpophalangeal joint in 10° more flexion than the point of instability. Each week thereafter it is extended 10° until terminal extension is obtained. Few studies have evaluated the long-term outcome of thumb metacarpophalangeal joint dislocation, but patients can expect to have a stable, albeit possibly stiff, joint. If, after reduction, the joint remains unstable and there is evidence to suggest complete collateral ligament rupture, operative repair is indicated, as discussed.

THUMB METACARPOPHALANGEAL JOINT ULNAR COLLATERAL LIGAMENT INJURIES

Commonly known as *skier's thumb*, acute injuries to the thumb metacarpophalangeal joint ulnar collateral ligament (UCL) can be partial or complete tears and are common in skiers and other sports that place the thumb at risk for forced radial deviation/abduction. Patients typically present complaining of pain with tenderness, swelling, and ecchymosis along the ulnar aspect of the thumb metacarpophalangeal joint.

Patients with suspected UCL injuries should undergo radiographic evaluation with standard posteroanterior and true lateral radiographs before physical examination to rule out associated fracture and prevent displacement of a nondisplaced fracture. Physical examination should include evaluation for the presence of a Stener lesion. Originally described in 1962, a Stener lesion presents as a palpable mass over the ulnar aspect of the joint and occurs as the distal insertion of the UCL avulses from the proximal phalanx and retracts proximal and dorsal to the adductor aponeurosis.[11] Present in 80% or more of cases, recognition of the presence of a Stener lesion is of paramount importance because it prevents reapproximation of the ligament to its insertion site and warrants surgical intervention.[12] Of note, however, inability to palpate a mass does not definitively rule out a Stener lesion[12] (Fig. 5).

Physical examination is of utmost importance to evaluate the stability of the joint and differentiate between sprains/partial tears and complete rupture of the ligament because sprains/partial tears can be treated nonoperatively with immobilization, whereas complete tears and those with a Stener lesion require operative intervention. Evaluation of joint stability is performed by applying a radial stress to the joint in full extension and 30° of flexion. Testing in full extension evaluates the integrity of the accessory collateral ligament and volar plate whereas testing in 30° of flexion accesses the proper collateral ligament. Lack of a firm endpoint, greater than 30° to 35° laxity with radial deviation or greater than 15° when compared with contralateral, uninjured side in both flexion and extension are indicative of a complete rupture of the collateral ligament and warrant operative intervention.[12–16]

Although diagnosis is primarily clinical and based on accurate physical examination, both ultrasound imaging and MRI have proven useful in differentiating partial and complete UCL tears. Ultrasonography has the benefit of being relatively inexpensive and has 76% sensitivity and 81% specificity.[17,18] In contrast, MRI is relatively more expensive but has 100% sensitivity and specificity[19,20] (Fig. 6).

Treatment of partial tears of the UCL are treated with immobilization in a thumb spica splint or cast for a period of 4 to 6 weeks.[13,14,21,22] During immobilization, the thumb IP joint is left free to allow ROM exercises and prevent extensor tendon adhesions. After initial immobilization, a removable thermoplastic splint is applied and ROM activities are begun while avoiding radial deviation or stress. Grip and pinch strengthening is started after attaining full ROM or at 6 weeks. Return to sport is dictated by the demands of the sport and the ability of the athlete to participate with protective equipment. Athletes with minor injuries can return to play in 2 to 4 weeks with a protective splint. Patients with more significant injuries and those involved in high-contact sports or sports with significant risk of repeat injury should

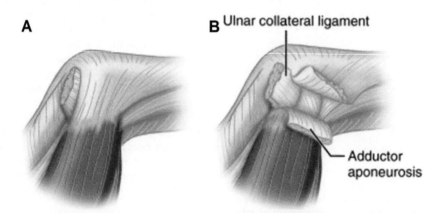

Fig. 5. Complete rupture of ulnar collateral ligament of metacarpophalangeal joint of thumb. (*A*) Ligament is ruptured distally and is folded back so that its distal end points proximally. (*B*) Adductor aponeurosis has been divided, exposing ligament and joint. (*From* Calandruccio JH. Fractures, dislocations, and ligamentous injuries. In: Canale ST, Beaty JH, editors. Campbell's operative orthopaedics. 12th edition. Philadelphia: Elsevier; 2013; with permission.)

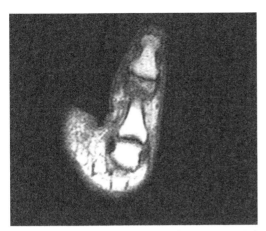

Fig. 6. MRI appearance of a Stener lesion. (*From* Calandruccio JH. Fractures, dislocations, and ligamentous injuries. In: Canale ST, Beaty JH, editors. Campbell's operative orthopaedics. 12th edition. Philadelphia: Elsevier; 2013; with permission.)

continue to protect the joint for a period of 6 more weeks during games and practice.

Complete tears of the UCL (ie, lack of a firm endpoint, greater than 30°–35° laxity with radial deviation or >15° when compared with contralateral, uninjured side in both flexion and extension, and presence of a Stener lesion) are best managed with acute surgical repair.[11,13,14,21,23,24] Midsubstance tears are treated with direct repair using nonabsorbable braided suture. In 90% of cases, the UCL avulses from the proximal phalanx.[25] Reattachment of the UCL to bone is typically achieved with a transosseous pullout suture tied over a button outside the skin over the radial aspect of the thumb or with suture anchors. Our preference is to use a suture anchor placed

3 mm distal to the articular surface and 3 mm dorsal to the volar cortex[26] (Fig. 7). Recent studies have demonstrated that, compared with a pullout suture, suture anchors allowed for shorter surgical time, fewer complications, lower cost, improved pinch strength, and better motion.[23,27–31] Temporarily pinning the metacarpophalangeal joint is probably unnecessary, unless the joint inadequately reduced after soft tissue repair.[14] However, complications with pinning the metacarpophalangeal joint for 3 to 4 weeks in full extension are rare and provides a measure of safety in tenuous repairs.

The thumb metacarpophalangeal joint is exposed through a midaxial or lazy S incision centered over the joint line taking care to protect the dorsal sensory branch of the radial nerve. If a Stener lesion is present, the UCL can be seen with its distal hemorrhagic end located proximal and dorsal to the adductor aponeurosis. The adductor aponeurosis is incised longitudinally and the failure site of the UCL is identified. The footprint of the ligament is debrided to bleeding bone and a suture anchor is placed at the site of insertion. We secure the ligament stump with either a Bunnell or Kessler stitch and tension the ligament with the joint in 15° of flexion and slight ulnar deviation.

Delay in diagnosis of more than 3 to 4 weeks results in fibrosis of the ligament and makes primary repair difficult. In this case, surgical reconstruction, typically with a free tendon graft, may be necessary. Our preferred graft material is the palmaris longus, but a strip of the flexor carpi radialis or a toe extensor may be used in its absence. Stability at long-term follow-up has been associated with "anatomic repairs" in

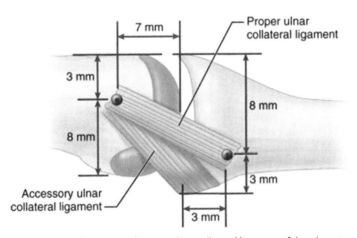

Fig. 7. Mean locations of origin and insertion of proper ulnar collateral ligament of thumb metacarpophalangeal joint. (*From* Calandruccio JH. Fractures, dislocations, and ligamentous injuries. In: Canale ST, Beaty JH, editors. Campbell's operative orthopaedics. 12th edition. Philadelphia: Elsevier; 2013; with permission.)

which the graft is used to reconstruct both the proper and accessory UCL. Although multiple methods of reconstruction have been reported, we recommend a modified anatomic reconstruction as described by Glickel and colleagues using a palmaris graft.[32,33]

The thumb metacarpophalangeal joint is exposed as previously described. The UCL stumps are excised and the joint is inspected for arthritic changes. If the joint is arthritic, reconstruction is precluded and an arthrodesis is performed. If the joint is not arthritic, 2 bone tunnels are created in the proximal phalanx at the anatomic footprint of the UCL. The first is located palmarly at 7 o'clock and the second more dorsally at 11 o'clock (right thumb) or 1 o'clock and 5 o'clock (left thumb). These are connected in the intramedullary canal preserving the overlying bone bridge. A single transverse bone tunnel from ulnar to radial is created in the metacarpal head ligament fossa. The graft is passed through the proximal phalangeal tunnels using either a stainless steel wire, suture passer, or small curved needle. The graft is then passed under the sagittal band and through the metacarpal tunnel from ulnar to radial. We hold the metacarpophalangeal joint in 15° of flexion and slightly overcorrected to take tension off the graft. The graft is then secured in the metacarpal with either a biotenodesis screw or by suturing it to the periosteum on the radial side of the thumb. If necessary, we protect the construct with a Kirschner wire transfixing the joint in 15° to 20° of flexion (Fig. 8).

Postoperatively, both repairs and reconstructions are protected in a cast for 6 weeks, after which therapy and ROM exercises are begun avoiding radial stress at the metacarpophalangeal joint. After cast immobilization, patients are transitioned to a removable splint. Strengthening begins approximately 8 weeks postoperatively or after full ROM has been obtained. Unrestricted activity without splint protection is allowed once the patient is pain free and ROM and strength are restored, generally between 12 and 16 weeks. Athletic participation is acceptable early on if immobilization is allowed and participation is possible without the use of the thumb. The most common complication after UCL repair is decreased motion at the metacarpophalangeal and IP joints.[21,34,35] Other complications include injury/neurapraxia to the dorsal sensory branches of the radial nerve, decreased pinch strength and persistent instability.[32,36,37]

Outcomes after acute repair and reconstruction are favorable. Most patients report good to excellent results and can expect to have a stable joint with minimal pain as well as well-preserved ROM and pinch and grip strength.[23,30,32,36–41]

Thumb Radial Collateral Ligament Injuries

Radial collateral ligament (RCL) injuries are far less common than ulnar collateral injuries and occur with forced adduction or torsion of the flexed thumb. Evaluation, diagnosis, and management is similar to UCL injuries. However, there are several key differences between UCL and RCL injuries. In contrast with the adductor aponeurosis, the abductor aponeurosis on the

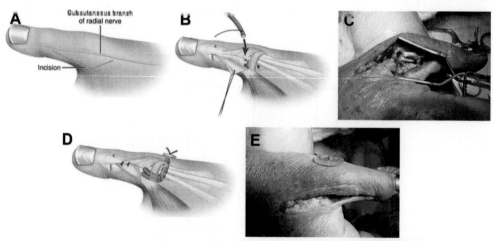

Fig. 8. Ulnar collateral ligament reconstruction described by Glickel and colleagues. (A) Incision. (B) Two gouge holes made on the ulnar side of the proximal phalangeal base and 1 across the metacarpal neck. (C–E), Passage and fixation of the tendon graft. (From Calandruccio JH. Fractures, dislocations, and ligamentous injuries. In: Canale ST, Beaty JH, editors. Campbell's operative orthopaedics. 12th edition. Philadelphia: Elsevier; 2013; with permission.)

radial side of the thumb is broad and does not become interposed between the ligament ends. As such, there is no equivalent to the Stener lesion. Likewise, the location of RCL injury is more variable. Most frequently, the ligament is avulsed from its proximal origin as opposed to its distal insertion.[25] Midsubstance tears of the RCL are also more common than midsubstance tears of the UCL.

As with UCL injuries, differentiation between partial tears/sprains and complete injuries is of paramount importance. Partial tears/sprains are typically treated with immobilization in a thumb spica splint or cast for 4 to 6 weeks followed by a removable splint for 2 more weeks while performing higher demand activities. Volar subluxation of the metacarpophalangeal joint, lack of a firm endpoint, greater than 30 to 35° laxity with ulnar deviation or greater than 15° when compared with the contralateral, uninjured side in both flexion and extension are indicative of a complete rupture of the RCL and warrant consideration of operative repair.

Although the literature is less clear than with UCL injuries, our preference is to repair complete tears of the RCL. Anatomic repair of the RCL affords greater joint stability because it neutralizes the ulnar pull of the adductor pollicis and extensor pollicus longus on the proximal phalanx and may result in ligament healing in an elongated fashion.[38,42] We repair the ligament with a suture anchor in a similar fashion to that described for UCL repair. Even in the instance of delayed presentation/diagnosis, rarely is ligamentous reconstruction required. The postoperative protocol is the same as UCL repair.

Similar to UCL repair, results after surgical repair of RCL injuries are favorable. Catalano and colleagues[38] reported 96% with good to excellent results in their series. Patients can expect minimal pain and near full restoration of ROM, grip and pinch strength.

THUMB INTERPHALANGEAL JOINT INJURIES

The thumb IP joint is a hinge joint stabilized by proper and accessory collateral ligaments and volar plate. Thumb IP joint dislocations are usually dorsal or lateral. Evaluation includes standard posteroanterior and true lateral radiographs to rule out associated fracture. Reduction is accomplished under digital block anesthesia with application of longitudinal traction and application of direct pressure on the dorsum of the distal phalanx. Inability to reduce the thumb IP joint rarely occurs and is most often secondary to interposition of the volar plate. After reduction, stability of the joint should be assessed and postreduction radiographs should be obtained to evaluate for concentric reduction. Treatment consists of immobilization for 2 to 3 weeks in a dorsal blocking splint. Instability after reduction is uncommon.

Chronic or irreducible thumb IP joint dislocations require open reduction through a dorsal approach. The extensor pollicus longus terminal slip is protected and the interposed volar plate can be reduced over the proximal phalanx head after scar excision. Sometimes partial excision of the or longitudinal splitting volar plate is required for joint congruency. Pinning the joint in full extension for 2 to 3 weeks is usually adequate for this injury if after reduction joint instability is appreciated.

SUMMARY

In many sports, the thumb is commonly injured. Ligamentous injuries to the thumb include thumb carpometacarpal dislocations, thumb metacarpophalangeal dislocations, and collateral ligament injuries and IP dislocations. Appropriate management requires knowledge of the type of injury, demands of the specific sport and position played, competitive level of the athlete, future athletic demands and expectations, and the role of rehabilitation and protective splints for return to play. In contrast with the nonathlete, management of the athlete often times requires more aggressive and expedient diagnostic intervention and treatment to minimize time away from sport while also ensuring safe return to competition.

REFERENCES

1. Rettig AC. Epidemiology of hand and wrist injuries in sports. Clin Sports Med 1998;17:401–6.
2. Patel D, Dean C, Baker RJ. The hand in sports: an update on the clinical anatomy and physical examination. Prim Care 2005;32:71–89.
3. Rettig AC. Athletic injuries of the wrist and hand. Part I: traumatic injuries of the wrist. Am J Sports Med 2003;31:1038–48.
4. Strauch RJ, Behrman MJ, Rosenwasser MP. Acute dislocation of the carpometacarpal joint of the thumb: an anatomic and cadaver study. J Hand Surg Am 1994;19:93–8.
5. Eaton RG, Lane LB, Littler JW, et al. Ligament reconstruction for the painful thumb carpometacarpal joint: a long-term assessment. J Hand Surg Am 1984;9:692–9.

6. Simonian PT, Trumble TE. Traumatic dislocation of the thumb carpometacarpal joint: early ligamentous reconstruction versus closed reduction and pinning. J Hand Surg 1996;21A:802–6.

7. Takwale VJ, Stanley JK, Shahane SA. Post–traumatic instability of the trapeziometacarpal joint of the thumb. J Bone Joint Surg Br 2004;86(4): 541–5.

8. Lane LB, Henley DH. Ligament reconstruction of the painful, unstable, nonarthritic thumb carpometacarpal joint. J Hand Surg Am 2000;26(4): 686–91.

9. Kaplan EB. Dorsal dislocation of the metacarpophalangeal joint of the index finger. J Bone Joint Surg Am 1957;39A:1081–6.

10. Gerrand CH, Shearer H. Complex dislocation of the metacarpophalangeal joint of the index finger with sesamoid entrapment. Injury 1995;26:574–5.

11. Stener B. Displacement of the ruptured ulnar collateral ligament of the metacarpo-phalangeal joint of the thumb: a clinical and anatomical study. J Bone Joint Surg Br 1962;44(4):869–79.

12. Heyman P, Gelberman RH, Duncan K, et al. Injuries of the ulnar collateral ligament of the thumb metacarpophalangeal joint: Biomechanical and prospective clinical studies on the usefulness of valgus stress testing. Clin Orthop Relat Res 1993; 292:165–71.

13. Posner MA, Retaillaud JL. Metacarpophalangeal joint injuries of the thumb. Hand Clin 1992;8(4): 713–32.

14. Heyman P. Injuries to the ulnar collateral ligament of the thumb metacarpophalangeal joint. J Am Acad Orthop Surg 1997;5(4):224–9.

15. Palmer AK, Louis DS. Assessing ulnar instability of the metacarpophalangeal joint of the thumb. J Hand Surg Am 1978;3(6):542–6.

16. Malik AK, Morris T, Chou D, et al. Clinical testing of ulnar collateral ligament injuries of the thumb. J Hand Surg Eur Vol 2009;34(3):363–6.

17. Papandrea RF, Fowler T. Injury at the thumb UCL: is there a Stener lesion? J Hand Surg Am 2008;33(10): 1882–4.

18. Hoglund M, Tordai P, Muren C. Diagnosis by ultrasound of dislocated ulnar collateral ligament of the thumb. Acta Radiol 1995;36:620–5.

19. Spaeth HJ, Abrams RA, Bock GW, et al. Gamekeeper thumb: differentiation of nondisplaced and displaced tears of the ulnar collateral ligament with MR imaging. Radiology 1993;188:553–6.

20. Hergan K, Mittler C, Oser W. Ulnar collateral ligament: differentiation of displaced and nondisplaced tears with US and MR imaging. Radiology 1995;194(1):65–71.

21. Smith RJ. Post-traumatic instability of the metacarpophalangeal joint of the thumb. J Bone Joint Surg Am 1977;59(1):14–21.

22. Camp RA, Weatherwax RJ, Miller EB. Chronic post-traumatic radial instability of the thumb metacarpophalangeal joint. J Hand Surg Am 1980;5(3):221–5.

23. Gerber C, Senn E, Matter P. Skier's thumb: surgical treatment of recent injuries to the ulnar collateral ligament of the thumb's metacarpophalangeal joint. Am J Sports Med 1981;9(3):171–7.

24. Melone CP Jr, Beldner S, Basuk RS. Thumb collateral ligament injuries: an anatomic basis for treatment. Hand Clin 2000;16(3):345–57.

25. Coyle MP Jr. Grade III radial collateral ligament injuries of the thumb metacarpophalangeal joint: treatment by soft tissue advancement and bony reattachment. J Hand Surg Am 2003;28(1):14–20.

26. Bean CH, Tencer AF, Trumble TE. The effect of thumb metacarpophalangeal ulnar collateral ligament attachment site on joint range of motion: an in vitro study. J Hand Surg Am 1999;24(2): 283–7.

27. Katolik LI, Friedrich J, Trumble TE. Repair of acute ulnar collateral ligament injuries of the thumb metacarpophalangeal joint: a retrospective comparison of pull-out sutures and bone anchor techniques. Plast Reconstr Surg 2008;122(5):1451–6.

28. Baskies MA, Tuckman D, Paksima N, et al. A new technique for reconstruction of the ulnar collateral ligament of the thumb. Am J Sports Med 2007; 35(8):1321–5.

29. Tsiouri C, Hayton MJ, Baratz M. Injury to the ulnar collateral ligament of the thumb. Hand (N Y) 2009;4(1):12–8.

30. Zeman C, Hunter RE, Freeman JR, et al. Acute skier's thumb repaired with a proximal phalanx suture anchor. Am J Sports Med 1998;26(5):644–50.

31. Moharram AN. Repair of thumb metacarpophalangeal joint ulnar collateral ligament injuries with microanchors. Ann Plast Surg 2013;71(5):500–2.

32. Glickel SZ, Malerich M, Pearce SM, et al. Ligament replacement for chronic instability of the ulnar collateral ligament of the metacarpophalangeal joint of the thumb. J Hand Surg Am 1993;18(5): 930–41.

33. Glickel SZ. Thumb metacarpophalangeal joint ulnar collateral ligament reconstruction using a tendon graft. Tech Hand Up Extrem Surg 2002; 6(3):133–9.

34. Bowers WH, Hurst LC. Gamekeeper's thumb: evaluation by arthrography and stress roentgenography. J Bone Joint Surg Am 1977;59(4):519–24.

35. Weiland AJ, Berner SH, Hotchkiss RN, et al. Repair of acute ulnar collateral ligament injuries of the thumb metacarpophalangeal joint with an intraosseous suture anchor. J Hand Surg Am 1997;22(4): 585–91.

36. Derkash RS, Matyas JR, Weaver JK, et al. Acute surgical repair of the skier's thumb. Clin Orthop Relat Res 1987;216:29–33.

37. Saetta JP, Phair IC, Quinton DN. Ulnar collateral ligament repair of the metacarpo-phalangeal joint of the thumb: a study comparing two methods of repair. J Hand Surg Br 1992;17(2):160–3.

38. Catalano LW III, Cardon L, Patenaude N, et al. Results of surgical treatment of acute and chronic grade III [corrected] tears of the radial collateral ligament of the thumb metacarpophalangeal joint. J Hand Surg Am 2006;31(1):68–75.

39. Jackson M, McQueen MM. Gamekeeper's thumb: a quantitative evaluation of acute surgical repair. Injury 1994;25(1):21–3.

40. Mitsionis GI, Varitimidis SE, Sotereanos GG. Treatment of chronic injuries of the ulnar collateral ligament of the thumb using a free tendon graft and bone suture anchors. J Hand Surg Br 2000;25: 208–11.

41. Oka Y, Harayama H, Ikeda M. Reconstructive procedure to repair chronic injuries to the collateral ligament of metacarpophalangeal joints of the hand. Hand Surg 2003;8:81–5.

42. Edelstein DM, Kardashian G, Lee SK. Radial collateral ligament injuries of the thumb. J Hand Surg Am 2008;33(5):760–70.

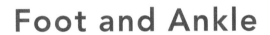

Foot and Ankle

Foot and Ankle Stress Fractures in Athletes

Michael C. Greaser, MD

KEYWORDS

- Stress fracture • Stress reaction • Foot • Ankle • Athlete

KEY POINTS

- Stress fractures of the foot and ankle are common in running and jumping athletes, and can result in significant disability and time away from sport.
- Bone scintigraphy and MRI are highly sensitive in evaluating athletes with suspected stress fracture, with the latter displaying higher specificity.
- Relative rest and gradual return to play is successful in treating most low-risk stress fractures.
- High-risk stress fractures often require operative treatment and can result in significant time away from sport.
- Bone stimulators and shock wave therapy have garnered significant interest, but have yet to be proved efficacious in the treatment of bone stress injuries.

INTRODUCTION

Epidemiology

Foot and ankle stress fractures are a major cause of disability in athletes of all types. Although the incidence of stress fractures in the general athletic population is less than 1%, the incidence may be as high as 15% in runners.[1] Stress fractures in military recruits have been studied extensively. The military recruit population is at particular risk because of the abrupt and rigorous nature of basic training. In a systematic review of the military literature, Wentz and colleagues[2] found a stress fracture incidence of 3% and 9.2%, in men and women respectively. The most common sites of stress fracture in both the military and athletic population are the leg and ankle. In a study of division I collegiate athletes over a 5-year period, the incidence of stress fracture was 1.4%. Foot, ankle, and tibia stress fractures were the most common, and sports with the highest rate of stress fracture were cross-country and track.[3] In a recent study of stress fractures in high school athletes, Changstrom and colleagues[4] reported a 0.8% incidence of stress fractures over a 7-year period, including more than 25 million athlete exposures. They reported a higher rate of stress fractures in women, and the lower leg and foot accounted for 40.3% and 34.9% of stress fractures respectively. Sports with the highest rates of stress fractures were girls' cross-country, girls' gymnastics, and boys' cross-country.

Causes and Pathogenesis

Stress fractures of bone result from submaximal, repetitive loading resulting in an imbalance between bone resorption and formation. Athletes at highest risk are those who abruptly increase the duration, intensity, or frequency of physical activity without adequate periods of rest. These phenomena result in increased osteoclastic activity, leading to increased bone resorption and lagging bone formation. Ultimately the bone fatigues, and if there are intense and repetitive activities, microfractures may result. Stress injuries occur along a continuum, and a stress reaction is a bone stress injury resulting from microfracture without a defined fracture line on imaging. Continued stress to the bone results in

Disclosure: The author has nothing to disclose.
Department of Orthopedic Surgery, University of Texas Health Science Center Houston, McGovern Medical School, 6400 Fannin Street, Suite 1700, Houston, TX 77030, USA
E-mail address: Michael.C.Greaser@uth.tmc.edu

coalescences of multiple microfractures, leading to a visible and defined stress fracture.[5–7]

Intrinsic and extrinsic factors affect the development of stress fractures. Intrinsic factors related to stress fractures include age, sex, bone mineral density, malalignment, hormonal imbalance, and poor vascular supply. Extrinsic factors are more easily modifiable and include activity type, intensity of training, training surface, improper technique or equipment, and poor nutrition.[8,9] Decreased bone mineral density has been correlated with increased stress fracture risk and may be related to diet, age, and hormone imbalance.[8,10,11] The female athlete triad (eating disorder, amenorrhea, and osteoporosis) refers to the phenomena most commonly seen in competitive female athletes involved in long-distance running, gymnastics, and figure skating. Barrack and colleagues[10] showed that the cumulative risk for bone stress injuries increased with increasing number of triad-related risk factors. Particular attention must be paid to these modifiable risk factors, and a dietary and menstrual history should be obtained when interviewing a female athlete.

History, Physical Examination, and Imaging

Athletes presenting with foot and ankle stress fractures often describe a progressive and insidious onset of pain and swelling. A thorough history should include details on the athletes: intensity of training, duration of training, and changes in training surface or footwear. General medical information, including diet, nutrition, and in female athletes menstrual cycles, should be gathered. Physical examination focuses on weight-bearing alignment and range of motion Areas of pain, tenderness, and swelling indicate areas of possible bone stress injury.

Imaging studies, including radiographs, computed tomography (CT), MRI, and bone scan, are helpful in evaluating patients for foot and ankle stress injuries. Initial and follow-up radiographs may be negative in as many as 85% and 50% of patients respectively.[12]

Bone scintigraphy is highly sensitive in evaluating bone stress injuries, and until the advent of MRI it was considered the gold standard.[13,14] Three-phase bone scan is recommended rather than other methods of bone scintigraphy because it allows differentiation between soft tissue and bony uptake. The sensitivity of bone scan is close to 100%, but it lacks specificity, with false-positive results possible with tumors, infections, and infarction.

MRI has become increasingly popular in the evaluation of bone stress injuries because of its high sensitivity and specificity. The added benefit of being able to evaluate the surrounding soft tissues for other pain-generating disorders makes MRI particularly attractive when evaluating patients with suspected bone stress injuries.[12,15] CT lacks the sensitivity of MRI, but is useful in defining fracture characteristics. The high-quality cross-sectional imaging produced with CT allows better definition of fracture lines, areas of sclerosis, and comminution.

High-risk and Low-risk Stress Fractures

Stress fractures can be categorized as either high risk or low risk based on their propensity to heal. High-risk stress fractures have a greater risk of complete fracture or nonunion, and often require prolonged periods of non–weight-bearing immobilization or surgical treatment. Stress fractures, including navicular, medial malleolus, talus, hallucal sesamoid, and proximal fifth metatarsal, are considered high risk. Low-risk stress fractures, such as calcaneus, lateral malleolus, and metatarsal shafts, are generally treated successfully with relative rest and symptomatic relief. Patients with low-risk stress fracture typically make a full recovery without long-term adverse effects.[5,6,16]

LOW-RISK STRESS FRACTURES

Fibular Stress Fractures

Fibular stress fractures are rare in the athletic population. These fractures, termed runners fractures, are most commonly seen in running athletes. In a study of 320 athletes, stress fractures of the fibula accounted for 6.6% of all stress fractures.[17]

Stress fractures of the fibula may occur along the entire length of the fibula, but are most commonly seen in the distal third in the athletic population. In Burrows'[18] study of fibula stress fractures, he noted that most fractures in runners occurred in the cortical area of the distal fibula just proximal to the syndesmotic ligaments, approximately 50 mm (2 inches) or more above the tip of the malleolus. In a later study of 50 fibular stress fractures in athletes, Devas and colleagues[19] reported similar findings, with the most common location of fracture being 4 to 7 cm above the tip of the lateral malleoli (Fig. 1).

Fibula stress fractures are thought to result from a combination of muscular forces and repetitive axial loading. Axial force transmission through the fibula during weight-bearing activities varies between 2.3% and 10.4% depending on ankle position and limb orientation.[20] Muscular forces during running are thought to play a role in fibular stress fractures; namely,

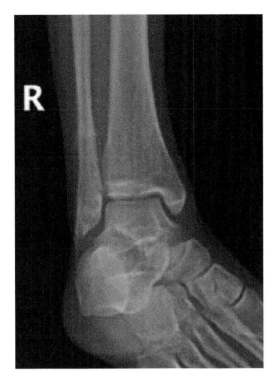

Fig. 1. Stress fracture of the distal fibula in a cross-country athlete. Note the typical location of the fracture 4 to 7 cm above the tip of the lateral malleolus.

strong contraction of the ankle flexors is thought to result in approximation of the distal tibia and fibula, with resultant increased stress in the area superior to the distal tibia-fibular syndesmosis.[19] Other factors, including shoe wear, training surface, and metabolic disease, have been implicated in causing these fractures.[19,21]

Evaluation of a patient with a potential fibular stress fractures should involve a thorough history, including change in footwear, running surface, or intensity of training. Patients often describe increased pain and swelling in the area of the distal fibula with an insidious onset or an acute episode of pain without specific trauma.

Radiographs are often negative for up to 3 weeks after the initiation of pain. Three-phase bone scan is the most sensitive test to identify early stress fractures or stress reaction when radiographs are negative. MRI has become popular in the imaging of stress fracture because of its high sensitivity and specificity. In addition, MRI can be used to evaluate other conditions in the differential diagnosis. Conditions included in the differential diagnosis of fibular stress fracture are tendonitis, neoplasm, osteochondral lesion of the tibia or talus, peroneal tendon dislocation, exertional compartment syndrome, and fascial hernias.

Stress fractures of the distal fibula respond favorably to nonoperative treatment. Most investigators recommend a period of relative rest and activity modification.[18,19,22] Athletes are allowed to cross-train during this period. In patients who present with a limp, a short period of non–weight-bearing immobilization may be indicated. Return to activity is allowed when tenderness at the fracture site abates and signs of radiographic healing are present. Contact athletes usually return to play 6 to 8 weeks from the initiation of symptoms. The author is unaware of any reports of operative treatment of these fractures.

Calcaneus Stress Fracture

Stress fractures of the calcaneus most commonly affect military recruits and long-distance runners. The 2 largest series of calcaneus stress fractures published to date involved a population of military recruits. Symptoms typically presented insidiously, and were worsened by activity and relieved with rest. Examination of the affected foot may reveal swelling, and pain may be present with compression of the heel. In both of these series, stress fractures were most commonly localized to the posterior tuberosity along the trabecular stress lines.[23,24] Radiographs typically reveal a sclerotic line after 2 to 3 weeks of symptoms, but may initially be negative, often leading to a delay in diagnosis. The differential diagnosis includes plantar fasciitis, Baxter neuritis, insertional Achilles tendonitis, retrocalcaneal bursitis, and calcaneal apophysitis in adolescents.

In cases of suspected stress fracture, MRI helps to delineate the diagnosis. In a recent MRI study of Finnish military recruits, 56% of fractures were localized to the posterior tuberosity (Fig. 2) and 44% of stress fractures were located at the anterior and middle portions of the calcaneus.[25] MRI seems to have a significant advantage in diagnosing stress fractures in the anterior part of the calcaneus, and often identifies other associated tarsal stress injuries. MRI is recommended because of its high sensitivity and specificity and its usefulness in the evaluation of other soft tissue disorders.

Calcaneus stress fractures are treated successfully with rest and protected weight bearing followed by reintroduction to training in most patients.[23,24] Leabhart[23] noted that reintroduction to training before 8 weeks of convalescence led to a recurrence of symptoms.

More recently in the literature several case reports have detailed stress fractures of the anterior process of the calcaneus in athletes.[26–28]

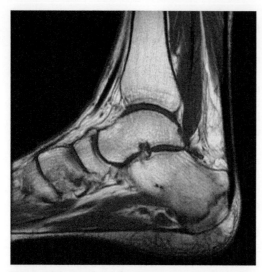

Fig. 2. Midsagittal cut from T1-weighted MRI of the ankle showing a stress fracture of the posterior tuberosity of the calcaneus.

In 2 of these case reports the fractures were associated a calcaneonavicular coalition.[27,28] In 1 case a calcaneonavicular bar was resected with screw fixation across the stress fracture at the anterior process.[27] Further evidence is needed to support operative versus nonoperative treatment of stress fracture of the anterior process of the calcaneus.

Stress fractures of the calcaneus may be more frequent than is reported in the literature, and are likely misdiagnosed as more common ailments of the hindfoot and ankle. Nonoperative treatment including rest and protected weight bearing is effective in treating most cases.

Metatarsal Shaft Stress Fractures

Stress fractures of the metatarsals are common in running athletes and represent up to 20% of stress fractures in the athletic population.[17,29,30] Metatarsal shaft stress fractures are most common at the second and third metatarsals, and are often referred to as march fractures because of the high incidence in military trainees. These fractures typically occur after an increase in exercise intensity or change in training surface. Physical examination often reveals swelling, point tenderness at the fracture site, and tenderness with metatarsal stress testing. Differential diagnosis includes Morton neuroma, metatarsophalangeal joint synovitis, metatarsalgia, infection, or rarely neoplasm.

Radiographs are typically negative for up to 3 weeks. Empiric treatment is typically initiated with suspected stress fractures, and radiographs repeated 2 to 3 weeks after initiation of symptoms confirm the diagnosis, with callus and fracture line typically noted (Fig. 3). In athletes who are unable or unwilling to interrupt their training, MRI is indicated because of its increased sensitivity.

Treatment of nondisplaced metatarsal stress fracture is nonoperative with weight bearing to tolerance in a postoperative shoe or prefabricated walker boot. Patients are allowed to gradually return to activity when tenderness and swelling have resolved and radiographic evidence of healing is present, typically 4 to 6 weeks after initiation or symptoms.[6,31–33]

HIGH-RISK STRESS FRACTURES
Medial Malleolar Stress Fracture

Stress fractures of the medial malleolus are rare, with an incidence of 0.6% to 4.1% reported in the literature.[29,30] Stress fractures of the medial malleolus are typically seen in running and jumping athletes, and are thought to result from torsional forces imposed on the medial malleolus during repetitive loading.[34] More recently an association between anterior impingement

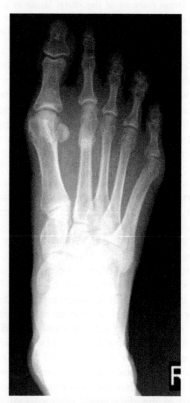

Fig. 3. Anteroposterior (AP) radiograph of a runner 4 weeks after initiation of forefoot pain showing a second metatarsal shaft stress fracture. Typical features, including surrounding callus formation and visible fracture line, are shown.

lesions has been suggested as a potential cause for these rare fractures.[35]

Medial malleolus stress fractures typically present with vague anterior medial ankle pain. Patients may complain of minor preceding trauma, with continued tenderness at the anterior medial ankle with activity. The pain is often relieved with rest, but persists with activity. Inspection may reveal swelling about the medial ankle. Anterior medial ankle impingement is associated with the condition and stress fractures may be difficult to discern from anterior medial ankle impingement symptoms. Palpation over the medial malleolus may elicit tenderness and increases the index of suspicion. The differential diagnosis includes posterior tibial tendonitis, deltoid ligament injuries, ankle arthritis, impingement, and tarsal tunnel syndrome.

Medial malleolar stress fractures present in a characteristic pattern: arising from the medial shoulder of the tibial plafond, the fracture line runs either obliquely or vertically to the medial tibial cortex (Fig. 4A). This pattern is similar to the typical supination-adduction pattern of fracture described by Lauge-Hansen.[36] Initial radiographs of the ankle may be negative in up to 70% of cases.[37–42] If stress reaction or occult stress fracture is suspected, an MRI or bone scan should be obtained, with the latter reported to have close to 100% sensitivity. Although bone scan remains the gold standard for diagnosis of stress-related injuries, MRI has the advantage of increased specificity, is noninvasive, and provides multiplanar images that may help guide treatment. In addition, MRI allows the differentiation of stress reactions and stress fractures.[43] CT provides excellent resolution and is useful in defining the extent of the fracture, areas of sclerosis, and associated impingement lesions (Fig. 4B, C).

Initial treatment of patients with stress reactions of the medial malleolus is a short period of immobilization and activity modification.[38] Return to activity is gradual and is based on resolution of swelling and tenderness. Nonoperative and operative treatment strategies have been advocated for stress fractures of the medial malleolus. In high-level or in-season athletes with a radiographically detectable fracture line, or in patients with displaced fractures, operative treatment has been recommended.[34,44,45] A variety of operative treatment strategies have been described, including isolated drilling, percutaneous fixation with 4-mm cannulated screws, and open reduction internal fixation with 4-mm cannulated screws.[34,35,38,44,45] Associated disorders should be addressed, including

ankle instability, bony impingement lesions, and malalignment.[35] Postoperative protocols vary widely in published studies of operatively treated patients, with a period of non–weight bearing of 1 to 3 weeks observed in most patients followed by gradual return to activity.

The author's review of the literature produced only 1 report of a medial malleolar stress fracture nonunion. The patient presented 2 years after seeking initial treatment with a hypertrophic nonunion of the medial malleolus. The patient was treated with open reduction and internal fixation and bone grafting. The patient returned to activity at 4.5 months, and achieved union of the fracture on radiographs at 7 months postoperatively.[46]

Current literature lacks consistent treatment protocols for operative and nonoperative management of medial malleolar stress fractures. In general, both operative and nonoperative treatment have been successful in treating these fractures. In a systematic review of the literature, Irion and colleagues[47] reported an average return to play of 7.6 and 2.4 weeks for nonoperatively treated and operatively treated patients respectively. In patients desiring an expedited return to activity, surgical management may be more effective based on the current literature.

Navicular Stress Fractures

Stress fractures of the tarsal navicular are uncommon in the general athletic population, but may account for 15% to 32% of stress-related fractures in track and field athletes.[29,48] The tarsal navicular lies between the talar head and the 3 cuneiforms at the medial midfoot. The blood supply to the navicular is derived from the medial tarsal branch of the dorsalis pedis artery and a branch of the tibialis posterior artery.[49] A watershed area exists at the central third of the bone and has been implicated in stress injuries to the tarsal navicular.[50] Anatomic variation, including a short first ray and long second metatarsal, have been proposed as potential risks factors as well.[41,51] Fitch and colleagues[52] expanded on this concept, relating that the compression forces exerted by the second metatarsal and middle cuneiform at the lateral navicular create an area of maximal shear stress at the central third of the navicular. The high level of force transmission at the central third of the navicular, together with the tenuous blood supply at the central third of the navicular, is postulated to predispose this area of the bone to stress injuries.

Navicular stress fractures can be difficult to identify and examiners should have a high index

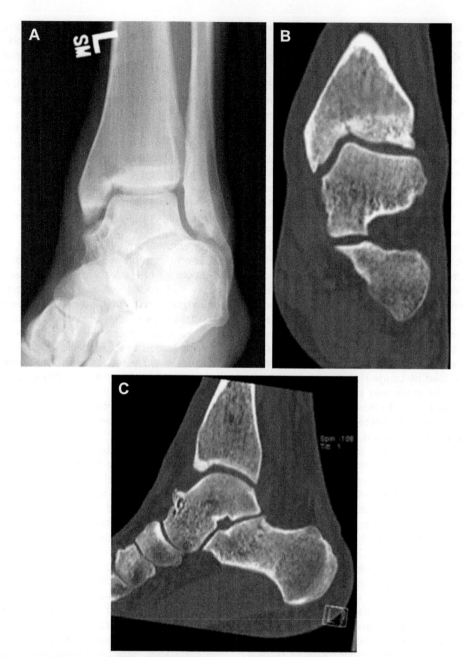

Fig. 4. (A) AP radiograph of a collegiate basketball player showing the typical vertical fracture line seen with medial malleolar stress fractures. (B) Coronal CT cut showing a complete medial malleolar stress fracture. (C) Sagittal CT cut reveals large bony anterior impingement lesions at the tibia and talus.

of suspicion in athletes involved in high-risk sports; namely football, rugby, track and field, and basketball.[41,52–55] Typical presentations involve an insidious onset of pain without swelling or an inciting event. These injuries can be difficult to detect, and frequently go undiagnosed for several months after the initiation of symptoms.[41,55] Examiners must have a high index of suspicion in athletes with medial foot and ankle pain. Tenderness at the proximal dorsal potion of the navicular, termed the N spot, is present in 81% of patients with navicular stress fracture.[55] Athletes with tenderness at the N spot should have a further work-up to rule out a stress fracture.

Plain radiographs are initially obtained, but lack sensitivity in diagnosing even complete fractures of the tarsal navicular. Khan and colleagues[54] reported a 76% false-negative rate for incomplete fracture and 19% false-negative rate for complete fractures in his review of the literature. Bone scan is inexpensive and has long been the gold standard for initial evaluation of the navicular stress fracture. Sensitivity of triple-phase bone scans is close to 100%, but specificity is low.[41,51,54] Bone scans indicating a stress injury should be further evaluated with a follow-up CT scan or MRI. CT scans differentiate stress reaction from stress fracture, and provide detailed imaging of the fracture, including potential comminution, sclerosis, or degenerative changes. Navicular stress fractures typically arise in the central third of the bone starting proximal dorsal and progressing in a distal plantar direction (Fig. 5).[56] Saxena and colleagues[57] proposed a CT-based classification system based on the propagation of the fracture line through the navicular body (Table 1).

A decision for operative versus nonoperative management of these fractures remains controversial. For nondisplaced fractures, conservative treatment with 6 to 8 weeks of non–weight bearing in a short leg cast is recommended. Patients treated with weight-bearing versus non–weight-bearing cast have shown significantly worse outcomes.[54] Patients undergoing nonoperative treatment are reexamined at 6 to 8 weeks with specific attention placed on tenderness at the N spot. In patients without tenderness, functional rehabilitation begins. However, if tenderness persists then a walker boot is used with low-impact activity allowed for an additional 6

Table 1 Saxena and colleagues' CT-based classification of tarsal navicular stress fractures	
Type I	Dorsal cortical break
Type II	Propagation of the fracture line into the navicular body
Type III	Fracture penetrates another cortex (dorsal, medial, or lateral)

From Saxena A, Fullem B, Hannaford D. Results of treatment of 22 navicular stress fractures and a new proposed radiographic classification system. J Foot Ankle Surg 2000;39(2):97; with permission.

to 8 weeks. If no improvement is realized within 3 to 4 months of the initiation of treatment, then some investigators have recommended a repeat CT scan be obtained.[58] Note that CT scan is only useful in assessing for progression of fracture lines and development of sclerosis of the cancellous margins indicating nonunion. Khan and colleagues[55] noted that CT scans at 3 months after initiation of treatment only show blurring of the fracture line and minor cortical bridging. In addition, it is important to point out that persistent sclerosis is typical at the proximal dorsal cortical margin even in healed asymptomatic fracture. This pattern of sclerosis should not be confused with nonunions, which have sclerosis extending into the trabecular margins of the fracture.[56,59]

Surgical management of these fractures may be considered in patients who have displaced

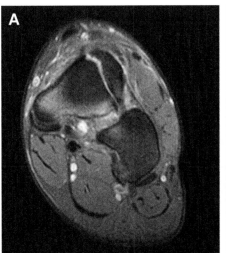
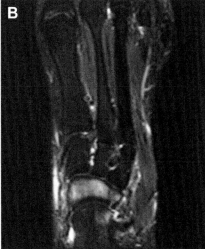

Fig. 5. (A) Axial MRI short tau inversion recovery sequence showing typical increased edema throughout the navicular with a lateral stress fracture evident. (B) T2-weighted coronal sequence showing a complete tarsal navicular stress fracture line.

fractures, nondisplaced complete fractures with sclerotic changes, and those who have failed conservative management or cannot tolerate the prolonged recovery of nonoperative treatment.[52,58,60] Recommended treatment typically consists of two to three 4.0-mm or 4.5-mm partially threaded screws placed from lateral to medial, with autogenous bone graft recommended for type III fractures or type II fractures with sclerosis. Postoperatively patients are treated with non–weight-bearing immobilization until tenderness has resolved at the N spot. Fracture severity (complete vs incomplete) has been shown to correlate with time to return to activity, with higher-grade fractures taking the longest to recover.[57]

Despite continued enthusiasm for operative treatment of navicular stress fractures, there remains a lack of high-quality evidence to support surgical management. Torg and colleagues[61] reviewed 250 navicular stress fractures and found that surgical intervention had no advantage compared with cast immobilization and complete non–weight bearing. They reported a trend favoring successful outcomes and return to activity with nonoperative management (96%) compared with surgery (82%), although this was not significant. In Mallee and colleagues'[16] meta-analysis of high-risk stress fractures, they noted a trend toward earlier return to play with operative (16.4 weeks) versus nonoperative (21.7 weeks) treatment of navicular stress fractures; however, a significant difference could not be calculated. The investigators noted that, given the limitations of the current literature, appropriate advice for standard of care could not be given.[16]

Talus Stress Fracture

McGlone[62] first reported on stress fracture of the talus in 1965. These injuries are rare, with most reports in the literature being case reports. Talus stress fracture have been reported in military recruits and athletes subjected to repetitive axial loading of the foot and ankle.[63–65] Symptoms are nonspecific and include ankle pain, swelling, and joint effusion. Pain is typically worsened with activity and radiographs are not commonly diagnostic.[65,66]

In the 2 largest studies published on a Finnish military population, stress injuries were found most commonly in the head of the talus, with the talar body and posterior process being a less common area of injury. These stress injuries were typically only visible on MRI, and stress injuries to surrounding tarsal bones were commonly found in conjunction with talus stress fractures.[65,66]

The lateral process of the talus has also been reported to be an area of stress fracture in athletes. Two case reports have been published on runners with stress injuries to the lateral talar process.[67,68] These fractures are typically evaluated with CT scan and may be associated with a persistent fracture line and mild degenerative changes. Based on these case reports patients may have long-term persistent low-grade symptoms.

The most commonly reported treatment of stress injuries to the talus involve a period of relative rest and gradual resumption of activity. Sormaala and colleagues[66] reported on the outcomes of 9 talar stress fractures in Finnish military recruits. Patients were suspended from military training for an average of 39 days, but no patients were treated in a cast or with surgery. All patients healed without osteonecrosis or collapse, but 4 of 8 patients developed degeneration around the area of injury with mild to moderate persistent symptoms. Further investigation of these rare injuries is needed to provide a reliable treatment algorithm and prognostic guidance.

Sesamoid Stress Fractures

Hallucal sesamoid stress injuries are most common in the medial sesamoid.[69] It is postulated that the position of the medial sesamoid directly under the first metatarsal head leads to increased force transmission through this bone.[70,71] Sesamoid stress fractures have been described in dancers, jumpers, and runners.[69,70,72] The presentation is often nonspecific, and elusive because of the many conditions causing pain in this area of the foot. The differential diagnosis is expansive and may include sesamoiditis, gout, osteonecrosis of the sesamoid, acute fracture, turf toe injury, nerve impingement, arthritis, and osteochondritis. Symptoms arise insidiously, with increased pain at the first metatarsal phalangeal joint with activity, especially activities involving forced dorsiflexion. Examination may reveal swelling, tenderness at the sesamoid, and pain with forced dorsiflexion.[70]

Bilateral foot anteroposterior radiographs are initially obtained and may be used to differentiate bipartite from a fractured sesamoid. A medial bipartite sesamoid is present in 5% to 15% of the population and is present bilaterally in 25% of patients.[71,73–76] Sesamoid stress fractures are differentiated from bipartite sesamoids by the characteristic sharp edges, comminution, sometimes wide separation, and the fact that fractures are rarely bilateral as with bipartite sesamoids. Bone scan is highly sensitive and can be used to detect stress injuries, but, as with all stress fractures, it lacks specificity. MRI and CT are recommended for further evaluation of a positive bone scan.[70,72,77] MRI is expensive but is most helpful to evaluate other causes of pain in the area.

Initial treatment of sesamoid stress fracture includes rest, nonsteroidal antiinflammatory drugs, and immobilization for 6 to 12 weeks.[69,70,76] Orthotics designed to offload the sesamoid and restrict excessive dorsiflexion may also be helpful.[77] Failure of 2 to 3 months of nonoperative treatment is an indication for surgical treatment.

Several treatment strategies have been described for sesamoid nonunions and sesamoid stress fractures. Biedert and Hinterman[70] reported on 5 athletes treated with excision of the proximal fragment of the medial sesamoid stress fracture. All 5 athletes returned to play within 6 months of treatment.[70] In another case series, 2 medial and 2 lateral sesamoid stress fractures were treated with complete excision. All patients returned to their previous levels of activity at an average of 10 weeks postoperatively.[69] Furthermore, Anderson and McBryde[78] thought the sesamoid should be preserved in competitive athletes. They recommended autogenous bone grafting of sesamoid nonunions and reported successful union in 19 of 21 patients with their technique.[78] All studies to date regarding operative treatment of these fractures are of poor quality and further prospective studies are need to recommend a standard of care for these fracture.

Proximal Fifth Metatarsal Stress Fractures

Stress fractures of the proximal fifth metatarsal differ in radiographic appearance and typical clinical presentation from acute fractures of the fifth metatarsal base. Many patients have a history of pain, followed by an acute injury. The cause of these fractures is thought to be repetitive vertical and mediolateral force on the bone.[79] A cavus foot structure and larger fifth metatarsal abduction angle may also play a role in development of fifth metatarsal stress fractures, although some investigators have shown that static foot position may be less important than dynamic foot position.[80,81] These fractures are frequently seen in American football, basketball, and soccer players, but may occur in any running and jumping athlete.

Treatment of these fractures requires examiners to have knowledge of the radiographic features that portend an unpredictable and guarded prognosis. Dameron[82] and Stewart[83] were two of the first investigators to make a distinction between the radiographic location of at-risk proximal fifth metatarsal stress fractures and acute fractures that typically healed uneventfully.[82,83] Dameron[82] noted that fractures occurring 1.5 cm distal to the metaphyseal flare of the metatarsal base healed less predictably, with 25% of these fractures requiring surgery.[82] Torg and colleagues[84] proposed a classification of the proximal fifth metatarsal stress fracture based on radiographic findings of 46 patients treated in his series (Table 2). Typical radiographic features including periosteal new bone formation and beaking at the fracture site are hallmarks of proximal fifth metatarsal stress fractures (Fig. 6).

The decision to treat proximal fifth metatarsal fractures must account for fracture type, the patient's level of activity, and the desire of the athlete to expedite return to play. Type I fractures are generally low risk and have been treated successfully with non–weight-bearing cast immobilization for 6 weeks, followed by gradual return to activity. In Torg's series of 15 type I fractures, 14 of 15 patients treated with 6.5 weeks of non–weight-bearing cast immobilization healed at an average of 7.4 weeks (range, 6–12 weeks).[84] Zogby and Baker[85] reported on 10 Torg type I fractures in 9 patients treated with non–weight-bearing cast immobilization for 6 weeks followed by gradual return to activity

Table 2	
Torg classification of proximal fifth metatarsal fractures	
Type I	Acute fracture with sharp fracture lines and absence of intramedullary sclerosis
Type II	Fracture line displays characteristics of delayed union, with periosteal new bone formation and intramedullary sclerosis
Type III	Resembles a nonunion with wide fracture lines and complete obliteration of the medullary canal. Patients present with a history of repetitive trauma and recurrent symptoms

From Torg JS, Balduini FC, Zelko RR, et al. Fractures of the base of the fifth metatarsal distal to the tuberosity. Classification and guidelines for non-surgical and surgical management. J Bone Joint Surg Am 1984;66(2):209–14; with permission.

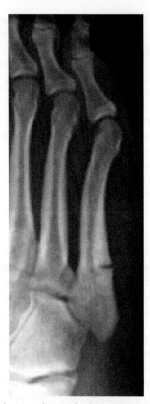

Fig. 6. Oblique radiograph showing cortical beaking and hypertrophy at the site of the fifth metatarsal fracture. This finding is typical of a Torg type I fracture.

over 6 weeks. All patients returned to preinjury levels of activity by 12 weeks. Based on these findings, a trial of 6 to 8 weeks of cast immobilization is recommended for type I fractures in most patients.

Operative treatment has been recommended for Torg type II fractures based on a high rate of delayed unions, nonunions, and refractures.[79,84,86] Operative treatment with tension band wiring or intramedullary screw fixation has yielded excellent results for the treatment of type II fractures.[87–90] Delee and colleagues[87] reported on 10 proximal fifth metatarsal fractures treated with intramedullary screws. Patients were allowed to weight bear to tolerance at 2 weeks. All fractures united at an average of 6.5 weeks and patients returned to play at an average of 8.5 weeks. Portland and colleagues[90] reported similar results with intramedullary screw fixation of Torg type II fracture, noting 100% union at 8.3 weeks. Patients were allowed to weight bear at 2 weeks postoperatively. Early weight bearing and expedited return to play with surgically treated fracture has led many investigators to promote operative treatment as an alternative to prolonged non–weight-bearing immobilization in active patients

with type I and II fractures.[87,89,90] Lee and colleagues[86,91] noted an increase in delayed unions and nonunions after treatment of proximal fifth metatarsal fracture with tension band wiring when the plantar gap was greater than 1 mm. Based on these findings they noted that fractures with greater than 1 mm of plantar gap may portend a more guarded prognosis. Surgical management of proximal fifth metatarsal stress fractures is technically challenging, and technical errors can result with intramedullary screw placement, including distal cortical perforation, intraoperative shaft fracture, and screw head impingement of the fifth metatarsal cuboid articulation. Complications such as nerve irritation at the screw insertions site, donor site morbidity with bone grafting, and hardware irritation have also been reported.

Torg type III fractures seem to be less common, with a paucity of recent studies to support treatment decisions. In Torg's original article, autogenous inlay grafting was used with a 95% healing rate at 12 to 16 weeks postoperatively.[84] Surgical stabilization of the nonunion was not performed in this study. Lee and colleagues[91] reported on 13 Torg type III fractures treated with inlay graft and tension band wiring, with an average time to union of 122 days and 1 nonunion. Surgical treatment is recommended for all type III fractures, including curettage, bone grafting, and fixation.[84,86,91,92]

OTHER TREATMENT CONSIDERATIONS
Calcium and Vitamin D
Calcium and vitamin D play a crucial role in bone turnover and remodeling. High levels of bone turnover are observed during the initial months of training in both athletes and military recruits.[93–95] Stress fractures are common in this population and optimization of calcium and vitamin D has been a subject of study to prevent these fractures. Several studies have documented a high rate of vitamin D deficiency in young healthy Americans.[96,97] Vitamin D deficiency is particularly prevalent in winter months at higher latitudes. In McCabe and colleagues'[98] review of vitamin D and stress fractures, 5 studies including more than 10,000 patients were identified. Three of these studies showed a positive correlation between vitamin D and protection against stress fractures, whereas the other 2 did not show an association. High-risk patients should be educated on the potential benefits of combined calcium and vitamin D supplementation. Supplementation during the winter and spring, when vitamin D stores are lowest, is of particular importance if an increase

in training is intended. Prophylactic supplementation with up to 2000 IU of vitamin D and 1200 mg of calcium daily is recommended in high-risk patients.[98]

Bone Stimulators

Electromagnetic stimulators and low-intensity pulsed ultrasound stimulators have been promoted to assist in fracture healing. Pulsed ultrasound administration potentially results in positive effects on tissues by promoting angiogenesis, increased growth factor release, and other markers of bone metabolism.[99] Low-intensity pulsed ultrasound has primarily been studied in acute fractures. There are no high-quality studies reporting on the use of ultrasound bone stimulation for treatment of stress fractures. Rue and colleagues[100] reported results of 43 tibia stress fractures treated with ultrasound bone stimulation and found no significant difference in return to activity.

Electromagnetic stimulators generate electromagnetic fields around fractures, inducing fluid flow through bones, which produces electrical currents in cell membranes. This process in turn produces calmodulin, which promotes cell proliferation.[101]

In a randomized controlled trial of tibia stress fractures, electromagnetic stimulation did not produce a significant difference in healing time compared with placebo controls. However, the investigators did note faster healing times for the more severe stress fracture.[102]

Few high-quality studies exist for evaluation of bone stimulators in stress fracture healing. Needle and Kaminski,[103] in their systematic review of the effectiveness of bone stimulation and shock wave therapy for acceleration of stress fracture healing, noted that current evidence is inconclusive. Further high-quality studies of these modalities are needed to determine the efficacy in treating stress fractures.

Extracorporeal Shock Wave Therapy

Shock wave therapy uses high-energy (>0.2 mJ/mm^3) or low-energy (<0.2 mJ/mm^3) acoustic waves to produce a healing response. High-energy treatment is painful and requires anesthesia, but has the advantage of deeper soft tissue penetration and requires fewer treatments. Basic science research on shock wave therapy has provided insight into the many positive effects on tissues, including enhanced neovascularity, increased growth factor release, and accentuated osteogenic stem cell recruitment.[104] These beneficial effects have resulted in the use of shock wave therapy for avascular necrosis,

nonunions, and stress fractures. Two case series have been reported using medium-energy to high-energy shock waves to treat stress fracture.[105,106] In one series 5 patients who failed 6 to 12 months of traditional treatment, subsequent treatment with high-energy shock wave therapy resulted in all patients achieving union between 2 and 3.5 months after treatment.[106] Further high-quality studies are needed to further delineate the role of shock wave therapy in the treatment of stress fractures.

SUMMARY

Stress fractures of the foot and ankle account for almost half of all stress fractures in athletes. These injuries can result in significant disability and time away from sport. Low-risk stress fractures are effectively treated with relative rest and nonoperative treatment modalities with good outcomes. However, high-risk stress fractures portend a more guarded prognosis, and in many cases require surgical management. Further high-quality studies are needed to define the optimal treatment strategies for high-risk stress fractures. The use of bone stimulators, shock wave therapy, and vitamin supplementation for treatment of bone stress injuries has garnered increased interest in recent years, but has yet to be proved efficacious.

REFERENCES

1. Hulkko A, Orava S. Stress fractures in athletes. Int J Sports Med 1987;8(3):221–6.
2. Wentz L, Liu PY, Haymes E, et al. Females have a greater incidence of stress fractures than males in both military and athletic populations: a systemic review. Mil Med 2011;176(4):420–30.
3. Hame SL, LaFemina JM, McAllister DR, et al. Fractures in the collegiate athlete. Am J Sports Med 2004;32(2):446–51.
4. Changstrom BG, Brou L, Khodaee M, et al. Epidemiology of stress fracture injuries among US high school athletes, 2005-2006 through 2012-2013. Am J Sports Med 2015;43(1):26–33.
5. Boden BP, Osbahr DC. High-risk stress fractures: evaluation and treatment. J Am Acad Orthop Surg 2000;8(6):344–53.
6. Boden BP, Osbahr DC, Jimenez C. Low-risk stress fractures. Am J Sports Med 2001;29(1):100–11.
7. Stanitski CL, McMaster JH, Scranton PE. On the nature of stress fractures. Am J Sports Med 1978;6(6):391–6.
8. Korpelainen R, Orava S, Karpakka J, et al. Risk factors for recurrent stress fractures in athletes. Am J Sports Med 2001;29(3):304–10.

9. Maitra RS, Johnson DL. Stress fractures. Clinical history and physical examination. Clin Sports Med 1997;16(2):259–74.

10. Barrack MT, Gibbs JC, De Souza MJ, et al. Higher incidence of bone stress injuries with increasing female athlete triad-related risk factors: a prospective multisite study of exercising girls and women. Am J Sports Med 2014;42(4):949–58.

11. Myburgh KH, Hutchins J, Fataar AB, et al. Low bone density is an etiologic factor for stress fractures in athletes. Ann Intern Med 1990;113(10):754–9.

12. Spitz DJ, Newberg AH. Imaging of stress fractures in the athlete. Radiol Clin North Am 2002;40(2):313–31.

13. Anderson MW, Greenspan A. Stress fractures. Radiology 1996;199(1):1–12.

14. Thrall JH, Ziessman HA. Nuclear medicine: the requisites. St Louis (MO): Mosby; 1995.

15. Arendt EA, Griffiths HJ. The use of MR imaging in the assessment and clinical management of stress reactions of bone in high-performance athletes. Clin Sports Med 1997;16(2):291–306.

16. Mallee WH, Weel H, van Dijk CN, et al. Surgical versus conservative treatment for high-risk stress fractures of the lower leg (anterior tibial cortex, navicular and fifth metatarsal base): a systematic review. Br J Sports Med 2015;49(6):370–6.

17. Matheson GO, Clement DB, McKenzie DC, et al. Stress fractures in athletes. A study of 320 cases. Am J Sports Med 1987;15(1):46–58.

18. Burrows HJ. Fatigue fractures of the fibula. J Bone Joint Surg Br 1948;30B(2):266–79.

19. Devas MB, Sweetnam R. Stress fractures of the fibula; a review of fifty cases in athletes. J Bone Joint Surg Br 1956;38-B(4):818–29.

20. Takebe K, Nakagawa A, Minami H, et al. Role of the fibula in weight-bearing. Clin Orthop Relat Res 1984;(184):289–92.

21. Burgess I, Ryan MD. Bilateral fatigue fractures of the distal fibulae caused by a change of running shoes. Med J Aust 1985;143(7):304–5.

22. Dugan RC, D'Ambrosia R. Fibular stress fractures in runners. J Fam Pract 1983;17(3):415–8.

23. Leabhart JW. Stress fractures of the calcaneus. J Bone Joint Surg Am 1959;41-A:1285–90.

24. Hullinger CW. Insufficiency fracture of the calcaneus. Similar to March fracture of the metatarsal. Journal of Bone and Joint Surgery 1944;26(4):751–7.

25. Sormaala MJ, Niva MH, Kiuru MJ, et al. Stress injuries of the calcaneus detected with magnetic resonance imaging in military recruits. J Bone Joint Surg Am 2006;88(10):2237–42.

26. Taketomi S, Uchiyama E, Iwaso H. Stress fracture of the anterior process of the calcaneus: a case report. Foot Ankle Spec 2013;6(5):389–92.

27. Pearce CJ, Zaw H, Calder JD. Stress fracture of the anterior process of the calcaneus associated with a calcaneonavicular coalition: a case report. Foot Ankle Int 2011;32(1):85–8.

28. Nilsson LJ, Coetzee JC. Stress fracture in the presence of a calcaneonavicular coalition: a case report. Foot Ankle Int 2006;27(5):373–4.

29. Brukner P, Bradshaw C, Khan KM, et al. Stress fractures: a review of 180 cases. Clin J Sport Med 1996;6(2):85–9.

30. Iwamoto J, Takeda T. Stress fractures in athletes: review of 196 cases. J Orthop Sci 2003;8(3):273–8.

31. Gehrmann RM, Renard RL. Current concepts review: stress fractures of the foot. Foot Ankle Int 2006;27(9):750–7.

32. Harrast MA, Colonno D. Stress fractures in runners. Clin Sports Med 2010;29(3):399–416.

33. Mayer SW, Joyner PW, Almekinders LC, et al. Stress fractures of the foot and ankle in athletes. Sports Health 2014;6(6):481–91.

34. Shelbourne KD, Fisher DA, Rettig AC, et al. Stress fractures of the medial malleolus. Am J Sports Med 1988;16(1):60–3.

35. Jowett AJ, Birks CL, Blackney MC. Medial malleolar stress fracture secondary to chronic ankle impingement. Foot Ankle Int 2008;29(7):716–21.

36. Lauge-Hansen N. Fractures of the ankle. II. Combined experimental-surgical and experimental-roentgenologic investigations. Arch Surg 1950;60(5):957–85.

37. Geslien GE, Thrall JH, Espinosa JL, et al. Early detection of stress fractures using 99mTc-polyphosphate. Radiology 1976;121(3 Pt. 1):683–7.

38. Orava S, Karpakka J, Taimela S, et al. Stress fracture of the medial malleolus. J Bone Joint Surg Am 1995;77(3):362–5.

39. Prather JL, Nusynowitz ML, Snowdy HA, et al. Scintigraphic findings in stress fractures. J Bone Joint Surg Am 1977;59(7):869–74.

40. Saunders AJ, El Sayed TF, Hilson AJ, et al. Stress lesions of the lower leg and foot. Clin Radiol 1979;30(6):649–51.

41. Torg JS, Pavlov H, Cooley LH, et al. Stress fractures of the tarsal navicular. A retrospective review of twenty-one cases. J Bone Joint Surg Am 1982;64(5):700–12.

42. Wilson ES Jr, Katz FN. Stress fractures. An analysis of 250 consecutive cases. Radiology 1969;92(3):481–6. passim.

43. Okada K, Senma S, Abe E, et al. Stress fractures of the medial malleolus: a case report. Foot Ankle Int 1995;16(1):49–52.

44. Kor A, Saltzman AT, Wempe PD. Medial malleolar stress fractures. Literature review, diagnosis, and treatment. J Am Podiatr Med Assoc 2003;93(4):292–7.

45. Shabat S, Sampson KB, Mann G, et al. Stress fractures of the medial malleolus–review of the literature and report of a 15-year-old elite gymnast. Foot Ankle Int 2002;23(7):647–50.

46. Reider B, Falconiero R, Yurkofsky J. Nonunion of a medial malleolus stress fracture. A case report. Am J Sports Med 1993;21(3):478–81.

47. Irion V, Miller TL, Kaeding CC. The treatment and outcomes of medial malleolar stress fractures: a systematic review of the literature. Sports Health 2014;6(6):527–30.

48. Bennell KL, Malcolm SA, Thomas SA, et al. The incidence and distribution of stress fractures in competitive track and field athletes. A twelve-month prospective study. Am J Sports Med 1996;24(2):211–7.

49. McKeon KE, McCormick JJ, Johnson JE, et al. Intraosseous and extraosseous arterial anatomy of the adult navicular. Foot Ankle Int 2012;33(10): 857–61.

50. Waugh W. The ossification and vascularisation of the tarsal navicular and their relation to Kohler's disease. J Bone Joint Surg Br 1958;40-B(4): 765–77.

51. Pavlov H, Torg JS, Freiberger RH. Tarsal navicular stress fractures: radiographic evaluation. Radiology 1983;148(3):641–5.

52. Fitch KD, Blackwell JB, Gilmour WN. Operation for non-union of stress fracture of the tarsal navicular. J Bone Joint Surg Br 1989;71(1):105–10.

53. Coris EE, Lombardo JA. Tarsal navicular stress fractures. Am Fam Physician 2003;67(1):85–90.

54. Khan KM, Brukner PD, Kearney C, et al. Tarsal navicular stress fracture in athletes. Sports Med 1994;17(1):65–76.

55. Khan KM, Fuller PJ, Brukner PD, et al. Outcome of conservative and surgical management of navicular stress fracture in athletes. Eighty-six cases proven with computerized tomography. Am J Sports Med 1992;20(6):657–66.

56. Kiss ZS, Khan KM, Fuller PJ. Stress fractures of the tarsal navicular bone: CT findings in 55 cases. AJR Am J Roentgenol 1993;160(1):111–5.

57. Saxena A, Fullem B, Hannaford D. Results of treatment of 22 navicular stress fractures and a new proposed radiographic classification system. J Foot Ankle Surg 2000;39(2):96–103.

58. Lee S, Anderson RB. Stress fractures of the tarsal navicular. Foot Ankle Clin 2004;9(1):85–104.

59. Potter NJ, Brukner PD, Makdissi M, et al. Navicular stress fractures: outcomes of surgical and conservative management. Br J Sports Med 2006;40(8):692–5 [discussion: 695].

60. Gross CE, Nunley JA 2nd. Navicular stress fractures. Foot Ankle Int 2015;36(9):1117–22.

61. Torg JS, Moyer J, Gaughan JP, et al. Management of tarsal navicular stress fractures: conservative versus surgical treatment: a meta-analysis. Am J Sports Med 2010;38(5):1048–53.

62. McGlone JJ. Stress fracture of the talus. J Am Podiatry Assoc 1965;55(12):814–7.

63. Bradshaw C, Khan K, Brukner P. Stress fracture of the body of the talus in athletes demonstrated with computer tomography. Clin J Sport Med 1996;6(1):48–51.

64. Rossi F, Dragoni S. Talar body fatigue stress fractures: three cases observed in elite female gymnasts. Skeletal Radiol 2005;34(7):389–94.

65. Sormaala MJ, Niva MH, Kiuru MJ, et al. Bone stress injuries of the talus in military recruits. Bone 2006;39(1):199–204.

66. Sormaala MJ, Niva MH, Kiuru MJ, et al. Outcomes of stress fractures of the talus. Am J Sports Med 2006;34(11):1809–14.

67. Black KP, Ehlert KJ. A stress fracture of the lateral process of the talus in a runner. A case report. J Bone Joint Surg Am 1994;76(3):441–3.

68. Motto SG. Stress fracture of the lateral process of the talus–a case report. Br J Sports Med 1993; 27(4):275–6.

69. Van Hal ME, Keene JS, Lange TA, et al. Stress fractures of the great toe sesamoids. Am J Sports Med 1982;10(2):122–8.

70. Biedert R, Hintermann B. Stress fractures of the medial great toe sesamoids in athletes. Foot Ankle Int 2003;24(2):137–41.

71. Hubay CA. Sesamoid bones of the hands and feet. Am J Roentgenol Radium Ther 1949;61(4): 493–505.

72. Biedert R. Which investigations are required in stress fracture of the great toe sesamoids? Arch Orthop Trauma Surg 1993;112(2):94–5.

73. Bizarro AH. On the traumatology of the sesamoid structures. Ann Surg 1921;74(6):783–91.

74. Burman MS, Lapidus PW. The functional disturbances caused by the inconstant bones and sesamoids of the foot. Arch Surg 1931;22(6): 936–75.

75. Powers JH. Traumatic and developmental abnormalities of the sesamoid bones of the great toe. Am J Surg 1934;23(2):315–21.

76. Richardson EG. Hallucal sesamoid pain: causes and surgical treatment. J Am Acad Orthop Surg 1999;7(4):270–8.

77. Cohen BE. Hallux sesamoid disorders. Foot Ankle Clin 2009;14(1):91–104.

78. Anderson RB, McBryde AM Jr. Autogenous bone grafting of hallux sesamoid nonunions. Foot Ankle Int 1997;18(5):293–6.

79. Kavanaugh JH, Brower TD, Mann RV. The Jones fracture revisited. J Bone Joint Surg Am 1978; 60(6):776–82.

80. Hetsroni I, Nyska M, Ben-Sira D, et al. Analysis of foot structure in athletes sustaining proximal fifth

metatarsal stress fracture. Foot Ankle Int 2010; 31(3):203–11.

81. Lee KT, Kim KC, Park YU, et al. Radiographic evaluation of foot structure following fifth metatarsal stress fracture. Foot Ankle Int 2011;32(8):796–801.

82. Dameron TB Jr. Fractures and anatomical variations of the proximal portion of the fifth metatarsal. J Bone Joint Surg Am 1975;57(6):788–92.

83. Stewart IM. Jones's fracture: fracture of base of fifth metatarsal. Clin Orthop 1960;16:190–8.

84. Torg JS, Balduini FC, Zelko RR, et al. Fractures of the base of the fifth metatarsal distal to the tuberosity. Classification and guidelines for non-surgical and surgical management. J Bone Joint Surg Am 1984;66(2):209–14.

85. Zogby RG, Baker BE. A review of nonoperative treatment of Jones' fracture. Am J Sports Med 1987;15(4):304–7.

86. Lee KT, Park YU, Jegal H, et al. Prognostic classification of fifth metatarsal stress fracture using plantar gap. Foot Ankle Int 2013;34(5):691–6.

87. DeLee JC, Evans JP, Julian J. Stress fracture of the fifth metatarsal. Am J Sports Med 1983;11(5): 349–53.

88. Lee KT, Park YU, Young KW, et al. Surgical results of 5th metatarsal stress fracture using modified tension band wiring. Knee Surg Sports Traumatol Arthrosc 2011;19(5):853–7.

89. Mindrebo N, Shelbourne KD, Van Meter CD, et al. Outpatient percutaneous screw fixation of the acute Jones fracture. Am J Sports Med 1993;21(5):720–3.

90. Portland G, Kelikian A, Kodros S. Acute surgical management of Jones' fractures. Foot Ankle Int 2003;24(11):829–33.

91. Lee KT, Park YU, Young KW, et al. The plantar gap: another prognostic factor for fifth metatarsal stress fracture. Am J Sports Med 2011;39(10):2206–11.

92. Lee KT, Park YU, Jegal H, et al. Factors associated with recurrent fifth metatarsal stress fracture. Foot Ankle Int 2013;34(12):1645–53.

93. Evans RK, Antczak AJ, Lester M, et al. Effects of a 4-month recruit training program on markers of bone metabolism. Med Sci Sports Exerc 2008; 40(11 Suppl):S660–70.

94. Friedl KE, Evans RK, Moran DS. Stress fracture and military medical readiness: bridging basic and applied research. Med Sci Sports Exerc 2008; 40(11 Suppl):S609–22.

95. Jones BH, Thacker SB, Gilchrist J, et al. Prevention of lower extremity stress fractures in athletes and soldiers: a systematic review. Epidemiol Rev 2002;24(2):228–47.

96. Tangpricha V, Pearce EN, Chen TC, et al. Vitamin D insufficiency among free-living healthy young adults. Am J Med 2002;112(8):659–62.

97. Constantini NW, Arieli R, Chodick G, et al. High prevalence of vitamin D insufficiency in athletes and dancers. Clin J Sport Med 2010;20(5):368–71.

98. McCabe MP, Smyth MP, Richardson DR. Current concept review: vitamin D and stress fractures. Foot Ankle Int 2012;33(6):526–33.

99. Khan Y, Laurencin CT. Fracture repair with ultrasound: clinical and cell-based evaluation. J Bone Joint Surg Am 2008;90(Suppl 1):138–44.

100. Rue JP, Armstrong DW 3rd, Frassica FJ, et al. The effect of pulsed ultrasound in the treatment of tibial stress fractures. Orthopedics 2004;27(11): 1192–5.

101. Brighton CT, Wang W, Seldes R, et al. Signal transduction in electrically stimulated bone cells. J Bone Joint Surg Am 2001;83-A(10):1514–23.

102. Beck BR, Matheson GO, Bergman G, et al. Do capacitively coupled electric fields accelerate tibial stress fracture healing? A randomized controlled trial. Am J Sports Med 2008;36(3):545–53.

103. Needle AR, Kaminski TW. Effectiveness of low-intensity pulsed ultrasound, capacitively coupled electric fields, or extracorporeal shock wave therapy in accelerating stress fracture healing: a systematic review. Athletic Training & Sports Health Care 2009;1(3):133–9.

104. Furia JP, Rompe JD, Cacchio A, et al. Shock wave therapy as a treatment of nonunions, avascular necrosis, and delayed healing of stress fractures. Foot Ankle Clin 2010;15(4):651–62.

105. Moretti B, Notarnicola A, Garofalo R, et al. Shock waves in the treatment of stress fractures. Ultrasound Med Biol 2009;35(6):1042–9.

106. Taki M, Iwata O, Shiono M, et al. Extracorporeal shock wave therapy for resistant stress fracture in athletes: a report of 5 cases. Am J Sports Med 2007;35(7):1188–92.

Index

Note: Page numbers of article titles are in **boldface** type.

Orthop Clin N Am 47 (2016) 823–828
http://dx.doi.org/10.1016/S0030-5898(16)30098-0
0030-5898/16/$ – see front matter

UNITED STATES POSTAL SERVICE ®

Statement of Ownership, Management, and Circulation
(All Periodicals Publications Except Requester Publications)

1. Publication Title	2. Publication Number	3. Filing Date
ORTHOPEDIC CLINICS OF NORTH AMERICA	950 – 920	9/18/2016

4. Issue Frequency	5. Number of Issues Published Annually	6. Annual Subscription Price
JAN, APR, JUL, OCT	4	$310.00

7. Complete Mailing Address of Known Office of Publication (Not printer) (Street, city, county, state, and ZIP+4®)
ELSEVIER INC.
360 PARK AVENUE SOUTH
NEW YORK, NY 10010-1710

Contact Person: STEPHEN R. BUSHING
Telephone (Include area code): 215-239-3688

8. Complete Mailing Address of Headquarters or General Business Office of Publisher (Not printer)
ELSEVIER INC.
360 PARK AVENUE SOUTH
NEW YORK, NY 10010-1710

9. Full Names and Complete Mailing Addresses of Publisher, Editor, and Managing Editor (Do not leave blank)

Publisher (Name and complete mailing address)
LINDA BELFUS, ELSEVIER INC.
1600 JOHN F KENNEDY BLVD. SUITE 1800
PHILADELPHIA, PA 19103-2899

Editor (Name and complete mailing address)
JENNIFER FLYNN-BRIGGS, ELSEVIER INC.
1600 JOHN F KENNEDY BLVD. SUITE 1800
PHILADELPHIA, PA 19103-2899

Managing Editor (Name and complete mailing address)
ADRIANNE BRIGIDO, ELSEVIER INC.
1600 JOHN F KENNEDY BLVD. SUITE 1800
PHILADELPHIA, PA 19103-2899

10. Owner (Do not leave blank. If the publication is owned by a corporation, give the name and address of the corporation immediately followed by the names and addresses of all stockholders owning or holding 1 percent or more of the total amount of stock. If not owned by a corporation, give the names and addresses of the individual owners. If owned by a partnership or other unincorporated firm, give its name and address as well as those of each individual owner. If the publication is published by a nonprofit organization, give its name and address.)

Full Name	Complete Mailing Address
WHOLLY OWNED SUBSIDIARY OF REED/ELSEVIER, US HOLDINGS	1600 JOHN F KENNEDY BLVD. SUITE 1800 PHILADELPHIA, PA 19103-2899

11. Known Bondholders, Mortgagees, and Other Security Holders Owning or Holding 1 Percent or More of Total Amount of Bonds, Mortgages, or Other Securities. If none, check box. ▶ ☐ None

Full Name	Complete Mailing Address
N/A	

12. Tax Status (For completion by nonprofit organizations authorized to mail at nonprofit rates) (Check one)
The purpose, function, and nonprofit status of this organization and the exempt status for federal income tax purposes:
☐ Has Not Changed During Preceding 12 Months
☐ Has Changed During Preceding 12 Months (Publisher must submit explanation of change with this statement)

13. Publication Title	14. Issue Date for Circulation Data Below
ORTHOPEDIC CLINICS OF NORTH AMERICA	JULY 2016

15. Extent and Nature of Circulation

			Average No. Copies Each Issue During Preceding 12 Months	No. Copies of Single Issue Published Nearest to Filing Date
a. Total Number of Copies (Net press run)			561	534
b. Paid Circulation (By Mail and Outside the Mail)	(1)	Mailed Outside-County Paid Subscriptions Stated on PS Form 3541 (Include paid distribution above nominal rate, advertiser's proof copies, and exchange copies)	130	152
	(2)	Mailed In-County Paid Subscriptions Stated on PS Form 3541 (Include paid distribution above nominal rate, advertiser's proof copies, and exchange copies)	0	0
	(3)	Paid Distribution Outside the Mails Including Sales Through Dealers and Carriers, Street Vendors, Counter Sales, and Other Paid Distribution Outside USPS®	140	221
	(4)	Paid Distribution by Other Classes of Mail Through the USPS (e.g., First-Class Mail®)	0	0
c. Total Paid Distribution (Sum of 15b (1), (2), (3), and (4))		▶	270	373
d. Free or Nominal Rate Distribution (By Mail and Outside the Mail)	(1)	Free or Nominal Rate Outside-County Copies Included on PS Form 3541	50	106
	(2)	Free or Nominal Rate In-County Copies Included on PS Form 3541	0	0
	(3)	Free or Nominal Rate Copies Mailed at Other Classes Through the USPS (e.g., First-Class Mail)	0	0
	(4)	Free or Nominal Rate Distribution Outside the Mail (Carriers or other means)	0	0
e. Total Free or Nominal Rate Distribution (Sum of 15d (1), (2), (3) and (4))		▶	50	106
f. Total Distribution (Sum of 15c and 15e)		▶	320	479
g. Copies not Distributed (See Instructions to Publishers #4 (page #3))		▶	241	55
h. Total (Sum of 15f and g)		▶	561	534
i. Percent Paid (15c divided by 15f times 100)		▶	84%	78%

* If you are claiming electronic copies, go to line 16 on page 3. If you are not claiming electronic copies, skip to line 17 on page 3.

16. Electronic Copy Circulation

	Average No. Copies Each Issue During Preceding 12 Months	No. Copies of Single Issue Published Nearest to Filing Date
a. Paid Electronic Copies ▶	0	0
b. Total Paid Print Copies (Line 15c) + Paid Electronic Copies (Line 16a) ▶	270	373
c. Total Print Distribution (Line 15f) + Paid Electronic Copies (Line 16a) ▶	320	479
d. Percent Paid (Both Print & Electronic Copies) (16b divided by 16c × 100) ▶	84%	78%

☒ I certify that 50% of all my distributed copies (electronic and print) are paid above a nominal price.

17. Publication of Statement of Ownership
☒ If the publication is a general publication, publication of this statement is required. Will be printed in the OCTOBER 2016 issue of this publication. ☐ Publication not required.

18. Signature and Title of Editor, Publisher, Business Manager, or Owner

STEPHEN R. BUSHING - INVENTORY DISTRIBUTION CONTROL MANAGER

Date: 9/18/2016

I certify that all information furnished on this form is true and complete. I understand that anyone who furnishes false or misleading information on this form or who omits material or information requested on the form may be subject to criminal sanctions (including fines and imprisonment) and/or civil sanctions (including civil penalties).

PS Form **3526**, July 2014 [Page 3 of 4] PSN: 7530-01-000-9931   PRIVACY NOTICE: See our privacy policy on www.usps.com.

PS Form **3526**, July 2014 (Page 1 of 4 (see instructions page 4)) PSN: 7530-01-000-9931   PRIVACY NOTICE: See our privacy policy on www.usps.com.

Moving?

Make sure your subscription moves with you!

To notify us of your new address, find your **Clinics Account Number** (located on your mailing label above your name), and contact customer service at:

Email: journalscustomerservice-usa@elsevier.com

800-654-2452 (subscribers in the U.S. & Canada)
314-447-8871 (subscribers outside of the U.S. & Canada)

Fax number: 314-447-8029

Elsevier Health Sciences Division
Subscription Customer Service
3251 Riverport Lane
Maryland Heights, MO 63043

*To ensure uninterrupted delivery of your subscription, please notify us at least 4 weeks in advance of move.

ELSEVIER

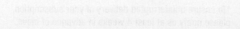

Printed and bound by CPI Group (UK) Ltd, Croydon, CR0 4YY

08/05/2025

01864686-0009